Field Guide to Global Health and Disaster Medicine

Field Guide to Global Health and Disaster Medicine

JAMES A. CHAMBERS, MD, MPH&TM, FACS, FCS(ECSA), CPE

Colonel, US Air Force, MC, SFS
Uniformed Services University
Bethesda, Maryland;
Brigham and Women's Hospital
Harvard Medical School
Boston, Massachusetts

ELSEVIER

ELSEVIER

1600 John F. Kennedy Blvd.
Ste 1800
Philadelphia, PA 19103-2899

FIELD GUIDE TO GLOBAL HEALTH AND DISASTER MEDICINE   ISBN: 978-0-323794121

Library of Congress Control Number: 2021932695

Content Strategist: Charlotta Kryhl
Content Development Specialist: Deborah Poulson
Publishing Services Manager: Deepthi Unni
Project Manager: Beula Christopher
Design Direction: Amy Buxton

Printed in India.

Last digit is the print number: 9   8   7   6   5   4   3   2   1

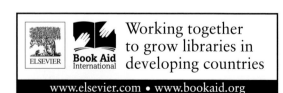

Working together to grow libraries in developing countries

www.elsevier.com • www.bookaid.org

To the vulnerable and suffering and those who care about and for them.

In memory of those who lost their lives in the fight against COVID-19,
including Walt Chambers, Pharm.D.
You will always be loved and missed for the joy you shared with others.
I wish I could tell you again today how proud I am of you.

Rahma Aburas, MBBS, ABOG, SBOG, MAS
Leadership for Healthcare Organizations,
    UCSD
MAS, Health Policy and Law, UCSD;
Consultant Obstetrician and Gynecologist
Alhabib Medical Group, Arrayan
Riyadh, Saudi Arabia

Rocio del Pilar Garzón Ayala, MD, MSc
Colonel
Aerospace Medicine and Ocupational Health
    Specialist, Flight Physiology Instructor
Aerospace Medical Center, Colombian Air
    Force;
Deputy, Diretorate-General of Military
    Health Services
Bogotá, Colombia

Saif Al-Bedwawi, MBBS, DTMH, FRCPC, FACP
Director, Public Health Department
United Arab Emirates Medical Service Corps
Abu Dhabi, UAE

Bradley Boetig, MD, MPH, MA
Director
Global Health Distance Learning Program
Uniformed Services University of the Health
    Sciences
Bethesda, Maryland

Margaret Ellis Bourdeaux, MD, MPH
Research Director
Program in Global Public Policy
Harvard Medical School;
Associate Physician
Brigham and Women's Hospital
Division of Global Health Equity
Boston, MA

Susan Miller Briggs, MD, MPH, FACS
Associate Professor of Surgery
Harvard Medical School;
Director
International Trauma and Disaster Institute
Massachusetts General Hospital
Boston, Massachusetts

Daniel S. Burns, BM, BCh, MRCP, DTM&H
Lieutenant Colonel
Infectious Diseases Consultant
Royal Centre for Defence Medicine
University Hospitals Birmingham
Birmingham, United Kingdom

Dennis T. Cherian, BHMS, MS, MHA
Senior Director
New Programs Development
Jhpiego, an affiliate of Johns Hopkins
    University
Herndon, Virginia

Alexandra Mejía Delgado, MD
Colonel (Ret.) Colombian Air Force
Aerospace Medicine Specialist and Flight
    Physiology Instructor
Aerospace Medical Deputy, Colombian Civil
    Aviation Authority
Bogotá, Colombia

Frédéric Dorandeu, BG, PharmD, PhD
Associate Professor of Val-de-Grâce
Technical Advisor to the Central Director
    of the Armed Forces Health Service for
    Chemical Defence Issues
Paris, France

Elizabeth A. Erickson, MD, MPH
Lieutenant Colonel, US Air Force
Assistant Professor
Uniformed Services University of the Health
    Sciences
Bethesda, Maryland

Fidel Angel Núñez Fernández, MD, MSc, PhD
Institute for Tropical Medicine Pedro Kourí
    (IPK)
Havana, Cuba;
Professor of Clinical Microbiology and
    Parasitology
Latin-American School for Medicine (ELAM)
La Habana, Cuba

Andrew Isaac Geller, MD
Commander, United States Public Health
  Service;
Medical Officer
Division of Healthcare Quality Promotion
US Centers for Disease Control and
  Prevention
Atlanta, Georgia

Christian Haggenmiller, PhD
Research Coordinator, Health and Biosecurity
German Institute for Defence and Strategic
  Studies (GIDS)
Hamburg, Germany

Amanda Huston, MPH
Major, USAF, BSC
Chief of Public Health
380th Expeditionary Medical Group
Al Dhafra Air Base, UAE

Lucas A. Johnson, MD, MTM&H, FACPM
Commander, Medical Corps, United States
  Navy
Preventive Medicine Physician
US Naval Hospital Okinawa, Japan
Okinawa, Japan

George G. Johnston, MD, FACS
Director/Quality Management
Bureau of Medical Services
US Department of State
Washington, DC

Chetan U. Kharod, MD, MPH, FAEMS
Associate Professor
Military and Emergency Medicine
Uniformed Services University
Bethesda, Maryland

Nathan Kinder, DO
Emergency Medicine Physician
Inova Health System
Alexandria, Virginia

Jan Ilhan Kizilhan, Prof Dr, Dr Dipl Psych
Institute for Transcultural Health Science
Baden-Wuerttemberg, Germany;
Institute for Psychotherapy and
  Psychotraumatology
University of Dohuk
KRI, Iraq

**Lucy Lamb, MB, BChir, MA, MRCP
(Infectious Diseases), DTM&H, PhD**
Consultant Infectious Diseases and General
  Medicine
Royal Free Hospital and the Academic
  Department of Military Medicine
London, United Kingdom

Joseph K. Maddry, MD, FACEP, FACMT
Associate Professor
Military and Emergency Medicine
Uniformed Services University
Bethesda, Maryland

Diego Leonel Malpica Hincapié, MD
Aerospace Medicine and Occupational Health
  Specialist
Aerospace Medical Center
Colombian Air Force
Bogotá, Colombia

Donald E. Meier, MD, FACS, FWACS
Professor Emeritus
Pediatric Surgery
Texas Tech University Health Sciences
  Center
Paul L. Foster School of Medicine
El Paso, Texas

Melinda S. New, MD
Associate Professor and Vice Chair for
  Education
Department of Obstetrics and Gynecology
Vanderbilt University
Nashville, Tennessee

Richard Pilch, MD, MPH
Director, Chemical and Biological Weapons
  Nonproliferation Program
James Martin Center for Nonproliferation
  Studies
Middlebury Institute of International Studies
  at Monterey
Monterey, California

Lorna Renner, MD, MPH, FRCPCH, FGCPS
Associate Professor and Consultant
  Paediatrician
Department of Child Health
University of Ghana Medical School
Accra, Ghana

Katrina Roper, PhD, MAppEpid
Honorary Senior Lecturer
Research School of Population Health
Australian National University
Acton, ACT, Australia

Alfonso C. Rosales, MD, MPH&TM
Senior Advisor for Maternal and Child
   Health
Senior Advisor for COVID-19 Global
   Response
World Vision US/International
Washington, DC

Lina Maria Sanchez Rubio, MD, PhD
Colonel (Ret.)
Past Director, Aerospace Medical Center
Past Chief, Health Services
Colombian Air Force
Bogotá, Colombia

Adam T. Soto, MD
Anesthesiologist
Department of Anesthesiology
Walter Reed National Military Medical
   Center;
Assistant Professor of Anesthesiology
Uniformed Services University of the
   Health Sciences
Bethesda, Maryland

Kaku Tamura, MD
CPT(O-6)
JMSDF MoD Japan;
Chief, Second Department of Internal
   Medicine
Self-Defense Force Central Hospital
Tokyo, Japan

John L. Tarpley, MD, FWACS, FACS
Professor and Head of Department, Surgery
Faculty of Medicine, University of Botswana
Gaborone, Botswana

Juan I. Ubiera, MPH, MS
Chief, Integrated Biosurveillance
Armed Forces Health Surveillance Division
   (AFHSD)
Public Health Directorate (PHD);
Assistant Director
Combat Support (AD-CS)
Defense Health Agency
Silver Spring, Maryland

Catherine T. Witkop, MD, MPH
Colonel (Ret), US Air Force
Professor
Uniformed Services University of the Health
   Sciences
Bethesda, Maryland

Ellen Yard, PhD, MPH
Commander, United States Public Health
   Service
Epidemiologist
National Center for Environmental
   Health
US Centers for Disease Control and
   Prevention
Atlanta, Georgia

María Alejandra Corzo Zamora, MD, Msc
Captain (Ret.) Colombian Air Force
Researcher and Lecturer
Aviation, Space and Extreme Environment
   Physiology
Bogotá, Colombia

ACKNOWLEDGMENTS

Thank you to the following individuals who helped organize and format material in the earliest stages of this book: Mia Snow, Ricardo Oliver, and Lance Mabry. Thank you also to the following persons for helping identify and recruit experts for this book and review their submissions: Dr. Keith Martin (Canada/USA), Dr. Niranjan "Tex" Kissoon (Canada), Dr. Charles Stratton (USA), Dr. Shuichi Kawano (Japan), Dr. Andrew Green (UK), Dr. Rudy Cachuela (USA), Dr. Vinay Gupta (USA), Dr. Christian Haggenmiller (Germany), Dr. Nicolas Brossard (France), Maj Gen Lansing Pilch (USA), and Dr. Janine Tillott (Australia).

Michael Earley, FRCS (Plast Surg), MCh, FRCSI, drew the cover art to emphasize the importance of the local community in global public health and disaster medicine. Dr. Earley graduated from University College Dublin medical school before specializing in plastic surgery with a focus on head and neck reconstruction as well as craniofacial and cleft surgery. He has an honorary doctorate from the National University of Ireland in recognition of over two decades of global volunteer leadership and support for organizations including Operation Smile, Chernobyl Children International, the Christina Noble Foundation. Dr. Earley enjoys painting as well as teaching anatomy with the Royal College of Surgeons in Ireland, and he has illustrated several books on craniofacial surgery and neuroanatomy. He is married with three children and two grandchildren.

Just over a century ago, World War One was drawing down. Forty million lives had been lost, economies bankrupted, infrastructures dissipated. A war-weary world needed to rebuild. Catastrophically, into that milieu the Spanish Flu brought death even faster and more widespread than the industrial war machines of Europe, killing an additional 50 million around the globe, dwarfing simultaneous tragedies such as the Fujian earthquake of 1918. Conflict, contagion, and natural disaster have decimated communities since the beginning of recorded history. When they coincide, civilizations are especially threatened.

The World Health Organization declared COVID-19 a pandemic on March 11, 2020. Already, SARS-CoV-2 has infected tens of millions and severely impacted economies worldwide. Governments and healthcare professionals must continue to prepare for the next 3/11, the next 9/11, and other baleful scenarios to protect against the harm of infectious diseases, violence, and natural disasters, as well as the chronic factors that undermine universal human aspirations.

In the last century, humanity achieved breathtaking advances in reducing global poverty and extending life expectancy and quality.[1] However, many challenges persist even as new ones arise in an increasingly interconnected world facing common threats such as climate change. US President Dwight Eisenhower shared his conviction with the United Nations that "if a danger exists in the world, it is a danger shared by all; and equally… if hope exists in the mind of one nation, that hope should be shared by all."[2] Current leaders echo these thoughts in the midst of a pandemic.[3] We fail to act on them at our own peril.

Hippocrates observed, "the physician must be ready, not only to do his duty himself, but also to secure the cooperation of the patient, of the attendants and of externals."[4] Global health is a complicated and complex arena with a myriad of well-intentioned stakeholders and actors, each with their own culture, goals, and resources. To serve the most important of these, the patient, all must work to understand how they can contribute in a coordinated fashion to achieve appropriately prioritized equitable and sustainable goals.

The contributors to this book hope the following chapters will support efforts to advance health security for all. *Field Guide to Global Health and Disaster Medicine* shares the training and experience of diverse, dedicated health professionals from six continents, representing academia, government, and non-government organizations. The majority of the chapters address primarily practitioner-level concerns, whereas the last ones explore organization- and systems-level challenges. Proceeds will be donated to UNICEF to protect the health of our world's children.

Your feedback is welcome at: global.health.disaster.med@gmail.com. Thank you for your commitment to making our world a healthier and more secure one for all.

James A. Chambers
August 31, 2020
Washington, DC

1. Pinker S. *Enlightenment Now*. Penguin Books, NY, 2019:53–68.
2. Eisenhower DD. "Atoms for Peace," United Nations, New York City, December 8, 1953.
3. Burns N. *Foreign Affairs*, 25 March 2020; Ngozi Okonjo-Iweala, *Foreign Affairs*, April 30, 2020. https://www.foreignaffairs.com/articles/2020-03-25/how-lead-time-pandemic. https://www.foreignaffairs.com/articles/world/2020-04-30/finding-vaccine-only-first-step.
4. Hippocrates. *Aphorisms*. In: *Hippocrates*. Jones WHS, trans. Harvard University Press, Cambridge, MA, 1931;4:99.

Wherever the art of medicine is loved,
there is also a love of humanity.
Hippocrates

CONTENTS

CHAPTER 1

Before You Leave Home: Immunizations and Preventive Measures for Travel

Elizabeth A. Erickson ■ Catherine T. Witkop

Introduction

When disaster strikes, time is of the essence. Disaster responders, including medical personnel, who travel to respond to a disaster may not dedicate the same amount of time and diligence to personal preparation that they would for planned travel. Inadequate preparation and preventive measures, however, can result in illness or injuries and loss of mission effectiveness—even utilization of medical resources intended for disaster victims. The importance of pretravel health preparation before departing for a disaster response cannot be overstated (Box 1.1). Many elements of pretravel health can be maintained over time, so that just-in-time measures can be implemented quickly.

This chapter will use a travel medicine framework, focusing on measures to prevent conditions and diseases that are associated with a change in physical and geographic environment. Travel medicine is dynamic, so it is important to use up-to-date resources to guide pretravel clinical decisions. This chapter will outline general considerations, but not attempt to be a comprehensive reference for location-specific recommendations. Some trusted travel medicine resources include:

1. World Health Organization (WHO) International Travel and Health (http://www.who.int/ith/en/)

   The WHO's International Travel and Health website includes up-to-date information on outbreaks of concern to travelers and policies on travel-related vaccinations, disease distribution maps, vaccine and disease information, and travel health topics.

2. US Centers for Disease Control and Prevention (CDC) Health Information for International Travelers (The Yellow Book) (https://wwwnc.cdc.gov/travel/page/yellowbook-home)

   The Yellow Book has been a trusted resource for travel health since 1967 (Yellow Book, 2020). The full text is available free of charge online. It includes information on many travel health topics and guidelines for prevention and management of travel-related illnesses. The

---

BOX 1.1 ■ Before You Go Checklist

- Review health insurance policies, obtain travel/evacuation insurance as needed, carry insurance cards/documents
- Obtain adequate supply of routine/daily medications
- Review location-specific health and security risks
- Review routine, required, recommended vaccinations; schedule healthcare visit to obtain needed vaccines
- Obtain malaria chemoprophylaxis medication, if indicated
- Insect repellent, >30% DEET or picaridin
  - Treat clothing with permethrin
  - Travel bed net, if indicated (e.g., if potentially sleeping outdoors)
- Obtain self-treatment medications for travelers' diarrhea
- Water filtration system and/or iodine tablets
- Sunscreen, sun protection factor of at least 15
- Obtain prophylactic medication for altitude illness, if indicated
- Pretravel screening for tuberculosis with tuberculin skin test or interferon-gamma release assay, if indicated

---

CDC website also includes destination-specific travel health recommendations and mobile apps related to travel health topics.

3. International Society for Infectious Disease ProMED Mail (http://www.promedmail.org/)

    ProMED mail's website lists infectious disease-related health alerts worldwide, and individuals can subscribe to receive email notifications free of charge.

4. Shoreland Travax (www.travax.com)

    Travax maintains up-to-date, country-specific travel health information that can be customized to provider and traveler reports that comprehensively list preventive measures that should be considered before travel. Use of Travax requires a fee-based subscription.

5. Global Infectious Disease and Epidemiology Online Network (GIDEON) (https://www.gideononline.com/)

    GIDEON web app and ebooks provide information on infectious disease threats by disease and by country. Use of GIDEON resources requires a fee-based subscription.

Health and Evacuation Insurance

An important consideration before leaving home is access to health care both at home and abroad. Those who may respond on short notice to disasters should have reliable access to medical care at home to receive routine preventive services, maintain optimal control of any medical conditions, and obtain timely pretravel care. Individuals who require routine medications or medical supplies must have adequate supplies available for short-notice travel. Before going overseas, all travelers should consider various scenarios requiring medical care for themselves, and in some cases for fellow travelers, and have plans in place for those contingencies. All travelers should have travel health insurance and are also advised to have means to pay at point-of-care for any required medical services. Some health insurance policies include coverage of care received abroad, but there may be caveats. It is important that travelers closely examine their health insurance policies before traveling, to determine if supplemental travel-specific health insurance may be necessary.

An additional consideration is the potential need for evacuation because of medical problems, or transport of remains in the event of death. Depending on the location, the local available level of care may not be adequate to manage complex medical situations and transport to a higher level of care may be necessary. Insurance that covers medical evacuation is recommended, as evacuation costs can be very high. Some travel health insurance policies include, or can be purchased concurrently with, medical evacuation insurance.

In additional to confirming travel health and medical evacuation insurance, one should become familiar with the names and locations of medical facilities in the travel destination. Health insurance providers may have specific recommended facilities. Embassies in the foreign country may maintain a list of recommended facilities. The traveler should be sure to have all necessary health insurance cards readily available during travel. Finally, all bills and receipts for medical care should be carefully retained.

Vaccinations

A key component of preparation for travel abroad is determining the need for vaccinations before travel. Characteristics of both the individual and the travel should be included in decision-making about pretravel vaccinations. One way to approach the multitude of vaccines that might be needed is to consider them within categories of routine, required, and recommended. Routine vaccinations include those that should be administered regardless of travel, such as childhood vaccines (e.g., polio, measles), age-, time-, or risk-based vaccines for adults (e.g., pneumococcal, tetanus boosters), and annual influenza vaccine. Required vaccines are those legally required for travel to certain locations, such as yellow fever. Recommended vaccines are those specifically indicated based on the travel location, environment or anticipated activities.

This chapter is not a comprehensive reference of all potential pretravel vaccines and does not include comprehensive details about administration, but rather provides an overview of vaccines that may be considered. This overview focuses primarily on pretravel vaccinations for adults, but some specific considerations relevant to children are included. Individual characteristics such as medical history, medications, immune status, age, and immunization history should be considered carefully within a pretravel medical encounter. Detailed, current information can be found at: https://wwwnc.cdc.gov/travel/page/yellowbook-home.

Vaccine Overview

ROUTINE

This list is not comprehensive of all routinely provided vaccinations, but is focused on the routine immunizations that are important to consider before travel:

1. Diphtheria, tetanus and pertussis: Diphtheria is a bacterial infection (*Corynebacterium diphtheriae*) that can cause respiratory disease. Transmission is typically via oral or respiratory droplets or close contact. Diphtheria is endemic in many countries in Asia, the South Pacific, Eastern Europe, and the Middle East, and on the island of Hispaniola (Haiti and Dominican Republic) in the Caribbean Sea. Tetanus is caused by the bacteria *Clostridium tetani*, which is ubiquitous in the environment worldwide. Transmission occurs via direct contamination of wounds or nonintact skin. Tetanus infection presents as muscle rigidity and spasms, and has a high case fatality ratio. Pertussis is a bacterial infection (*Bordetella pertussis*) that can cause respiratory disease known as "whooping cough." Pertussis is endemic worldwide. Each of these bacterial infections are preventable with vaccination, therefore vaccination against these pathogens are a cornerstone of childhood and adult vaccination recommendations.

   These three pathogens are often combined within vaccine products, with different combinations most suitable for certain ages and circumstances. Diphtheria vaccine is an inactivated bacterial toxoid. Tetanus vaccine is also a toxoid. Vaccines against pertussis may be whole cell (wP) based on killed *Bordetella pertussis* organisms, or acellular (aP) based on bacterial antigens. In many countries only acellular pertussis vaccines are used. Childhood immunization schedules worldwide recommend a primary series of three doses of a combined product containing these three vaccines, starting as early as 6 weeks of age. Two boosters are recommended during childhood, usually between 12 and 23 months and 4 and 7 years. These childhood immunizations are typically delivered as DTaP or DTwP.

Adolescents who have completed the five-shot childhood series should receive a Tdap (tetanus, reduced diphtheria, and acellular pertussis) vaccine between ages 11 and 18. Only acellular pertussis vaccines should be used at or above the age of 7 years. The adolescence dose should be followed by a Td (tetanus and reduced diphtheria) or Tdap vaccine every 10 years. Pregnant women should receive Tdap in the second or third trimester. Individuals with high risk wounds for tetanus should receive a Td vaccine if it has been 5 years or more since their last Td.

It is important to review diphtheria, tetanus, and pertussis immunization status before travel. Various activities during travel may increase risk of all these pathogens. Healthcare workers may be at increased risk of exposure to diphtheria and pertussis. Immunity from acellular pertussis vaccine wanes over time, so a Tdap may be considered before travel regardless of the interval from the last Td or Tdap vaccine. Any adults who have not had primary immunization against diphtheria, tetanus, and pertussis should complete an appropriate catch-up schedule.

Td or Tdap should not be given to those with a prior severe allergic reaction to any tetanus, diphtheria or pertussis-containing vaccine. Common adverse reactions include pain and redness at the injection site, and mild fever, headache, and tiredness. These vaccines are generally well tolerated.

2. Hepatitis A: Hepatitis A is an RNA virus that is typically spread by fecal-oral transmission, often via contaminated food or water. Hepatitis A vaccination is now a routinely recommended childhood vaccination in many countries. It is recommended for use in children aged 12 months or older, but can be given safely to infants as young as 6 months old when indicated for travel. For unvaccinated adults, it is a commonly recommend vaccine before travel to developing nations. The hepatitis A vaccine is an inactivated virus vaccine that is administered intramuscularly. The vaccine is given in a two-shot series. The first dose provides protective immunity in 94% to 100% of adults 1 month after administration. The second dose is provided at 6 to 18 months, depending on the vaccine given. Hepatitis A and B may be combined into a single vaccine for administration to adults. Individuals who receive a complete series of hepatitis A vaccinations as children or adults do not require boosters. The hepatitis A vaccine is generally safe and well tolerated, with few contraindications. The most commonly reported side effects include injection site tenderness and headache.

3. Hepatitis B: Hepatitis B is a partially double-stranded DNA virus that is spread by contact with infected blood and other body fluids. Hepatitis B vaccination is recommended as a routine childhood vaccination, with administration starting at birth. Unvaccinated adults should also be vaccinated, especially healthcare workers and travelers. Hepatitis B vaccines are inactivated virus vaccines administered intramuscularly. The vaccine is typically administered as a three-shot series, although two-shot versions may be used for unvaccinated older children and adults. Hepatitis A and B may be combined in vaccine products. Hepatitis B vaccination is generally safe and well tolerated, with few contraindications. The most common side effects are injection site soreness and low-grade fever.

4. Influenza: Influenza viruses are RNA viruses classified into four types: A, B, C, and D. Types A and B cause disease in humans. Within the types, there are combinations of surface proteins called hemagglutinins and neuraminidase that result in many different influenza virus

subtypes that can cause disease (e.g., influenza A [H3N2]). Influenza occurs worldwide, with seasonality in the winter months (depending on hemisphere). Influenza is spread via respiratory droplets. Seasonal influenza vaccines are developed annually based on anticipated predominant strains. Different vaccines are made for the flu seasons in the northern and southern hemispheres. Seasonal influenza vaccine has become a recommended annual vaccination for nearly all populations greater than 6 months of age.

Influenza vaccines are grouped into three categories: inactivated influenza vaccine (IIV), live attenuated influenza vaccine (LAIV), and recombinant influenza vaccine (RIV). Children 6 months to 8 years of age receiving influenza vaccine for the first time require two doses, more than 4 weeks apart. All others need a single vaccine each year. The most commonly used vaccines are IIV, which can be delivered intramuscularly, transdermally, or intradermally. RIV is labeled for persons 18 years or older. LAIV is given via nasal spray, and may be used for individuals 2 to 49 years of age.

Influenza vaccines may be trivalent or quadrivalent. Trivalent vaccines provide protection against two influenza A subtype viruses and one influenza B virus. Quadrivalent vaccines provide protection against two influenza A subtype viruses and two influenza B viruses—one each of the B-Yamagata and B-Victoria lineages.

There are few contraindications to receiving the influenza vaccine. Those who have had a prior anaphylactic reaction to an influenza vaccine should not be vaccinated. A history of egg allergy requires consideration of the type of prior response to eggs and type of vaccine to be given. The LAIV should not be used in children aged 2 to 4 years with history of wheezing in the past year or diagnosis of asthma. LAIV should also not be used in pregnant women or those with immunocompromising conditions. Caretakers of severely immunocompromised people should also not receive LAIV. Adverse reactions are rare and vary depending on the vaccine type. The most common complaints in those who receive the IIV are soreness and redness at the injection site. Those who receive LAIV may experience a mild flu-like illness, which is generally well tolerated.

Travelers who have not already received the current annual influenza vaccine for their hemisphere should be vaccinated before travel to areas with ongoing influenza activity, ideally at least 2 weeks before departing.

5. Measles, mumps, and rubella: These three viral illnesses are very contagious and have potential for significant morbidity and mortality. They can be effectively prevented with vaccination and are therefore a key component of childhood vaccine programs around the world. The measles (or rubeola) virus belongs to the Paramyxovirus family, *Morbillivirus* genus. Measles infection causes fever, rash, and respiratory symptoms, and in rare cases can result in encephalitis or other complications that can be fatal. Measles is one of the most contagious diseases known, spread by direct contact with respiratory droplets or airborne transmission of aerosolized virus. Measles can remain in the air for up to 2 hours after an infected person has left a room. Mumps virus also belongs to the Paramyxovirus family, genus *Rubulavirus*. Mumps causes a viral syndrome that often includes infection of the salivary or parotid glands, called parotitis. Although mumps infection is most often mild and well tolerated, it can cause complications such as orchitis, meningitis, and deafness. Mumps is spread by airborne transmission. Rubella virus is of the Togavirus family, genus *Rubivirus*. Infection with the rubella virus may cause a rash and lymphadenopathy, and a mild viral syndrome. Infections may be asymptomatic. A significant concern is rubella infection in pregnant mothers within the first trimester, which can cause miscarriage, fetal death, or congenital rubella syndrome (CRS). CRS can result in congenital defects including cataracts, heart defects, and hearing impairment. Infants with CRS can transmit virus for up to 1 year. Rubella is spread by airborne transmission. All these infections are rare in developed nations with high levels of vaccination; however, they continue to circulate

in some regions and countries. Outbreaks may be more likely in the setting of disasters or crises that interrupt vaccination efforts.

Vaccines for measles, mumps, and rubella (MMR) are all live attenuated virus vaccines and are given together in a combination product. As a childhood vaccine, the first dose is usually given at 12 to 15 months, although may be given as early as 9 months in places with ongoing transmission. A second dose is usually given at age 4 years, although in areas with ongoing transmission the interval between doses can be as short as 4 weeks. Adults who are planning to travel overseas should be assessed for evidence of immunity, which can be either documentation of having received two doses of MMR vaccine or antibody test results indicating immunity. Those born before 1957 are considered immune and do not require any catch-up or pretravel vaccination. If there is no evidence of immunity, adults preparing to travel should receive two MMR vaccines at least 4 weeks apart.

There are some contraindications to the MMR vaccine. Because it is a live attenuated virus vaccine, it should not be given to pregnant women or those attempting to become pregnant, and women who receive the vaccine should be advised not to attempt to become pregnant for 4 weeks after receiving the vaccine. Individuals who are severely immunocompromised should not receive the MMR vaccine. MMR should not be given to those who have previously had a severe allergic reaction to the MMR vaccine, or have a severe allergy to gelatin or neomycin. The vaccine should not be given to those who have recently received blood transfusions or other blood products. Individuals with tuberculosis (TB) should not receive MMR vaccine. The vaccine should not be given within 4 weeks of other live virus vaccines.

Adverse reactions to MMR vaccine can include mild injection site soreness or redness, rash, fever, pain and stiffness of the joints, and swelling of lymph nodes or salivary glands. More serious, but rare, reactions include thrombocytopenia, seizures, or severe allergic reactions.

6. Pneumococcal: Pneumococcal disease is spread by person-to-person transmission of the gram-positive coccus *Streptococcus pneumoniae* via respiratory droplets. The 13-valent vaccine conjugate vaccine (PCV13) protects against 13 serotypes and is recommended for all people 65 years and older and some immunocompromised adults 19 to 64 years of age. The 23-valent polysaccharide vaccine (PPSV23) is recommended for adults 65 years and older and those 2 to 64 years with underlying medical conditions. Intervals for administration for each of the types of vaccine vary by age and risk group and guidelines should be followed.

7. Polio: Polioviruses (serotypes 1, 2, and 3) are nonenveloped, single-stranded RNA viruses (genus *Enterovirus*). Transmission is person to person, through oral and fecal-oral routes. Inactivated polio vaccine (IPV) is the only polio vaccine available in the United States, although oral polio vaccine (OPV) is used in much of the world. Primary vaccination of adults in the United States should occur if they are: travelers to areas of polio epidemicity/endemicity (even adults who have received a three-dose primary series and booster should receive an additional one-time booster dose of OPV/IPV before travel to areas of high risk); lab workers who handle specimens which may contain poliovirus; healthcare workers who care for possible excreters of wild poliovirus; or unvaccinated adults whose children will be receiving OPV. Adults who never finished a complete series should be given their final shot regardless of interval since most recent dose or type of vaccine.

All infants and children should receive four doses of IPV (ages 2 months, 4 months, 6–18 months, 4–6 years). If it appears the routine series cannot be completed before travel is anticipated, an alternative is to give the first dose at age 6 weeks or above, the second dose at least 4 weeks later, the third dose 4 weeks after that, with the fourth dose at least 6 months after the third. Unvaccinated adult travelers should receive three doses (two doses of IPV administered 4–8 weeks apart, third dose 6–12 months later). If the whole series cannot be completed in time for travel, continue as feasible in the interval prescribed. Vaccines given outside the United States can be accepted with valid evidence of vaccination, but caveats apply (see www.cdc.gov/mmwr for details).

See the requirements for polio vaccine before travel in the Required Vaccines section.

The most common side effects are minor local reactions (pain, redness). Hypersensitivity reactions can occur in people allergic to streptomycin, polymyxin B, and neomycin. If indicated, IPV can be administered to women who are pregnant or breastfeeding.

REQUIRED

Documentation of vaccination may be required for entry into certain countries:

1. Yellow fever. Yellow fever (YF) virus, a single-stranded RNA virus of genus *Flavivirus*, is transmitted through the bite of a mosquito (typically *Aedes* or *Haemagogus* spp.). There is currently one YF vaccine (YF-Vax), a live attenuated viral vaccine, licensed in the United States. Vaccination is recommended for those at least 9 months of age who are traveling to areas with evidence of persistent or periodic YF transmission (e.g., high risk areas in South America and Africa). Recommendations for vaccination should be guided by itinerary, season, duration of exposure, occupation, and activities, as well as local rate of virus transmission. Requirements for entry should be checked before travel and a completed International Certificate of Vaccination or Prophylaxis ("yellow card") with proof of a single dose of vaccine should be sufficient. A single 0.5-mL dose (administered subcutaneously) provides protection for life and booster is not needed; countries cannot require proof of booster, regardless of how long ago vaccination was administered.

   Additional doses of YF vaccine may be indicated for (1) women who were pregnant when receiving their initial dose (one more dose when indicated); (2) those who received hematopoietic stem cell transplant subsequent to a dose of YF (one more dose when at risk, if immunocompetent); (3) those infected with human immunodeficiency virus (HIV) when they last received YF vaccine and still at risk for YF (dose every 10 years). Booster should also be considered in travelers who received YF vaccine more than 10 years prior who are going to higher-risk environments, such as regions with a current outbreak or endemic areas during peak transmission.

   Mild reactions such as low-grade fever, headache, and myalgia occur in 10% to 30% of people vaccinated. Severe reactions are rare but can include immediate hypersensitivity reactions (rash, urticarial, bronchospasm), YF vaccine-associated neurologic disease (YEL-AND; meningoencephalitis, Guillain-Barré syndrome, acute disseminated encephalomyelitis, and cranial nerve palsies), and YF vaccine-associated viscerotropic disease (YEL-AVD; similar to YF disease). Contraindications to YF vaccine include: being under 6 months of age, hypersensitivity to vaccine components, altered immunity (thymus disorder, acquired immunodeficiency syndrome [AIDS] or clinical manifestations of HIV, immunodeficiencies, immunosuppressive or immunomodulatory therapies). People with contraindications should not receive YF vaccine.

   There are others who are considered higher risk for receiving vaccination and the decision to vaccinate should be weighed against risk of complication. Precautions include: 6 to 8 months of age, aged 60 years or older, pregnancy, breastfeeding, and asymptomatic HIV infection with moderate immunosuppression.

2. Polio (see also "Polio" under Routine). Travelers should know that there may exist a requirement for documentation of appropriate polio vaccine to depart from any states with wild poliovirus (WPV1) or circulating vaccine-derived poliovirus (cVDVP1 or cVDPV3) transmission. All residents or visitors for 4 weeks or more should receive a dose of IPV or

bivalent oral poliovirus vaccine (bOPV) 4 to 12 weeks before international travel. If travel is urgent (<4 weeks), individuals should still receive a dose of polio vaccine. Travelers from states with circulating cVDPV2 transmission should also be immunized and documented as such. Proof of vaccination may also be required from some individual polio-free countries and travelers should confirm individual requirements by contacting the consulate or embassy.

RECOMMENDED

These vaccines may be recommended before travel, depending on location, duration, and types of activities:

1. Cholera: Cholera is a diarrheal (dysentery) illness caused by toxigenic *Vibrio cholerae* O-group 1 or O-group 139. These bacteria are found in fresh or brackish water, and may be associated with aquatic plants and life forms. Outbreaks of cholera are often associated with drinking water contaminated with the bacteria, frequently caused by contamination with the feces of infected individuals. Cholera outbreaks may occur in settings where sanitation and hygiene are inadequate and untreated water is consumed. Cholera is a concern in disasters and crises where the bacteria is endemic and water, hygiene, and sanitation (WaSH) systems are ineffective to prevent infection. Cholera illness is characterized by diarrhea (called "rice-water stools"), nausea, and vomiting. It can quickly cause significant dehydration if fluids are not replenished either via oral rehydration solution (ORS) or intravenous fluids.

   Travelers to areas with endemic cholera who follow routine guidance to prevent travelers' diarrhea (discussed later in this chapter), such as only drinking bottled water, are not at risk of cholera disease and typically do not require vaccination. Travelers who are responding to disasters and/or may work in healthcare settings with infected patients may have increased risk of cholera infection. Those with blood type O and low gastric acidity may be at risk of more severe disease if they become infected.

   There are cholera vaccines available, but they are generally not part of routine vaccination recommendations. The WHO recommends vaccination only as a complementary measure after aggressive WaSH preventive efforts. Cholera vaccination may be used in the setting of a cholera outbreak, or as a preexposure prophylactic measure for individuals at higher risk. All currently available cholera vaccines are delivered orally. In the United States, the live attenuated CVD 103-HgR vaccine, marketed as Vaxchora, may be used in adults aged 18 to 64 traveling to areas with active cholera transmission. Specific areas that are considered to have active transmission can be found at https://wwwnc.cdc.gov/travel/diseases/cholera.

   The Vaxchora vaccine is given as a single oral dose. It should be administered in a healthcare setting, with no eating or drinking 60 minutes before or after administration. It should be administered at least 10 days before potential exposure to cholera. Contraindications to the vaccine include history of allergy to a cholera vaccine or any severe, life-threatening allergy. The vaccine should not be given to those with a compromised immune system, or anyone who is pregnant or trying to become pregnant. The vaccine may be less effective in those who have recently (within last 14 days) received antibiotics or are currently taking chloroquine or plan to start it within 10 days. Vaccine may be shed in the stool for 7 days after administration. Care should be taken to avoid any contamination of immunocompromised close contacts. Adverse reactions are rare, but may include mild fatigue, headache, abdominal pain, nausea, vomiting, and diarrhea.

2. Japanese encephalitis: Japanese encephalitis (JE) virus is a single-stranded RNA virus, belonging to the genus *Flavivirus*, which is transmitted via the bite of an infected mosquito. Ixiaro

is an inactivated Vero cell-culture-derived vaccine for those 2 months of age and older and is the only vaccine licensed in the United States. Vaccine recommendation should be guided by itinerary and length of stay in JE-endemic areas, time spent with unprotected evening or outdoor exposure, and the possibility (low) of serious adverse effects. The CDC's Advisory Committee on Immunization Practices recommends JE vaccine for longer-term ($\geq$1 month) travelers or frequent travelers to JE-endemic areas, or for shorter-term (<1 month) travelers with an increased risk of JE (based on location, activity, lodging, season).

The primary vaccination dose and schedule varies by age. The two-dose series should be completed at least 1 week before travel. If ongoing exposure is expected, a booster dose should be given at least 1 year after the primary Ixiaro series is complete.

Pain and tenderness at the injection site are the most commonly reported side effects, with headache, myalgia, fatigue, influenza-like illness, and fever (in children) also possible. Serious adverse effects are rare. No studies have been conducted in pregnancy and generally administration of vaccine for pregnant women should be deferred, unless the risk of infection outweighs the risk.

3. Meningococcal: *Neisseria meningitidis* is a gram-negative diplococcus, spread through respiratory secretions by either asymptomatic carriers or those with meningococcal disease. Four meningococcal vaccines are available in the United States: Menveo, Manactra, Trumenba, and Bexero. A quadrivalent meningococcal conjugate vaccine (MenACWY) is recommended routinely for all between 11 and 18 years of age (first dose at age 11 or 12 years, followed by booster at age 16 years). Routine immunization is not recommended for other age groups except in those with persistent complement component deficiency or functional, anatomic asplenia, or HIV. Vaccination with serogroup B meningococcal (MenB) series may be recommended for those aged 16 to 23 years or those at increased risk (note: MenB vaccine is not routinely recommended for travel unless an outbreak of MenB is reported.)

   Travelers to the "meningitis belt" of sub-Saharan Africa (from Senegal and Guinea to Ethiopia) during the dry season (December–June) and areas of recent outbreaks (information can be found at www.cdc.gov/travel) should be vaccinated with meningococcal vaccine. Travelers to the Kingdom of Saudi Arabia (KSA) for Umrah or the Hajj or for seasonal work are requested to document meningococcal vaccination within the last 3 years (polysaccharide vaccine) or 5 years (conjugate vaccine), but no more recently than 10 days before arrival. Visa requirements should be checked with the KSA embassy.

   Infants less than 9 months should be vaccinated with MenACWY-CRM (Menveo). At 2 months of age, MenACWY-CRM should be administered as a four-dose series (2, 4, 6, and 12 months). If initiating vaccination at 7 to 23 months of age, MenACWY-CRM should be administered as a two-dose series (second dose administered at $\geq$12 months of age and $\geq$3 months after the first dose). If needed for travel itinerary, the second dose can be administered as early as 8 weeks following the first.

   MenACWY-CRM or MenACWY-D (Menactra) may be used in travelers from 9 months of age through age 55 years. For travelers 9 to 23 months of age, two doses of MenACWY-D should be administered at least 3 months between doses, unless needed for travel (can administer 8 weeks apart to precede travel). A single dose of a MenACWY vaccine (MenACWY-CRM or MenACWY-D) is recommended for most travelers 2 years of age and over.

   International travelers previously vaccinated with a quadrivalent vaccine should receive a booster (children: after 2 years and every 5 years; those $\geq$7 years: after 5 years and every 5 years).

   Injection site pain, swelling, and low-grade fevers may be side effects after MenACWY vaccination, but severe adverse reactions are rare.

4. Rabies: Rabies is caused by neurotropic viruses in the family Rhabdoviridae, genus *Lyssavirus*, and the most common mode of transmission is inoculation of saliva secondary to an animal bite. Preexposure vaccination is recommended based on occupation of traveler (hunters, forest rangers, taxidermists, laboratory workers, stock breeders, abattoir workers, veterinarians, and spelunkers), occurrence of animal rabies in the destination country, activity of the traveler, duration of stay, and availability of treatments. Persons planning to stay over 30 days in a rabies-endemic area, such as most countries in Latin America, Africa, and Asia (except Taiwan and Japan) should be vaccinated.

   Preexposure vaccination includes three pretravel intramuscular injections given on days 0, 7, and 21 or 28 in the deltoid with human diploid cell rabies vaccine (HDCV) or purified chick embryo cell (PCEC) vaccine. If three doses of rabies vaccine cannot be completed before travel, the traveler should not start the series.

   Travelers who have completed a three-dose preexposure rabies immunization series or have received full postexposure prophylaxis (PEP) are considered previously vaccinated and do not require routine boosters. Routine testing for rabies virus-neutralizing antibody is not recommended for international travelers who are not otherwise in the frequent or continuous risk categories.

   PEP is recommended for all persons exposed to rabies virus, irrespective of immunization history. See Rabies in Chapter 3 for details about PEP.

   Local reactions such as pain, erythema, swelling, or itching, or mild systemic reactions such as headache, nausea, abdominal pain, muscle aches, and dizziness, may occur. Booster vaccinations with HDCV may result in systemic hypersensitivity reactions (urticaria, pruritus, and malaise). Once initiated, rabies PEP should not be interrupted or discontinued because of local or mild systemic reactions to rabies vaccine. If an adverse event occurs with one of the vaccine types, consider switching to the alternative vaccine for the remainder of the series. PEP is not contraindicated in pregnant women.

   Chloroquine phosphate or mefloquine may weaken the antibody response to HDCV when HDCV is given intradermally—if giving the vaccination any time near the taking of these medications, consider IM route; corticosteroids, chemotherapy, antimalarials (chloroquine, mefloquine), and immunosuppressive agent usage may warrant testing for antibody response.

   Other: preexposure immunization does not eliminate the need for the treatment with more vaccine after an exposure to rabies; any person exposed to rabies should always contact local or state health authorities and a personal physician for guidance – if the state epidemiologist is unavailable, call the CDC during Eastern working hours at (404) 639-1050 or (404) 639-2888 at any other time; for travelers abroad, if the availability of safe, effective postexposure products are in question, one should contact the nearest US embassy or consulate.

5. Typhoid: Typhoid and paratyphoid fever are potentially life-threatening illnesses caused by *Salmonella enterica* serotypes typhi and paratyphi A, B, and C. Transmission is by consumption of water or food contaminated by feces of an ill person or an asymptomatic carrier.

   Typhoid vaccine is recommended for travelers to areas at high risk for typhi exposure. The two vaccines available in the United States are Vi capsular polysaccharide vaccine (ViCPS) (Typhin Vi) or oral live attenuated vaccine (Vivotif). One 0.5-mL IM dose of ViCPS should be administered at least 2 weeks before travel to those 2 years of age or older, with a booster every 2 years for those who continue to be at risk. Oral Ty21a vaccine administration for those 6 years of age or older is one capsule every other day for 4 days (taken with cool liquid no warmer than 98.6°F), taken at least 2 hours after a meal and 1 hour before a meal. A booster is recommended every 5 years for those who remain at risk.

ViCPS vaccine may cause headache and injection site reactions. Reactions reported following Ty21a include abdominal discomfort, nausea, headache, fever, diarrhea, vomiting, and rash. Vaccination with Ty21a should be delayed for 72 hours following antibiotic treatment and antibiotics should not be administered within 72 hours of last dose of Ty21a vaccine. For pregnant women at high risk for typhoid exposure, ViCPS administration may be considered.

Prevention and Chemoprophylaxis of Vector-Borne Disease

The next important travel health consideration is whether the travel destination increases risk of vector-borne diseases, and what forms of prevention and prophylaxis are recommended. Vectors such as mosquitoes and other insects can transmit diseases caused by bacteria, viruses, and parasites. The first line of defense against vector-borne diseases is to avoid bites from vectors using mechanical, chemical, behavioral, and environmental measures. Mechanical barriers include use of netting (ideally impregnated with insecticide) while sleeping, wearing long sleeves and long pants, and tucking pants into shoes or boots. Chemical barriers include use of insect repellents, such as DEET, picaridin, and permethrin. DEET and picaridin can be applied directly to the skin in sprays, liquids, lotions, and on wipes. Products should be at least 30% active ingredient. Repellents should be reapplied regularly, according to recommendations for the particular product used. When concurrently applied with sunscreen, sunscreen should be applied first followed by insect repellent. Clothing can be pretreated with permethrin, which will last through many washes, and some travel clothing can be purchased already treated. Military uniforms are often pretreated with permethrin. Treatment needs to be completed 24 to 28 hours before travel to ensure drying of the permethrin solution. Behavioral measures such as avoiding being outside at times of highest risk for bites may be implemented; however in a disaster response scenario one may have little control over when time is spent outdoors. Skin checks for ticks should be performed after time spent in an area at risk for ticks. Environmental measures such as spraying of insecticides can be very helpful to control vector populations, but also may not be available in a disaster response setting.

Malaria is the vector-borne disease typically of greatest concern for travelers. Malaria is caused by several species of *Plasmodium* parasites and is transmitted from person to person by mosquitoes of the *Anopheles* genus. The WHO estimated there were 214 million malaria cases and 438,000 malaria deaths worldwide in 2015. Transmission occurs in much of Africa, parts of Latin America and the Caribbean, parts of Asia, and some South Pacific islands. The distribution of *Plasmodium* species varies by geographic location.

Malaria causes a febrile illness that can be debilitating and sometime fatal if untreated. Most clinical cases are caused by *P. falciparum* or *P. vivax*; *P. falciparum* malaria causes severe disease and can be fatal, while *P. vivax* is often less severe. Additional species that can cause clinical malaria are *P. ovale*, *P. malariae*, and *P. knowlesi*. Prompt diagnosis and treatment with appropriate medication(s) are critical. Development of drug resistance has been a continual problem for treatment of malaria, with limited treatment choices remaining in some geographic areas. Details of clinical malaria infection, diagnosis and treatment will be covered in detail in Chapter 3.

Risk of malaria transmission can vary greatly depending on destination (including geographic variation within a country), season of travel, and anticipated activities. Recommendations for prevention of malaria should be tailored to the individual traveler. However, for travelers responding to a disaster or other contingency, a conservative approach to prevention may be advised since location and activities may change unexpectedly.

The best way to avoid infection with malaria is to avoid mosquito bites via the preventive measures covered above. The *Anopheles* mosquitoes tend to be nocturnal feeders, biting primarily between dusk and dawn. Sleeping under bed nets, avoiding outdoor activities at night, proper wear of clothing, and use of repellents should be practiced rigorously. Equally important is use of malaria chemoprophylaxis when appropriate. There are multiple regimens available, which should be selected based on information about the endemic species in the travel destination, local drug resistance patterns, and the medical history and preferences of the traveler. Current travel health resources should be consulted before travel, as recommendations may change over time. Here is a summary of commonly used chemoprophylaxis regimens:

1. Atovaquone-Proguanil (US trade name Malarone): This combination provides effective prophylaxis for all malaria parasite species. It is dosed 250 mg/100 mg (single tablet) once daily in adults, and should be started 1 to 2 days before entry into an area at risk for malaria. It should be continued for 7 days after departing the malaria risk area; however, some studies suggest effectiveness if continued just 1 day after departing the area. The half-life is longer than other daily prophylactic medications such as doxycycline, so a missed dose will not likely decrease prophylactic effectiveness. Atovaquone-proguanil is generally well tolerated without significant side effects when taken with food or a milky drink. This is a good choice for short-term travel, given the minimal dosing required pre- and posttravel. Atovaquone-proguanil cannot be used in pregnant or lactating women, children weighing less than 5 kilograms, or those with severe renal impairment. This is the newest option for malaria chemoprophylaxis and is usually of higher cost than other options.

2. Chloroquine (US trade name Aralen) or hydroxychloroquine (US trade name Plaquenil): Although it is a historically important malaria treatment, development of resistance has limited chloroquine's use for treatment and prophylaxis in much of the world. However, some areas of Mexico, Central America, and the Caribbean have malaria parasites that remain susceptible. Chloroquine is dosed 500 mg salt (300 mg base) once weekly in adults, starting 1 to 2 weeks before travel, and continuing until 4 weeks after departing the area at risk for malaria. Potential side effects include gastrointestinal upset, and long-term use can cause retinopathy. It can potentially exacerbate psoriasis. There are few contra-indications to chloroquine; it can be used in pregnant and lactating women and children. Hydroxychloroquine is a similar prophylactic option, and may be better tolerated in some individuals. It is dosed 400 mg (310 mg base) once weekly in adults, starting 1 to 2 weeks before travel and continuing until 4 weeks after departing the area at risk.

3. Doxycycline: The antibiotic doxycycline may be used to prevent malaria, and can be used in all geographic areas. It is dosed 100 mg once daily in adults, starting 1 to 2 days before entering the area at risk of malaria, and continued for 4 weeks after departing. Given its relatively short half-life, consistent daily dosing is critical. Some may experience side effects, including gastrointestinal problems such as dyspepsia, nausea/vomiting, esophageal ulcers, and inflammation. Doxycycline is also associated with increased photosensitivity and vaginal yeast infections. For individuals taking medications that may have risk of phototoxicity, doxycycline should be avoided. Doxycycline cannot be used in pregnant and lactating women or children under 8 years of age. An additional benefit of doxycycline use is that it also may prevent leptospirosis and rickettsial diseases.

4. Mefloquine (US trade name Lariam): Mefloquine was developed in response to growing chloroquine resistance. It is dosed 250 mg salt (228 mg base) once weekly in adults, starting 1 to 2 weeks before travel, and continuing until 4 weeks after departing the area at risk for malaria. Resistance to mefloquine is present in some areas of Southeast Asia, and monitoring is ongoing for spread of resistance to other geographic areas. Mefloquine is associated with neuropsychiatric side effects such as vivid dreams or nightmares, anxiety, depression, confusion, restlessness, and dizziness. There are also risks of cardiovascular conduction depression. Mefloquine should not be used in individuals with preexisting psychiatric disorders, seizure disorders, or cardiovascular disorders. Mefloquine can be used in pregnant

and lactating females and in children. The potential psychiatric side effects of mefloquine have received a great deal of media attention in the last decade, prompting a US Food and Drug Administration boxed warning, and it is no longer considered as a first line malaria prophylactic medication in the US military.

5. Primaquine: Primaquine is an option for primary malaria chemoprophylaxis in areas with more than 90% *Plasmodium vivax* malaria, and is used for presumptive antirelapse therapy, occasionally referred to as terminal prophylaxis, after departing areas with high levels of *Plasmodium vivax* and *ovale*. Primaquine treats hypnozoites in the liver, in contrast to all other chemoprophylactic agents that treat blood stages of the malaria parasite. For primary prophylaxis, primaquine is dosed 52.6 mg salt (30 mg base) daily in adults, starting 1 to 2 days before travel, and is continued for 7 days after departing the area at risk for malaria. For presumptive antirelapse therapy, the dosing is 15 to 30 mg base daily for 14 days after departing the area at risk. Presumptive antirelapse therapy is usually recommended in longer-term travelers. Primaquine can cause hemolysis in individuals with glucose-6-phosphate dehydrogenase (G6PD) deficiency, so it should not be prescribed in those not screened for G6PD deficiency. It is contraindicated in pregnancy, but can be used in lactating women if the infant has been screened and does not have a G6PD deficiency. It can be used in children without G6PD deficiency. Primaquine may cause gastrointestinal side effects, which can be lessened by taking it with food.

Additional vector-borne diseases of concern are arboviruses, or viruses spread by arthropod vectors, such as YF, dengue, Zika, chikungunya, West Nile, JE, and others. These viruses can cause a range of clinical syndromes from mild rash to hemorrhagic fever to encephalitis. The geographic distributions of these viruses and their vectors vary and are dynamic, especially given the impacts of climate change, land-use changes, and global transit and travel. For travelers, preventive measures to avoid insect bites are key to preventing these infections. Some of the mosquito vectors of these viruses breed rapidly in standing water, such as species of the *Aedes* genus. Avoiding the accumulation of water in tires, pots, containers, and other areas can help decrease the vector burden. There are vaccines widely available for YF and JE, and vaccines in development for dengue, Zika, and other viruses. A 2015 outbreak of Zika in Brazil brought worldwide attention to the virus as it spread elsewhere in the western hemisphere. Zika infection during pregnancy has been linked with microcephaly and other brain abnormalities in fetuses. Zika infections have also been associated with Guillain-Barre syndrome. Zika-related travel guidance includes a recommendation that pregnant women not travel to areas with active Zika transmission, and that couples use barrier contraception for 6 months after males have been in an area with active Zika transmission because the virus can remain in the semen for several months.

Ticks, fleas, lice, and mites are vectors for bacterial, viral, and parasitic pathogens. Ticks are usually found in wooded or grassy areas. Fleas, lice, and mites are often associated with animals and may be found in urban or rural environments. Rickettsial bacterial infections are spread by these vectors in most of the world. Tickborne encephalitis (TBE) is a viral infection spread by ticks in Europe and Asia. Vaccines for TBE are produced in Austria, Germany, and Russia. Travelers to endemic areas should consider receiving the vaccination if available in their home country, or when they arrive in the area at risk. Ticks can also spread the parasitic disease babesiosis. Prevention of diseases caused by ticks, fleas, lice, and mites includes typical insect bite prevention measures, as well as controlling rodent and other animal populations in areas of human habitation. Maintaining good hygiene and performing skin checks for ticks are also important preventive measures.

Flies and sandflies also serve as vectors for infectious pathogens. Flies can directly transmit bacteria or viruses, acting as fomites. Blackflies can transmit onchocerciasis, or river blindness. Sandflies can transmit leishmaniasis. Contact with flies and sandflies should be avoided with preventive measures discussed above. Sandflies are quite small (2–3 mm) and may be able to pass through an ordinary bed net, but insecticide treatment of bed nets will help improve effectiveness against these small insects.

Finally, animals also serve as vectors of disease. Bites and scratches can result in skin infections, or can transmit rabies virus. Bites of certain poisonous snakes or spiders can result in illness or death. Travelers should avoid close contact with animals to prevent bites. The pretravel medical encounter is the appropriate time to determine if tetanus vaccination is up to date and discuss the option of rabies preexposure prophylaxis. Typically, rabies preexposure prophylaxis is recommended for those traveling longer than 1 month to areas potentially at risk for rabies, especially rural areas in developing countries. Whether an individual has had preexposure prophylaxis or not, it is important to seek medical care after an animal bite for PEP with rabies immune globulin and/or rabies vaccine. Details of this management will be discussed further in Chapter 3. Those with snake or spider bites should also seek medical care, as antivenom may be available in some healthcare facilities. As part of preparation for travel, individuals may wish to investigate where there are local medical facilities with therapies that could be needed acutely for animal bite situations.

Travelers' Diarrhea

The most common affliction of travelers is gastrointestinal illness with diarrhea and other bothersome gastrointestinal symptoms, such as nausea, vomiting, cramps, abdominal pain, and bloating. Known as travelers' diarrhea (TD) in the setting of foreign travel, this may affect up to 10% to 40% of travelers, depending on itinerary and characteristics of the traveler (Steffen, 2015). Travel destination and travel style, including where food purchases are made and where consumed food is prepared, likely influence risk the most. Although the ultimate goal is prevention, this is often challenging for travelers, especially those traveling to low-income regions. Therefore, travelers need to be prepared to manage and treat TD if it occurs.

TD is often caused by ingestion of fecally contaminated food or water, and the etiologic agent is most often bacterial. TD is present if an individual has three or more unformed stools in a 24-hour period plus one or more additional symptoms, such as cramping, tenesmus, nausea, vomiting, fever, or fecal urgency (Steffen, 2015). Severity is variable, ranging from discomfort that does not impact activities to debilitating pain and other symptoms. Although most cases are self-limited and can be managed effectively, in some cases TD can result in life-threatening dehydration and even death.

The most common causes of TD that occur in developing regions include the following: ETEC (heat-labile and heat-stable toxin producing *Escherichia coli*), *E. coli* (enteroaggregative and diffusely adherent), noroviruses, rotavirus, *Salmonella* species, *Campylobacter jejuni*, *Shigella* species, *Aeromonas, Plesiomonas shigelloides, Bacteroides fragilis*, and *Vibrio* species; there are regions where parasites such as *Giardia duodenalis, Cryptosporidium* species, *Entamoeba histolytica*, and *Microsporidium* species are also potential culprits (Steffen, 2015). The average duration of untreated TD is 4 to 5 days and, although between 12% and 46% of patients may have short-term "disability," most report only 1 day of incapacitation (Steffen, 2015). TD is also sometimes linked with long-term sequelae such as irritable bowel syndrome (IBS) (Riddle, 2016; Steffen, 2015).

Travelers can learn the approximate risk of developing TD at their destination by examining historical data. Prevention of TD is primarily focused on avoiding consumption of contaminated liquids and foods, but this can be more challenging than the common advice "boil it, cook it, peel it, or forget it" implies. In some locations there is inadequate processing (including filtration, treatment, and testing) of municipal water at baseline. In a disaster scenario, even locations with adequate water processing infrastructure at baseline may have increased risk for contamination. It is best to avoid consuming local municipal water if the reliability of water processing infrastructure is unclear. Bottled water from a trusted processing company is typically safe for consumption.

Water purification with a reverse osmosis water purification unit (ROWPU) may be employed in a disaster setting, producing large volumes of safe-for-consumption water in a short amount of time. Individual water filtration devices may also be used; these may be in the form of a pumping-type device or a small water bottle that filters directly. Water may also be boiled (to rolling boil for at least 1 minute) or treated, to be safe for consumption.

Travelers may consider bringing along items to assist in purification of water, especially in areas with a higher risk of TD. Iodine tablets are a quick and easy way to purify water and can be easily transported. Low-concentration bleach products can also be used to treat water, although it is important to understand the products that should be used in such scenarios. The CDC and a social marketing nongovernment organization Population Services International worked together to produce and market the Safe Water System chlorination product (Lantagne, 2009). Before travel, a small personal filtration device may be a good investment.

Besides water, other liquids may become contaminated in processing or preparation. It is best to drink bottled products only when you have seen them opened and can confirm that there was a tight seal. Fruit juices that are prepared fresh may be at risk of contamination. Generally, hot beverages like coffee or tea are low risk; however, if they are made with contaminated water and not heated sufficiently, they may also carry risk. Finally, consumption of ice should be avoided as often ice is made using municipal water which may be contaminated.

Appropriate food selection can be even more challenging when attempting to prevent TD. Because many eating establishments may have sanitation and cooking practices that are inadequate and not readily apparent to travelers, even the most careful traveler may consume the pathogens that cause TD. Foods are often not brought to the correct temperature, may be left out at room temperature, or may be subject to insects when not covered appropriately (Steffen, 2015). Whereas travelers should exert caution in choosing eating establishments and the foods they eat, additional measure might be considered to protect from TD more fully.

In addition to liquid and food preventive measures, there is a high level of evidence that prophylactic use of bismuth subsalicylates have moderate effectiveness in preventing TD and may be considered in travelers who do not have contraindications to use and can adhere to the dosing requirement (Riddle, 2016). The recommended dose is two tablets, four times a day (mealtimes and at bedtime) for up to 3 weeks and individuals should be warned that their stools and tongues will turn black. It should not be taken as prophylaxis when other salicylates are being used or when a trip is longer than two weeks and should not be used by individuals with inflammatory bowel disease or HIV (Riddle, 2016).

Antibiotic chemoprophylaxis can also be considered to prevent TD, especially in high risk groups. Historically, concerns about antibiotic resistance and side effects and questions about effectiveness have precluded guidelines recommending the routine use of prophylactic antibiotics. However, the increasing recognition of postinfectious IBS as a public health issue and the availability of rifaximin, a nonabsorbable antibiotic with an improved safety profile, have led to more recent recommendations to consider rifaximin in certain populations (Riddle, 2016). A traveler who is at high risk for TD or for whom TD could pose serious medical consequence or a significant negative impact on the mission of the travel, might consider rifaximin.

Environmental Factors

Travel may involve rapid changes of environmental conditions, which can have health impacts. Travelers should be prepared for potential temperature extremes. Environmental heat exposure may increase risk for heat illness. Classic heat illness occurs primarily in young children or the elderly, and exertional heat illness occurs more often in young adults. Heat illness occurs when the physiologic responses to heat stress are inadequate and core body temperature rises, resulting in a spectrum of symptoms ranging from cramps to syncope to organ failure. Heat stroke, which includes mental status changes, is a medical emergency and will require contact with the local healthcare system.

Lack of adequate acclimatization is a risk factor for heat illness. Disaster responders may quickly become involved in strenuous duties upon arrival to a new location and put themselves at risk for heat illness. When traveling to a significantly warmer environment, individuals should limit strenuous physical activity in the initial days. Some acclimatization protocols recommend up to 2 weeks of gradual increase in activity. Additional risk factors include prior heat illness, obesity, poor physical fitness, sleep deprivation, illness, excessive alcohol use, dehydration, and certain medical conditions and medications. The medications that may increase risk of heat illness include anticholinergics, antihistamines, antiepileptics, tricyclic antidepressants, amphetamines, lithium, beta-blockers, and diuretics. Avoiding alcohol use, hydrating well, and getting adequate sleep can help avoid heat illness. There is no specific threshold of environmental heat that portends a greater risk of heat illness; each individual's physiology is unique and heat illness can occur at temperatures that might not be considered very extreme. It is important to be cognizant of potential heat-related symptoms, and act quickly to cool body temperature if there is any concern for heat illness.

Cold environments can also result in health problems, although this is uncommon with proper planning and gear. Most travel-related cold injuries are related to accidents or unexpected severe weather. Hypothermia can occur rapidly if an individual becomes wet or exposed in cool conditions. Those who will be traveling on or working around cold bodies of water should make sure to have personal flotation devices available, as immersion hypothermia can render a person unable to swim or tread water in less than 15 minutes. Other cold-related conditions include nonfreezing injuries such as trench foot, pernio (chilblains) and cold urticaria, and the freezing injuries of frostbite. Frostbite can result in loss of digits if not recognized and treated promptly. Severe hypothermia and frostbite will likely require contact with the local healthcare system and may necessitate medical evacuation depending on the treatment capabilities available locally.

Depending on the travel destination, the level of exposure to ultraviolet (UV) light may increase significantly. Higher elevation, tropical latitude, and increased reflection from snow or sand increase risk for sunburn and associated health risks. Also, some medications may increase sun sensitivity, including medications that may be only taken during travel (e.g., doxycycline for malaria chemoprophylaxis). Prevention of sunburn requires diligent preventive efforts. As much as possible, clothing should provide the first defense against UV rays. Some clothing items provide a specified level of sun protection factor (SPF). A wide-brimmed hat can help decrease exposure of the face and neck. Sunscreen with a SPF of at least 15 should be used routinely on any exposed skin and reapplied regularly, approximately every 2 hours. A waterproof or water-resistant sunscreen will provide longer duration of protection. Sunscreen should be applied before insect repellents and combination products should be avoided since sunscreen will need to be reapplied more frequently than the repellent. Severe sunburns are like thermal burns and may require medical care.

Rapid ascent to high altitude environments can result in acute mountain sickness (AMS), high altitude cerebral edema (HACE), and high altitude pulmonary edema (HAPE) in those not acclimatized. These conditions can be rapidly fatal if not promptly recognized and descent quickly initiated. There is no specific altitude at which all unacclimatized persons will have difficulty, as each individual's physiology and susceptibility differ, although rapid ascent from low altitude to above 9000 ft (2750 m) sleeping altitude should trigger consideration of preventive measures. Pretravel exposure to 9000 ft (2750 m) for 2 nights or more within 30 days of travel can be very helpful in preventing altitude illnesses. Gradual ascent to higher elevations, if possible, decreases risk of altitude illnesses. Spending a few days at 8000 to 9000 ft (2500–2750 m), and then moving sleep altitude no greater than an additional 1600 ft (500 m) per day is advised. If a gradual ascent is not possible, use of prophylactic medications may be considered. Acetazolamide (US trade name Diamox) is most commonly used for AMS/HACE prevention, at 125 mg twice a day (250 mg if weight >100 kg) starting 1 day before ascent and continuing the first 2 days at high altitude. Acetazolamide is contraindicated in individuals with a history of an anaphylactic reaction to a sulfa drug, although in those with nonanaphylactic reaction to sulfa the risk of a reaction to acetazolamide is quite low. Acetazolamide causes increased urination and paresthesias of the fingers and toes. Additional medications that are used for treatment of altitude illnesses (dexamethasone, nifedipine) can be considered for prophylactic use in those at high risk and not eligible for acetazolamide. This topic will be discussed further in Chapter 9.

Another environmental consideration is potential exposure to bodies of water. As mentioned above, submersion in cool or cold water can quickly result in hypothermia. Accidents of vessels of conveyance can result in drowning; travelers should be mindful of whether personal flotation devices are available on ferries, boats, or ships. When near the ocean, travelers should be aware of tides and surf because conditions can change quickly. Sand at the beach can be home to helminths; wearing footwear on the beach helps prevent infection. Freshwater exposure may increase risk of leptospirosis or schistosomiasis, depending on location. For those with anticipated freshwater exposure in an area known to be at risk for leptospirosis, doxycycline 200 mg once weekly starting 1 or 2 days before exposure and continued through the period of exposure, may be used as chemoprophylaxis. Flooding situations can increase risk for trauma and contact with water that is potentially contaminated with pathogens and chemicals.

Air pollution is increasingly a health threat for travelers. In some large cities, the particulate matter in the air frequently reaches unhealthy levels. Those with preexisting respiratory or cardiovascular conditions, such as asthma, chronic obstructive pulmonary disease, and heart disease, may wish to monitor air quality measures before travel. The WHO provides historical information on air pollution by country (gamapserver.who.int/gho/interactive_charts/phe/oap_exposure/atlas. html) and some US embassies provide real-time air quality information on their websites. Those at risk should avoid strenuous exercise when air pollution levels are elevated. Additionally, travelers may be at risk of indoor air pollution from cigarette smoking and cooking fuels (e.g., charcoal, wood, kerosene). Carbon monoxide poisoning can occur because of unvented cooking stoves and space heaters, or improper placement of generators.

Finally, a travel-related change in environment may increase risk for accidents and injuries. An unfamiliar environment, different safety standards, hazardous traffic, and limitations of communication can all contribute to this increased risk. Injuries are the leading cause of preventable death in travelers. Travelers should use common sense approaches to decrease injury risk, such as using seat belts in vehicles (or choosing not to ride in vehicles that do not have seat belts), avoiding driving at night or peak traffic hours, exercising caution when crossing roads, and not using cellular telephones when driving (or allowing drivers to use them while driving). The Association for Safe International Road Travel (www.asirt.org) provides specific information about road safety for some countries (requires no-fee registration to access). It is important to maintain situational awareness while traveling. Travelers should not consume excessive alcohol or any other substances that may impair alertness or decision-making ability.

Other Infectious Risks

Sexually transmitted infections (STIs) are common worldwide. Travelers who engage in casual sex while in foreign countries increase their risk of acquiring STIs, including HIV. Prevalence of certain infections vary by country, so a traveler may be exposed to infections not common in his or her home country. Commercial sex workers often have high rates of certain STIs. Prevention includes abstinence from sex with new partners during travel, or use of male latex condoms. Consistent use of condoms can prevent transmission of some, but not all, STI pathogens. Pretravel vaccination for hepatitis A and B is also preventive because both viruses can be spread sexually. Posttravel testing for STIs including HIV may be indicated for those at increased risk. Certain travelers at high risk for HIV exposure may consider preexposure prophylactic treatment.

Travelers may be at risk for exposure to blood and bodily fluid-borne pathogens, especially travelers involved in patient care during responses to disasters or other contingencies. Healthcare workers should practice standard precautions and enhanced infection control precautions as indicated. Pretravel training on use of personal protective equipment can help prepare health-care personnel to protect themselves. Healthcare workers' immunization records should be carefully scrutinized to ensure protection from vaccine-preventable infections that may be encountered in the healthcare setting. These include measles, mumps and rubella, hepatitis B, varicella (immunization or prior infection), tetanus, diphtheria, and pertussis, and annual influenza. Contact with blood or bodily fluids by percutaneous exposures, such as needle sticks, puts healthcare workers at risk of infection with hepatitis B, hepatitis C, and HIV. Depending on the assessed risk of infection, the healthcare worker may opt to initiate PEP treatment for HIV. The regimen used most commonly in the United States is a three-drug regimen daily for 4 weeks; either tenofovir-emtricitabine (300/200 mg once daily) plus dolutegravir (50 mg once daily) or tenofovir-emtricitabine (300/200 mg once daily) plus raltegravir (400 mg twice daily). Laboratory testing for HIV should occur at baseline, 6 weeks, 3 months, and 6 months. Laboratory testing for hepatitis C should occur at baseline and three or more weeks after potential exposure. If susceptible to hepatitis B, there is also a regimen for PEP.

Another travel-related infectious risk that is heightened for healthcare workers is TB. This bacterial infection is most commonly spread through respiratory aerosols from individuals with active pulmonary TB. Healthcare workers should use respiratory protection, such as N-95 respirators, when working with patients known or suspected to have TB. Healthcare workers may be screened periodically with tuberculin skin test (TST) or interferon-gamma release assay (IGRA) for evidence of latent TB infection. Healthcare workers who may have increased risk of exposure to TB during travel should have pretravel screening with TST or IGRA before travel and again 8 to 10 weeks after return. TB will be covered further in Chapter 3.

CHAPTER 2

Global Infectious Diseases: Four Steps Toward a Differential Diagnosis

Saif Al-Bedwawi ▦ Amanda Huston

Symptoms and Signs

FEVER

1. Etiologies to think about
   a. Malaria, visceral leishmaniasis, African trypanosomiasis, Chagas' disease, relapsing fever, rickettsial infections, arboviral diseases (e.g., dengue fever), rabies, typhoid/para-typhoid, leptospirosis, tuberculosis, human immunodeficiency virus (HIV).

2. Things to do routinely
   a. Thick blood films to evaluate for malaria. In endemic areas, remember fever may be caused by something other than malaria in patients with (+) films. Malaria can cause acute, chronic, or relapsing fever. Malaria is highly suspicious when fevers occur every (q) 48–72 hours but may usually take 2 weeks for schizontocytes to become synchronized. *Plasmodium falciparum* rarely develops such a fever pattern.
   b. Complete blood count with differential (CBC with differential [w/ diff])
      i. Malaria will usually have normal or low white blood cell count (WBC), often with thrombocytopenia.
      ii. With leukocytosis (especially with left shift), even patients with a (+) film are very likely to have a cause other than malaria.
   c. Begin a fever chart: 4-hour intervals are most useful.
   d. Check for rash, lymphadenopathy (LAD), splenomegaly, anemia, jaundice, polyarthritis, and so on.

Acute Fevers (<2 Weeks)

1. Acute fever + negative malarial film
   a. Polymorphonuclear leukocytosis (PNL)?
      i. Yes: pyogenic infection, leptospirosis, relapsing fever, amebic hepatic abscess, collagen-vascular disease (collagenosis)
      ii. No: viral infection, rickettsial infection, typhoid
         - PNL often does develop after onset of severe viral infections such as Lassa fever.
         - Typhoid may be of gradual onset with remittent fever (never quite fully defervesces).
2. Acute fever + negative malarial film + PNL + localizing symptoms (sx)?
   a. Sore throat: various pharyngitis etiologies, remember *Corynebacterium diphtheriae*
   b. Pulmonary: various pneumonial etiologies
   c. Pain, swelling in joint: pyogenic arthritis
   d. Urinary tract infection (UTI) sx + flank/back pain: pyelonephritis
   e. Headache, neck stiffness: meningitis
   f. Bone pain: osteomyelitis
   g. Bloody diarrhea: bacterial dysentery (*Shigella*, *Salmonella*, *Campylobacter*, enteroinvasive *Escherichia coli*, *Yersinia*, etc.)
   h. Local lymphadenopathy: local infection, plague
   i. Sharply defined cutaneous inflammation: erysipelas
   j. Poorly defined subcutaneous inflammation: cellulitis
3. Acute fever + negative malarial film + leukocytosis but no localizing sx?
   a. Septicemia: *Staphylococcus*, *Streptococcus*, *Meningococcus*, endocarditis
   b. *Leptospira*, *Borrelia* spp.
      i. Leptospirosis: look for jaundice, renal involvement
      ii. Tick-borne relapsing fever
      iii. Louse-borne relapsing fever
   c. Nontyphoid *Salmonella* septicemia: may be paucity of gastrointestinal (GI) sx; rose spots, splenomegaly possible
4. Acute fever + negative malarial film, but no PNL?
   a. Consider virus, rickettsia, typhoid
      i. Double-humped fever pattern suggests virus, especially dengue.
         - First fever represents viremia; second fever represents antibody-mediated viral destruction, perhaps with cells.
      ii. Significant space-time clustering suggests nonspecific viral source.
         - With rickettsial diseases, look for adenopathy, possibly an eschar.
         - With typhoid, pay attention to abdominal sx.

5. Acute fever + right upper quadrant (RUQ) tenderness?
   a. Obtain CBC w/ diff, malarial film, liver function tests (LFTs).
   b. Ultrasound (U/S) liver, gallbladder
   c. Amebic sensitized particle agglutination test (SPAG); often (–) in early amebic liver abscess
      i. Typically, ALA with (w/) leukocytosis, increased erythrocyte sedimentation rate (ESR).
   d. ESR
   e. Hepatitides panel
6. Acute fever + hemorrhagic rash?
   a. Consider viral hemorrhagic fevers (dengue, Crimean-Congo, etc.) meningococcemia.
   b. Can be fatal w/in hours if meningococcemia; aspirate from spots should be examined for meningococci.

Note that cases of acute fevers may be accompanied by nonhemorrhagic rashes. A notable exception is malaria (rarely causes a rash); a drug eruption in treated malaria patients could still occur.

7. Acute fever + anemia?
   a. Although anemia is common in developing areas (diet, sickle cell diseases (SCDz), thalassemia, glucose-6-phosphate dehydrogenase [G6PD] deficiency), consider malaria, babesiosis, and bartonellosis specifically.

Chronic Fever (>2 Weeks)

1. Overlap
   a. *Borrelia* infections, typhoid, and malaria may be seen as acute or chronic.
2. Chronic fever + PNL
   a. Typically sustained fever
      i. Deep sepsis
      ii. ALA
      iii. Erythema nodosum leprosum
   b. Typically relapsing fever
      i. Cholangitis
      ii. Relapsing fever
3. Chronic fever + eosinophilia
   a. Invasive *Schistosoma mansoni*, *Schistosoma japonicum*
   b. Invasive *Fasciola hepatica*
   c. Acute lymphangitic exacerbations of *Wuchereria bancrofti*, *Brugia malayi*
   d. Gross visceral larva migrans (*Toxocara canis*)
4. Chronic fever + neutropenia
   a. Malaria
   b. Disseminated tuberculosis
   c. Visceral leishmaniasis
   d. Brucellosis
5. Chronic fever + normal WBC
   a. Localized tuberculosis
   b. Brucellosis
   c. Secondary syphilis
   d. Trypanosomiasis
   e. Toxoplasmosis
   f. Subacute bacterial endocarditis (SBE)
   g. Chronic meningococcal septicemia
6. Chronic fever + variable WBC
   a. Tumors

    b. Drug reactions

    c. Other fever of unknown origin differential diagnosis (FUO ddx)

7. Chronic fever w/ relapsing pattern

    a. Malaria

    b. Visceral leishmaniasis

    c. Trypanosomiasis, especially African

    d. Relapsing fever (*Borrelia* spp.)

    e. Brucellosis

    f. Filariasis

    g. Cholangitis

    h. Subacute bacterial endocarditis

Note that many other diseases may have a relapsing pattern; these frequently do.

8. Fever of unknown origin w/u for tropical and/or developing areas

    a. CBC w/ diff, repeated malarial films

    b. Chest x-ray (CXR)

    c. Urine analysis (U/A)

    d. Repeated blood culture (cx)

    e. Liver biopsy (bx), to include tuberculosis cx

    f. Marrow bx, to include cx and animal inoculation

    g. IVP

    h. Mantoux test to 1, 10, and 100 tuberculin units

    i. Brucella cx and antibody titers

    j. Toxoplasma dye test

    k. Rickettsial and viral antibodies

    l. Serum assays for systemic lupus erythematous (SLE), and antinuclear factor

    m. ESR

Note that disseminated tuberculosis is a common cause; remember it can manifest in the spine (Pott's dz), bowel (enteritis), abdominal viscera, and as ascites and/or peritonitis.

9. Chronic fever + normal WBC + normal ESR

    a. Consider spurious fever or toxoplasmosis

10. Chronic fever and HIV infection

    a. The virus itself can cause fever, but opportunistic organisms should be ruled out (R/O'd), especially *Salmonella*, *Pneumococcus*, and tuberculosis.

ABDOMINAL PAIN

1. Abdominal pain

    a. Amebiasis

    b. Anisakiasis

    c. Bacterial enteritis (*Salmonella, Shigella, Yersinia*; especially right lower quadrant [RLQ]), *Campylobacter* (can be very intense)

    d. Fascioliasis

    e. Giardiasis

    f. Hymenolepiasis

    g. Strongyloidiasis

    h. Taeniasis

    i. Typhoid

    j. Abscess (hepatic, splenic)

    k. Pancreatitis

    l. Hepatitis

    m. Other non-ID causes

DIARRHEA

1. Historical considerations
   a. Duration?
      i. Acute <2 w, chronic >2 w.
   b. Fever?
      i. May be resulting from enteritis, dehydration, or extraenteric source (i.e., malaria)
   c. Appearance? Blood? Mucous?
      i. Blood may signify colonic ulceration, especially in developing nations where hemorrhoids are less common.
   d. Frequency?
      i. Mainly ask to gauge need for hydration.
   e. Abdominal pain?
      i. Most acute with bacterial organisms (*Campylobacter, Shigella*, etc.), necrotizing toxin (*Clostridium perfringens*), or w/ electrolyte imbalances in cholera.
   f. Tenesmus?
      i. Suggests rectal inflammation, sometimes seen with shigellosis.
   g. Vomiting?
      i. May indicate systemic illness, preformed toxins, or intestinal infections. In nonimmune patients, may be a sx of malaria, especially *P. falciparum*.
   h. Others w/ similar sx?
      i. For obvious epidemiologic reasons
2. The three essential questions: Duration? Fever? Blood?
   a. Acute + Fever + Blood
      i. Bacterial dysentery/enterocolitis (*Campylobacter, Salmonella*, enteropathogenic *E. coli*, etc.)
         - Macrophages in stool may be mistaken for amoebae.
         - *Shigella*: suggested by sheets of PMNs in stained smears; antibiotic (abx) resistance is an increasing problem
         - *Campylobacter*: tends to be more painful and lasts longer than other bacteria and may be dx'd under dark-field microscopy of wet specimens (small spirillum-like organisms with characteristic movement)
         - *Salmonella*: increased risk if meat ingested; stool is only rarely grossly bloody as main pathology is in small bowel
         - Enterotoxigenic *E. coli* may be complicated by hemolytic-uremic syndrome.
         - Vomiting is common with any/all of these organisms.

   Note that in outbreaks with limited resources, it is reasonable to provide IV hydration to the very ill and oral rehydration to the mildly ill, and provide chemotherapy (tetracycline, ciprofloxacin) only selectively. Regardless of bacterial species, almost all cases are self-limiting, requiring only hydration/electrolyte management and supportive care. (See Chapter 3 for more details.)

   Note that Bacillary dysentery not uncommonly accompanies visceral leishmaniasis. Falciparum malaria has been reported to cause bloody diarrhea.

   b. Acute + fever, but no blood
      i. *Salmonella* enteritis.
         - Usually in food-borne outbreaks; food usually looks and tastes fine. In contrast to shigella, person-to-person spread rare because it is water-borne transmission.
         - Incubation period 12 to 48 hours. Onset usually w/ fever and chills, followed by vomiting and diarrhea. A zoonosis of mammals, reptiles, and birds, more than 100 spp. exist; invasive forms may mimic typhoid, especially in acquired immunodeficiency syndrome (AIDS); HIV (+) pts should get abx.

- Consider abx for anyone w/ invasive dz: fever >48 hours, rose spots (pink macules scattered over trunk), splenomegaly.
- Relapsing salmonellosis associated w/ *Schistosoma mansoni*, biliary dz
- Sickle-cell pts should always get abx at increased risk for *Salmonella* osteomyelitis.
 ii. Malaria, especially *P. falciparum.*
 iii. Almost any infection in a child
 iv. Mild (nonulcerating) shigellosis
 v. *Campylobacter* infection
 vi. In children especially, fever with diarrhea may be indicative of an infection elsewhere than in the gut.
c. Acute, no fever, but + blood
 i. *Entamoeba histolytica* (or other amoeba)
   - Most common cause
 ii. *Balantidium coli*
 iii. Acute schistosomiasis (*S. mansoni, S. japonicum*)
   - Check for eosinophilia: early on, fever may be present
 iv. Trichuriasis
   - Most common in children w/ pica or institutionalized adults.
 v. Ulcerative colitis or other inflammatory bowel disease
   - Rarer in developing nations than in Europe, United States.
 vi. Pseudomembranous colitis
   - From *Clostridium difficile*, usually after abx course.
d. Acute, but no fever, no blood
 i. Most often preformed toxins in food
   - *S. aureus*: usually from hands of food preparer, but occasionally from milk of cow w/ mastitis.

 Incubation period short: 2 to 6 hours. Vomiting is soon followed by *diarrhea* which can be almost as severe as in cholera. Intuitively, abx are useless.
 ii. Enterotoxigenic *E. coli*: most important cause of travelers' diarrhea, conferring prolonged immunity to victims; most often in children and tourists/visitors (becomes part of normal flora in residents after initial infection). Widespread antibiotics (abx) resistance except to newer fluoroquinolones.
 iii. Loperamide (Imodium) and other antimotility agents are often used for convenience but should never be given for bloody diarrhea or to children—even when used for properly selected pts, may delay elimination of pathogen. Some prophylaxis is afforded by taking bismuth subsalicylate two × 262 mg po, chewed, qid. Abx should not be used for prophylaxis routinely because of possible side effects and resistance induction; exceptional pts can use a regimen such as ciprofloxacin 500 mg po qd. (See Chapter 3 for more details.)

 C. perfringens: a significant inoculum is needed, but may occur with various foods, especially meats, left at ambient temperature. Heat-resistant spores can also cause sx in well-cooked foods. Type A strains produce a toxin which causes diarrhea with abdominal cramps. Type C strains are enteroinvasive and can produce full-thickness intestinal wall necrosis; these are the organisms responsible for "pig bel" in Papua New Guinea following communal pig feasts. Severe cases may present with abdominal pain and ileus rather than diarrhea, possibly leading to obstruction and/or peritonitis. A vaccine is available for type C strains.
   - Cholera
   - Consider with voluminous watery stool in the midst of a diarrheal outbreak or when diarrhea is associated w/ muscle cramps.
 Enterotoxigenic *E. coli* may mimic this as well.

    iv. Viral
- Rotaviral (and others) gastroenteritis is common in children worldwide. Treatment is supportive.

    v. Toxins
- Foods which are new to visitors may occasionally cause diarrhea (i.e., capsaicin), but enterotoxigenic *E. coli* or *S. aureus* are more commonly responsible. Incubation is very short, and the illness is short-lived.

e. Persistent (after an acute attack) diarrhea
    i. Disaccharidase deficiency following infectious diarrhea
    ii. Giardiasis, amebiasis
    iii. Tropical sprue
    iv. HIV, especially with *Cryptosporidium* or *Isospora* spp.
    v. Enteropathogenic *E. coli*, causing long-lasting damage to enterocyte brush border.
    vi. Inflammatory bowel disease. Infectious diarrhea may precede onset of ulcerative colitis.
    vii. Tuberculous enteritis

f. Chronic + fever
    i. Tuberculous enteritis
- May be marked wasting, acid-fast bacillus (AFB) (+) sputum

    ii. Visceral leishmaniasis
- May be caused by direct gut mucosa involvement or to variety of secondary infections

    iii. Schistosomiasis (*S. japonicum*, *S. mansoni*)
- Fever in early stages only; look for eosinophilia

    iv. Yersiniosis
    v. AIDS

g. Chronic: fever + blood
    i. Amebiasis
    ii. Balantidiasis
    iii. Schistosomiasis (*S. japonicum*, *S. mansoni*)
    iv. Trichuriasis

h. Chronic: fever–blood
Note that fatty diarrhea is common.
    i. Giardiasis
- Diarrhea resolves spontaneously in a few months.

    ii. Celiac dz.
- Gluten enteropathy: accompanying iron deficiency is common

    iii. Tropical sprue
- An accompanying megaloblastic anemia is common (low folate and/or B12)

    iv. Strongyloidiasis
- Upper abdominal pain early on, eosinophilia suggestive. Gradually becomes a commensal infection.

    v. *Capillaria philippinensis*
- Clinical pictures simulate severe strongyloidiasis and will often not resolve spontaneously. May lead to fatally severe malabsorption.
- Small bowel lymphoma
- Often diffusely infiltrates bowel walls, making intestine rigid. Often responds to chemotherapy.

    vi. Chronic pancreatitis or tropical pancreatitis
    vii. Cryptosporidiosis
- Usually self-limiting but can be fatal in immunocompromised pts.

ORGANOMEGALY

1. Hepatomegaly
   a. Amoebic liver abscess
   b. Clonorchiasis
   c. Echinococcosis
   d. Fascioliasis
   e. Histoplasmosis
   f. Malaria
   g. Leishmaniasis, visceral
   h. Opisthorchiasis
   i. Schistosomiasis
   j. Toxocariasis
   k. Trypanosomiasis, American
   l. Typhoid
2. Splenomegaly
   a. Leishmaniasis, visceral
   b. Malaria
   c. Schistosomiasis
   d. Trypanosomiasis, American
   e. Typhoid
3. Variable (may see hepatic tenderness instead of either or all three)
   a. Typhoid
   b. Brucellosis
   c. Relapsing fever
   d. Leptospirosis
   e. Rocky Mountain spotted fever
   f. Q fever (chronic)
   g. Psittacosis
   h. Hepatitis
   i. Yellow fever
   j. Malaria
   k. Toxoplasmosis
   l. Leishmaniasis, visceral (kala-azar)
   m. Amebic abscess
   n. Schistosomiasis
   o. Liver flukes
   p. Visceral larva migrans

JAUNDICE

1. Jaundice
   a. Hepatitis
   b. Leptospirosis
   c. Malaria (*P. falciparum*)

RESPIRATORY COMPLAINTS

1. Cough
   a. Ascariasis

    b. Bacterial or chlamydial pneumonia
    c. Lassa fever
    d. Paragonimiasis
    e. Pertussis
    f. Plague
    g. Psittacosis
    h. Tuberculosis
    i. Viral upper respiratory infection (URI), postnasal drip, etc.

2. CXR anomalies
    a. Blastomycosis
    b. Coccidioidomycosis
    c. Echinococcosis
    d. Histoplasmosis
    e. Melioidosis
    f. Pneumocystosis
    g. Tuberculosis

3. Pharyngitis
    a. Diphtheria
    b. Mycoplasma or chlamydia
    c. Streptococcus
    d. Viral

4. Pneumonia
    a. AIDS
    b. Anthrax
    c. Ascariasis
    d. Blastomycosis
    e. Coccidioidomycosis
    f. Histoplasmosis
    g. Legionellosis
    h. Paragonimiasis
    i. Plague
    j. Pneumococcosis
    k. Psittacosis
    l. Q fever
    m. Scrub typhus
    n. Strongyloidiasis
    o. Tuberculosis

HEADACHE, OTHER CENTRAL NERVOUS SYSTEM COMPLAINTS

1. Altered mental status
    a. Acute psychosis
    b. Trypanosomiasis, African (can coma)
    c. Relapsing fever
    d. Leptospirosis
    e. Rickettsial dz (esp. Rocky Mountain spotted fever)
    f. Psittacosis
    g. Tuberculosis
    h. Viral encephalitis (can coma)
    i. Malaria (*P. falciparum*—can coma)

    j. African trypanosomiasis
    k. Impending sudden unexplained adult death
    l. Meningococcal meningitis
    m. Rabies
    n. Tick-borne encephalitis
2. Neurologic lesion with localizing sign(s)
    a. Angiostrongyliasis
    b. Botulism
    c. Cryptococcosis
    d. Cysticercosis (seizures)
    e. Diphtheria
    f. Echinococcosis
    g. Gnathostomiasis
    h. Lyme disease
    i. Meningococcal meningitis
    j. *Naegleria/Acanthamoeba* infection
    k. Paragonimiasis (seizures)
    l. Poliomyelitis
    m. Schistosomiasis (seizures w/ *S. japonicum*)
    n. Strongyloidiasis, disseminated
    o. Tetanus

SKIN LESIONS

1. Analgesia
    a. Leprosy
2. Anal pruritis
    a. Enterobiasis
    b. Strongyloides
3. General pruritis
    a. Onchocerciasis
    b. Toxocariasis
    c. Any etiology of jaundice
    d. Filarial disease (Loa, Oncho, Mansonella)
4. Rash
    a. Chikungunya fever
    b. Childhood exanthems
    c. Dengue
    d. Enteroviral infections
    e. Filariasis (may cause recurrent cellulitis)
    f. Glanders
    g. Gonococcemia
    h. Leptospirosis
    i. Meningococcemia
    j. Melioidosis (multiple pustular or necrotic lesions)
    k. Plague
    l. Rat-bite fever
    m. Relapsing fever
    n. Rickettsial diseases
    o. Syphilis (secondary): especially on palms/soles, as does rubella and measles

      p. Toxoplasmosis
      q. Typhoid: 10% with "rose spots"
5. Swelling or erythema
      a. Gnathostomiasis (migratory)
      b. Loiasis (migratory)
      c. Lyme disease
      d. Pinta (?)
      e. Wuchereria
6. Ulcer, eschar, or abscess
      a. Anthrax (eschar with surrounding edema)
      b. Buruli ulcer (ulcer)
      c. Dracunculiasis
      d. Glanders
      e. Leishmaniasis, cutaneous (ulcer)
      f. Lymphogranuloma venereum
      g. Mycobacterial (*Mycobacterium ulcerans*, *M. marinum*) (ulcer)
      h. Mycosis (blastomycosis, coccidioidomycosis, sporotrichosis)
      i. Rickettsial—eschar—(scrub typhus, rickettsialpox, boutonneuse fever, Queensland tick typhus, North Asian tick typhus, etc.)
      j. Syphilis
      k. Tropical ulcer
      l. Trypanosomiasis, American
      m. Trypanosomiasis, African
      n. Tularemia
      o. Yaws
7. Nodules
      a. Bartonellosis
      b. *Cysticercosis*
      c. Onchocerciasis
      d. Myiasis
      e. Hansen's disease
      f. Elephantiasis
      g. Chromoblastomycosis
      h. Leishmaniasis
8. Hypopigmented
      a. Leprosy
      b. Onchocerciasis
      c. Tinea versicolor
      d. Vitiligo
      e. Mansonella streptocerca
      f. Pinta
9. Hyperpigmented
      a. Pinta
      b. Onchocerciasis (*sowda*)

HEMATOLOGIC ABNORMALITIES

1. Anemia
      a. Diphyllobothriasis (typically megaloblastic)
      b. Histoplasmosis

   c. Hookworm infection (typically microcytic)
   d. Iron deficiency, nutritional origin (typically microcytic)
   e. Malaria (typically microcytic)
   f. Tropical sprue
   g. Visceral leishmaniasis
   h. Pernicious anemia (typically megaloblastic)
2. Eosinophilia
   a. Filariasis
   b. Fascioliasis
   c. Schistosomiasis
   d. Strongyloidiasis
   e. Toxocariasis
   f. Trichinosis
   g. Coccidioidomycosis

LYMPHADENOPATHY

1. Lymphadenopathy (general vs. regional)
   a. Blastomycosis, South American
   b. Dengue
   c. Filariasis
   d. Glanders
   e. Histoplasmosis
   f. HIV infection
   g. Leishmaniasis, visceral (kala-azar)
   h. Lymphogranuloma venereum
   i. Onchocerciasis
   j. Plague
   k. Rubella (posterior auricular/cervical LAD + rash suggestive of rubella or toxoplasmosis)
   l. Scrub typhus
   m. Syphilis (secondary)
   n. Toxoplasmosis (posterior auricular/cervical LAD + rash suggestive of rubella or toxoplasmosis)
   o. Trypanosomiasis, African (occipital LAD = "Winterbottom's sign")
   p. Trypanosomiasis, American
   q. Tuberculosis
   r. Tularemia
   s. Sporotrichosis (chain of lymphadenitis extending proximally from lesion)
   t. Cat-scratch fever (chain of lymphadenitis extending proximally from lesion)
   u. Cutaneous leishmaniasis (chain of lymphadenitis extending proximally from lesion)
   v. Mycobacterial (chain of lymphadenitis extending proximally from lesion)

CARDIOVASCULAR FINDINGS

1. Heart murmur
   a. Trypanosomiasis, American
   b. Enteroviral carditis
   c. Rheumatic heart disease
2. Myocarditis
   a. Trypanosomiasis, American

    b. Rheumatic heart disease

    c. Trichinosis

    d. Trypanosomiasis, African (Rhodesian)

3. Paradoxical bradycardia

    a. Typhoid

    b. Psittacosis

    c. Dengue

    d. Yellow fever

    e. Q fever

    f. Scrub typhus

    g. Leptospirosis (anicteric)

4. Afebrile tachycardia

    a. Myocarditis (viral, bacterial, parasitic etiologies)

       i. Consider: trichinosis, toxoplasmosis, Chagas' disease, African trypanosomiasis

HEAD AND NECK FINDINGS

1. Periorbital swelling

    a. Bilateral: trichinosis, Rocky Mountain spotted fever, nephrotic syndrome

    b. Unilateral: Chagas' disease (Romaña sign)

2. Conjunctival abnormalities

    a. Injection: leptospirosis, Rocky Mountain spotted fever

    b. Conjunctivitis, ulcerating and/or purulent: oculoglandular tularemia (w/ regional lymphadenitis)

3. Throat complaints

    a. Tonsillitis w/ pseudomembranes/lymphadenopathy: tularemia, diphtheria

MUSCULOSKELETAL

1. Myalgia

    a. Dengue

    b. Trichinosis

    c. Rickettsial disease

    d. Bartonellosis

2. Bone/joint infection

    a. Tuberculosis

    b. Bartonellosis

    c. Brucellosis

    d. Other

GENITOURINARY

1. Dysuria

    a. Gonorrhea

    b. Chlamydia

    c. Candiru (males)

    d. Other

2. Pyuria

    a. Tuberculosis

    b. Hansen's disease

  c. Bartonellosis
  d. Other
 3. Epididymo-orchitis
  a. Tuberculosis
  b. Hansen's disease
  c. Filariasis
  d. Mumps
  e. Other

Incubation/Latency Period

LESS THAN 2 HOURS

Chemical exposure

2 to 6 HOURS

Staphylococcal preformed toxin

1 to 3 DAYS

Scabies
Influenza
Puerperal infection
Bacterial pneumonia

1 to 7 DAYS

Anthrax
Bacillary dysentery
Cholera (often 3 days)
Tularemia
Scarlet fever
Diphtheria
Chancroid
Gonorrhea
Plague
Yellow fever
Relapsing fever (tick)
Dengue
Paratyphoid
Infectious keratoconjunctivitis
Meningococcal meningitis
Rocky Mountain spotted fever
Legionellosis

7 to 14 DAYS

Pertussis
Relapsing fever (louse)
Trichinosis

Leptospirosis
Viral encephalitides
Psittacosis
Poliomyelitis
Typhoid
Lymphocytic choriomeningitis
Malaria
Mononucleosis
Mycoplasma pneumonia
Measles
Typhus
Coccidiomycosis
Chlamydia
Giardiasis
Trachoma

MORE THAN 14 DAYS

Tetanus
Malaria
Brucellosis
Chickenpox
Lymphogranuloma venereum
Q fever
Rubella
Mumps
Syphilis
Amebic dysentery
Hepatitis
Rabies
Granuloma inguinale
Yaws
Tuberculosis
HIV
Enterobiasis
Lyme disease

YEAR(S)

P. malariae
Onchocerciasis
Echinococcosis
Hansen's disease (6–10+ years)

Geography

Anthrax, Q fever, brucellosis, plague, botulism, tularemia are used as biological weapons: may not follow geographical boundaries.

For country-specific or new information, refer to the Centers for Disease Control and Prevention (CDC) Yellow Book, available on the Internet.

THE AMERICAS

1. North America
   a. Food/water-borne: E. coli, Salmonella spp, shigella spp, giadria, norovirus.
   b. Vector-borne: plague (primary), rabies, Rocky Mountain spotted fever, tularemia (primary), encephalitis (arthropod-borne), hantavirus (rodent-borne), Lyme disease, babesiosis, scrub typhus
   c. Interpersonal: plague (rare, only in pneumonic form), Q fever (rare)
   d. Environmental: tularemia (rare), hantavirus (rodent-borne), Q fever (primary)
2. The Caribbean islands
   a. Food/water-borne: amebiasis, ascariasis, fascioliasis, hepatitis A (primary), trichuriasis
   b. Vector-borne: dengue, filariasis, leishmaniasis (cutaneous), malaria, rabies, tularemia (primary)
   c. Interpersonal: hepatitis A (rare), yaws
   d. Environmental: amebiasis, hookworm, schistosomiasis, trichuriasis, tularemia (rare)
3. Mexico
   a. Food/water-borne: amebiasis, anisakiasis, ascariasis, campylobacter, cysticercosis, E. coli enteritis, echinococcosis, hepatitis A/E
   b. Vector-borne: American trypanosomiasis, campylobacter, dengue, leishmaniasis (cutaneous and visceral), malaria, rabies, relapsing fever, typhus
   c. Interpersonal: hepatitis B/C/D, leprosy, pinta, tuberculosis
   d. Environmental: hookworm, trichuriasis
4. Tropical South America (Bolivia, Brazil, Colombia, Ecuador, French Guiana, Guyana, Paraguay, Peru, Suriname, Venezuela)
   a. Food/water-borne: cholera, brucellosis, hepatitis A/E (esp. D in Amazon basin), amebiasis (esp. Colombia), cryptosporidium, giardia, ascariasis, echinococcosis (esp. Peru), fascioliasis (rare), taeniasis, trichinosis, paragonimiasis (rare, Ecuador, Peru, Venezuela)
   b. Vector-borne: Rocky Mountain spotted fever (Brazil, Colombia), tick-borne relapsing fever (sporadic), dengue, equine encephalitis (Eastern/Western/Venezuelan), yellow fever, Oropouche fever (rural Peru, Brazil), Chagas' disease, bancroftian filariasis (foci in Brazil, Guyana, Suriname), plague (foci in NE Brazil, Ecuador, Peru, Bolivia), onchocerciasis (foci in N Brazil, Colombia, Ecuador, Venezuela), trench fever (foci in Bolivia), louse-borne typhus (foci in highlands of Colombia, Peru, Ecuador, Bolivia), bartonellosis (foci in W Andes to 3000 m), cutaneous/mucocutaneous leishmaniasis (all, mucocutaneous esp. in Brazil), visceral leishmaniasis (esp. NE Brazil)
   c. Interpersonal: diphtheria (sporadic), leprosy (esp. Brazil), pertussis, meningococcus (sporadic, esp. Brazil), Q fever, measles (rare), mumps, rubella, hepatitis B (esp. Amazon basin), hepatitis C/D
   d. Environmental: anthrax, leptospirosis, psittacosis, hemorrhagic fever (sporadic, Venezuela, Bolivia), rabies, cat-scratch fever (rare), rat-bite fever (rare), intestinal schistosomiasis (Brazil, Suriname, N Venezuela)
5. Temperate South America
   a. Food/water-borne: cholera, echinococcosis, hepatitis A, salmonellosis, taeniasis, typhoid
   b. Vector-borne: arenavirus infection (primary), American trypanosomiasis, cutaneous leishmaniasis, rabies, typhus
   c. Interpersonal: arenavirus infection (rare, healthcare settings), hepatitis B, meningococcal meningitis (esp. Chile), typhoid
   d. Environmental: anthrax (animal skins, contaminated animal products)
6. Andes Mountains
   a. Food/water-borne: brucellosis, tapeworm

    b. Vector-borne: bartonellosis, rabies, plague, typhus
    c. Interpersonal: plague (rare, only in pneumonic form), tuberculosis
    d. Environmental: brucellosis

EUROPE

1. Northern Europe
    a. Food/water-borne: cholera (rare dz), diphyllobothriasis (Baltic Sea), fasciolopsiasis, hepatitis A (Eastern Europe), taeniasis, trichinellosis
    b. Vector-borne: Crimean-Congo hemorrhagic fever, hemorrhagic fever with renal syndrome (low risk), Lyme disease, rabies, typhus (tick-borne, Siberia, rare)
    c. Interpersonal: diphtheria (various Baltic nations and former Union of Soviet Socialist Republic [USSR] states and Poland), encephalitis (tick-borne, vaccine available) poliomyelitis (various former USSR states)
    d. Environmental: diphtheria (various Baltic nations and former USSR states)
2. Southern Europe
    a. Food/water-borne: brucellosis, cholera, echinococcosis, fasciolopsiasis, typhoid
    b. Vector-borne: encephalitis (tick-borne, vaccine available), hemorrhagic fever with renal syndrome (rodent-borne), leishmaniasis (cutaneous and visceral), Lyme disease, rabies, sandfly fever, typhus (murine and tick-borne), West Nile fever
    c. Interpersonal: hepatitis B
    d. Environmental: brucellosis

AFRICA AND THE MIDDLE EAST

1. North Africa
    a. Food/water-borne: ascariasis, brucellosis, cholera, dracunculiasis, *E. coli* enteritis, giardiasis, hepatitis A/E, hydatid disease, hymenolepiasis, taeniasis, typhoid
    b. Vector-borne: boutonneuse fever, Crimean-Congo hemorrhagic fever, dengue (Nile), filariasis (Nile), leishmaniasis, malaria, plague, rabies, relapsing fever, Rift Valley fever, sandfly fever, typhus, West Nile fever
    c. Interpersonal: giardiasis, poliomyelitis (rare), trachoma, tuberculosis
    d. Environmental: anthrax, brucellosis, giardiasis hookworm, schistosomiasis, trachoma
2. East, West, and Central Africa
    a. Food/water-borne: ascariasis, cholera, dracunculiasis, *E. coli* enteritis, echinococcosis, giardiasis, hepatitis A, paragonimiasis, schistosomiasis, taeniasis, trichinosis, typhoid
    b. Vector-borne: boutonneuse fever, Crimean-Congo fever, Ebola-Marburg hemorrhagic fever, filariasis, Lassa fever, leishmaniasis (cutaneous and visceral), loiasis, malaria (up to 2600 m), onchocerciasis, plague (primary), rabies, relapsing fever, Rift Valley fever, African trypanosomiasis (eastern and western variants), tungiasis, typhus (louse-, tick-, and flea-borne), yellow fever
    c. Interpersonal: HIV/AIDS, hepatitis B, giardiasis, leprosy, plague (rare, only in pneumonic form), poliomyelitis, meningococcal meningitis, trachoma, tuberculosis, yaws
    d. Environmental: anthrax, giardiasis, hookworm, strongyloidiasis, trichuriasis
3. South Africa
    a. Food/water-borne: amebiasis, ascariasis, hepatitis A, schistosomiasis, typhoid
    b. Vector-borne: African trypanosomiasis (Botswana, Namibia), Crimean-Congo hemorrhagic fever, malaria, plague, relapsing fever, Rift Valley fever, tick-bite fever, typhus (mostly tick-borne)

    c. Interpersonal: hepatitis B, plague (rare, only in pneumonic form), poliomyelitis (rare), tuberculosis

    d. Environmental: anthrax, hookworm, trichuriasis

4. Middle East

    a. Food/water-borne: ascariasis, brucellosis, dracunculiasis, *E. coli* enteritis, giardiasis, hepatitis A, hydatid disease, hymenolepiasis, schistosomiasis, taeniasis, typhoid

    b. Vector-borne: dengue fever, boutonneuse fever, Crimean-Congo hemorrhagic fever, filariasis, leishmaniasis (cutaneous and visceral), malaria, onchocerciasis (Yemen only), plague, rabies, relapsing fever, typhus (murine and tick-borne)

    c. Interpersonal: diphtheria (various former USSR states), giardiasis, hepatitis B, plague (rare, only in pneumonic form), poliomyelitis, trachoma, tuberculosis

    d. Environmental: anthrax, brucellosis, giardiasis, hookworm

ASIA

1. India, Bangladesh, Pakistan, and Sri Lanka

    a. Food/water-borne: amebiasis, ascariasis, brucellosis, cholera, dracunculiasis, echinococcosis, *E. coli* enteritis, giardiasis, hepatitis A, hymenolepiasis, shigellosis, trichinosis, typhoid

    b. Vector-borne: boutonneuse fever, dengue, filariasis, hemorrhagic fever (tick-borne), Japanese encephalitis, leishmaniasis (cutaneous and visceral), malaria, plague, rabies, relapsing fever, scrub typhus, typhus

    c. Interpersonal: giardiasis, hepatitis B, leprosy, meningococcal meningitis, plague (rare, only in pneumonic form), poliomyelitis, trachoma, tuberculosis

    d. Environmental: brucellosis, giardiasis, hookworm, strongyloidiasis, trichuriasis,

2. Southeast Asia

    a. Food/water-borne: amebiasis, angiostrongyliasis, clonorchiasis, *E. coli* enteritis, fasciolopsiasis, giardiasis, gnathostomiasis, hepatitis A/E, melioidosis, opisthorchiasis, paragonimiasis, schistosomiasis, shigellosis, taeniasis, trichinosis, typhoid

    b. Vector-borne: dengue, filariasis, Japanese encephalitis, malaria, plague, rabies, scrub typhus

    c. Interpersonal: giardiasis, hepatitis B, leprosy, plague (rare, only in pneumonic form), poliomyelitis, trachoma, tuberculosis

    d. Environmental: giardiasis, hookworm, strongyloidiasis, trichuriasis

3. China and Korea

    a. Food/water-borne: ascariasis, clonorchiasis, *E. coli* enteritis, hepatitis A/E, leptospirosis, paragonimiasis, schistosomiasis, trichinosis

    b. Vector-borne: dengue, filariasis, hemorrhagic fever with renal failure, Japanese encephalitis, leishmaniasis (cutaneous and visceral), malaria, plague, rabies, scrub typhus

    c. Interpersonal: hepatitis B, leprosy, meningococcal meningitis, plague (rare, only in pneumonic form), poliomyelitis, trachoma, tuberculosis

    d. Environmental: hookworm, leptospirosis, trichuriasis

OCEANA

1. Australia, New Zealand, and the Antarctic

    a. Food/water-borne: rare

    b. Vector-borne: encephalitis (viral), dengue (Northern Australia, occasional)

    c. Interpersonal: rare

    d. Environmental: rare

2. Melanesia and Micronesia-Polynesia/Pacific Islands
   a. Food/water-borne: angiostrongyliasis, ascariasis, ciguatera poisoning, hepatitis A, scombroid poisoning, trichinosis, typhoid
   b. Vector-borne: dengue, filariasis, malaria, Ross River fever, typhus (mite-borne, Papua New Guinea)
   c. Interpersonal: hepatitis B, leprosy, trachoma, tuberculosis, yaws
   d. Environmental: hookworm, strongyloidiasis, trichuriasis

Vectors and Environmental Exposures

SAMPLING STRATEGIES FOR ARTHROPOD VECTORS

1. Sampling methodology
   a. Presence-absence: As name suggests, provides determination if arthropod exists in environment
      i. Quick to complete
      ii. No quantitative information (i.e., no sense of population density)
   b. Direct counts/absolute estimates
      i. Generally too resource-intensive in large areas to be feasible
      ii. Most accurate because provides as accurate a count of population possible
   c. Relative estimate of population
      i. Best balance between generalities of presence-absence and absolute estimate
      ii. Results are influenced by method used
2. Random, systematic, serial sampling
   a. Random samples less useful because implies that animals have equal chance of being found throughout environment
      i. Least bias introduced in this method
      ii. Least reflective of animal behavior (i.e., animals prefer favorable habitats and will, generally, cluster in those habitats rather than randomly in environment)
   b. Systematic samples are easiest method to obtain samples from large population
      i. Pick samples via some predetermined rules (e.g., hang trap from every third tree; drag for ticks every second meter)
      ii. Can introduce bias via choice of sampling sites
   c. Serial samples are collected at same location
      i. Trapping at the same location(s) over time
      ii. Provides reasonable estimate of population changes over time (e.g., with seasonal variation)
3. Sampling/trapping methods vary by arthropod but general methods include
   a. Plastic dipper in standing water for larval stage mosquitoes
   b. Light traps
      i. Light trap with CO_2 or other attractant for mosquitoes
      ii. Without attractant can be used for sand flies
   c. Natural resting stations with white sheet on ground to collect arthropods after spraying aerosol pesticide
   d. Sticky/oil paper traps
      i. Used with many species of biting fly
      ii. Method varies by location (indoor/outdoor) and arthropod of interest
   e. Visual landing counts
      i. Used with aspirator to collect insect before biting
      ii. Technique may increase risk to personnel collecting arthropods

    f. Tick drags
      i. Done with soft, white cloth
      ii. Cannot be done in wet/damp conditions
    g. Direct observation
4. Sample size considerations
    a. Multiple samples (more than three) are general preferable for better accuracy of information
    b. Typically balanced with resource considerations (e.g., cost, available manpower to set, collect traps, review collected arthropods)

GENERAL PROTECTIVE MEASURES AGAINST VECTOR CONTACT

1. Arthropods
    a. Use of protective clothing impregnated with permethrin
    b. For flying insects, use of screened rooms a/o insecticide-impregnated bed netting
    c. Spray rooms with pyrethroids during evening
    d. Personal application of 35% nonabsorbable N,N-diethyl-metatoluamide (DEET)

TICKS AND MITES

1. *Sarcoptes scabei* (itch mite, scabies mite)
    a. Causes scabies in humans, mange in other mammals
2. Demodex (follicle mite)
    a. Extremely small, generally infests older persons, especially in areas of facial/nasal hair. Can cause dry erythema, occasionally blepharitis, or granulomatous acne. Dx by examining sebum for mites. Tx is gamma benzene hexachloride 0.5% in a cream.
3. Trombiculid mites (chiggers) (Fig. 2.1)

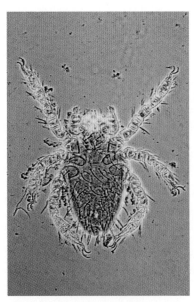

Fig. 2.1   Larvae of *Leptotrombidium*, vector for scrub typhus. (From Nabarro L, Morris-Jones S, Moore DAJ. Arthropod-borne diseases. In: Nabarro L, Morris-Jones S, Moore DAJ, eds. *Peters' Atlas of Tropical Medicine and Parasitology.* 7th ed. London, UK: Elsevier Ltd; 2019:1–108.)

    a. The larvae are "chiggers" which can cause a pruritic dermatitis. Cosmopolitan, females lay eggs in damp soil, usually in grassy areas. After hatching, larvae climb grass or debris until CO_2 from a host activates them. They partially digest tissue, and in humans tend to attach near areas of tight clothing (waist, scrotum). Dermatitis occurs typically 3 to 6 hours after exposure as pustules a/o wheals.

    b. Certain adult species (genus *Leptotrombidium*) are vectors for scrub typhus (caused by *Rickettsia tsutsugamushi*). Mites do not travel far independently, so disease is restricted to areas with high mouse concentration. Prevention of bite with DEET a/o permethrin recommended in high risk areas.

4. Dust mites
    a. Known cause of bronchial asthma/reactive airway disease. Appropriate usage of insecticides and vacuuming is needed.

5. Other domestic mites
    a. Only need to know that several species of mites have a strong preference for natural hosts (rat, chicken, etc.) but will attack humans if deprived of usual host. Rat mites are found in groceries, warehouses, and bird mites often in air-conditioning ducts and may be carried with air-conditioning currents.

6. Forage mites (*Acaridae*)
    a. Inhabit stored cheese, copra, vanilla pods, flour, and macaroni. Contact allergies may develop if exposed (grocer's itch, copra itch, baker's itch, etc.). GI or respiratory sx may also develop, depending on route of exposure.

7. Argasidae ticks (soft ticks)
    a. Feed rapidly at night, most often on wild animals, then return to home site.
    b. Exception is *Ornithodoros moubata* of East/Central/South Africa which is found in tents and readily attacks man.
    c. Most species found around cracks, crevices, nests, sheds, or, more rarely, houses.
    d. Argas species usually affect birds or bats but do cause painful bites for humans.
    e. *Ornithodoros* species transmit *Borrelia* spirochetes (relapsing fever). For such diseases, ticks are the main reservoir. In East Africa, vectors are night feeders and have a predilection for mud floors and cracks/crevices in mud walls. In arid parts of Sri Lanka, India, Arabia, and Africa, another species tends to habituate outdoor resting areas of livestock. Species in NW Africa and Spain/Portugal tend to be near pig sties and rodent habitats. Most other species around the world can be found near animal stables or rural housing. Two species are not known to be vectors of relapsing fever but are important: *O. rostratus* ("quanco") of southern South America has a painful, sometimes pruritic bite which may become secondarily infected; *O. muesebeck* of the Arabian Gulf normally feeds on marine birds of various islands but will aggressively bite humans, causing a pruritic bullae, headache, and fever, perhaps from a virus.

8. Ixodidae ticks (hard ticks) (Fig. 2.2)
    a. Feed slowly, often on domestic animals, remaining attached at times for days.
    b. Have much more extensive mouthparts than soft ticks, especially *A. americanum*; carefully remove these ticks to avoid leaving behind these potential sources of irritation/secondary infection. Use of 0.6% permethrin in methyl benzoate or of camphorated phenol makes detachment easier.
    c. Man usually bitten by larvae stages. May remain attached for days up to months, dependent upon several factors.
    d. If tick is removed before 36 to 48 hours, risk of transmission of Lyme disease is significantly reduced.
    e. Specifics

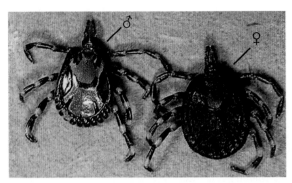

Fig. 2.2 *Amblyomma variegatum,* vector for *Rickettsia africae.* (From Nabarro L, Morris-Jones S, Moore DAJ. Arthropod-borne diseases. In: Nabarro L, Morris-Jones S, Moore DAJ, eds. *Peters' Atlas of Tropical Medicine and Parasitology.* 7th ed. London, UK: Elsevier Ltd; 2019:1–108.)

   i. *I. scapularis/dammini* (American deer tick) in United States and Canada is the vector for human babesiosis (*Babesia microti*), Lyme disease (*Borrelia burgdorferi*), and human granulocytic ehrlichiosis (*E. equi*).

  ii. *I. ricinus* (European sheep tick or castor bean tick) in Europe and N Iran is the vector for "louping ill" in United Kingdom (flavivirus), tick-borne viral encephalitis (TBE—flavivirus) in central Europe, and Lyme disease.

 iii. *I. persiculatis* (the taiga tick) from the Baltics to Japan, somewhat more cold-hardy than *I. ricinus* but with some overlap. Chief vector for Russian spring-summer encephalitis (flavivirus).

 iv. *I. holocyclus* in humid areas of Queensland and New South Wales (Australia). Bites often responsible for tick paralysis. Vector of Queensland tick typhus (*Rickettsia australis*).

  v. *Haemaphysalis spinigera* of Sri Lanka and southern India, often found in cleared forests, is the vector of Kyasanur Forest disease (flavivirus).

 vi. *H. leachi* is a widespread feeder on carnivores. Known to be an incidental vector of boutonneuse fever (*Rickettsia conori*) in individuals who become contaminated while removing ticks from dogs (eyes, skin, etc.).

 vii. *Rhipicephalus appendiculatus* is a vector of African tick typhus (*Rickettsia*) in the South African veld.

viii. *R. sanguineus* is a cosmopolitan dog tick and the chief vector of boutonneuse fever in the Mediterranean basin.

 ix. *Dermacentor andersoni* (Rocky Mountain wood tick) is a vector of Rocky Mountain spotted fever in the western United States and Canada; if the tick is promptly removed (may be as long as 24 hours), the risk of transmission of *Rickettsia rickettsi* greatly reduced. Also transmits Colorado tick fever and a vector for human monocytic ehrlichiosis (*E. chaffeensis*).

  x. *D. variabilis* (American dog tick) from Mexico to Canada is vector of Rocky Mountain spotted fever in the easternmost United States. Also a vector for human monocytic ehrlichiosis (*E. chaffeensis*).

 xi. Three species of *Dermacentor* are vectors for Siberian tick typhus (*Rickettsia sibirica*) from central Europe to China.

xii. *Amblyomma hebraeum* (South African bont tick) is the vector of boutonneuse fever in the South African veld.

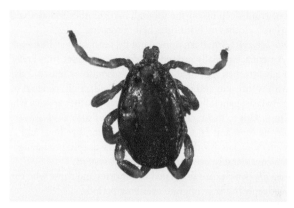

Fig. 2.3 *Hyalomma marginatum.* (From Nabarro L, Morris-Jones S, Moore DAJ. Arthropod-borne diseases. In: Nabarro L, Morris-Jones S, Moore DAJ, eds. *Peters' Atlas of Tropical Medicine and Parasitology.* 7th ed. London, UK: Elsevier Ltd; 2019:1–108.)

xiii. *A. americanum* (Lone-star tick) in South America and central/eastern United States is the principal vector of Rocky Mountain spotted fever in the United States— long mouth parts are particularly difficult to remove. May transmit tularemia (*F. tularensis*) and human monocytotropic ehrlichiosis (*E. chaffeensis*) and human granulocytotropic ewingii ehrlichiosis (*E. ewingii*).

xiv. *A. cajennense* (Cayenne tick) from South America to the Caribbean and southern Texas is the vector of Rocky Mountain spotted fever in Mexico, Panama, Colombia, and Brazil.

xv. *Hyalomma marginatum* found in many parts of Europe and Africa depends upon (usually migratory) birds in the immature stages and is the vector for Crimean-Congo hemorrhagic fever (arbovirus) (Fig. 2.3).

PENTASTOMIDS (LENGUATULIDS, "TONGUE WORMS")

1. Linguatulidae: arthropod-like worms normally found in nares of canines whose eggs, if ingested, lead to larval encysting in viscera (visceral linguatulosis). Ingested larvae may migrate to nasal passages (nasopharyngeal linguatulosis, "halzoun," marrara syndrome). Occasionally, nymphs may penetrate the anterior chamber of the eye, causing uveitis; this clears with surgical removal of the parasite. Worldwide.

2. Armilliferidae: various species in Africa, Malaysia, Java, Manila, Sumatra, and China. Man acquires by eating undercooked snake meat or water contaminated by snake feces. Almost always asymptomatic, the nymphs encyst in liver, intestinal tract, and lungs.

FLIES AND MYIASIS

1. Myiasis: an infestation of dipterous larvae that feed on the host's tissue. After recovery of worm from host, kill in hot water or alcohol.

2. Cutaneous myiasis (may be confused with tungiasis)

   a. *Cordylobia anthropophaga* (African tumbu fly, mango fly, ver du cayor) found throughout sub-Saharan Africa but may be taken to other parts of the world via air traffic of infested individuals. Females lay eggs on soil (esp. if contaminated with urine or feces) or clothing. Larvae hatch in response to heat or vibration and can survive up to 9 days. They painlessly penetrate intact skin, especially in the head and neck region. To prevent infestation, avoid sleeping on the ground, hang clothes indoors with windows/screens down, and iron clothes on both sides before wearing.

b. *Dermatobia hominis* (American human bot fly, ver macaque, Berne, el torsalo, beefworm) in Latin America, especially near edges of tropical forests, hilly areas 160 to 3000 MSL. Adult female attaches eggs to abdomen of mosquito or muscoid fly, which hatch upon contact with warm skin and penetrate. Ocular and, rarely, cerebral myiasis may occur.

c. Creeping myiasis: generally from endoparasites of other species which cannot develop in man. Important to distinguish from nematodes such as *Ancylostoma*.

   i. *Hypoderma bovis* and *H. lineatum* cause creeping swellings and eruptions, especially in persons associated with cattle. May burrow deeply, producing a boil-like lesion, or migrate considerably, even into the nervous system.

   ii. *Gasterophilus* species are associated with horses and those who care for them. Do not burrow deeply but may migrate over long periods.

d. Larvae attacking wounds and sores:

   i. Numerous genii will feed on devitalized tissue and may also attack healthy tissue. Other species that normally feed off soiled anus or genitalia may at times enter the rectum or vagina to become internal parasites.

   ▪ *Cochliomyia hominivorax* (New World screw-worm fly), an obligate parasite of the Americas which normally attacks cattle but can cause serious human disease. Near the smallest of wounds or abrasions, females lay eggs; larvae feed rapaciously on healthy tissue, often creating pockets. Alternately, eggs may be laid in ears, nasal passages, vulva, or vagina. Larvae grow rapidly and yield a reported 8% mortality.

   ▪ *Wohlfahrtia magnifica* (Old World flesh fly) is similar to the above organism. It dwells in warm Eurasia and is responsible for impressive disfigurement.

   ▪ Wohlfahrtia vigil (Nearctic flesh fly) of North America is similar to the above two organisms and will also lay eggs on uninjured skin. It is attracted by malodorous ear, nose, eye, or other secretions and is especially fond of children. They are found exclusively outside.

   ii. Sanguinivorous larvae *Auchmeromyia luteola* (Congo floor-maggot) is widely found throughout sub-Saharan Africa. The red larvae hides in the floor or soil (as deep as 7.5 cm) and surfaces to feed on blood at night. They retreat immediately when satisfied or disturbed.

3. Myiasis of body cavities

a. Several species that attack wounds described above may affect the eye, nasal cavities, and ear canal. Pain, nasal obstruction, epistaxis, and/or purulent/fetid nasal discharge may result from nasal/sinus infestation. Inhalation or packing with chloroform, weak carbolic acid, or turpentine has been described, but therapy may require surgical intervention.

   i. *Chrysomya bezziana* (Old World screw-worm) is found in Asia and sub-Saharan Africa. Females lay eggs along mucous membranes (inc. vagina), ears, and ulcers/wounds. Larvae burrow into tissues, sometimes into bone, resulting in fetid, disfiguring lesions. Treat with 15% chloroform in vegetable oil; this will cause larvae to surface for removal.

b. In Asia and North Africa, myiasis of the orbit and ocular apparatus occurs in up to 1/10,000 persons, with several species being responsible. Patients may report initial trauma to eye, followed by several days of inflammation. Responsible organisms may migrate (i.e., to nasal cavities) but will die within a few days as humans are not the natural host.

4. Myiasis of organ systems

a. Intestinal myiasis: species are only facultative or accidental parasites. If larvae are ingested from contaminated food, may cause intestinal lesions, damage to mucous membranes, or hemorrhagic infiltrations (clinically, vomiting/diarrhea/nausea, etc.). Caudad, flies attracted to feces may in extreme cases of poor hygiene deposit eggs near the anus, with larval penetration into the distal rectum.

    b. Urogenital myiasis: rarely, vaginal or vulvar infestation may lead to transient bladder infestation, but clinically this is of little importance.

PHLEBOTOMINE (PHLEBOTOMINAE SUBFAMILY) SANDFLIES

   1. Small (1.5–3.5 mm long: can get through standard mosquito netting) hairy flies found somewhat focally distributed around the world (Figs. 2.4 and 2.5). In the Americas, *Lutzomyia*

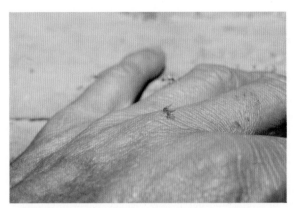

Fig. 2.4 Adult female *Lutzomyia longipalpis* (vector for leishmaniasis in Latin America), biting. (From Nabarro L, Morris-Jones S, Moore DAJ. Arthropod-borne diseases. In: Nabarro L, Morris-Jones S, Moore DAJ, eds. *Peters' Atlas of Tropical Medicine and Parasitology.* 7th ed. London, UK: Elsevier Ltd; 2019:1–108.)

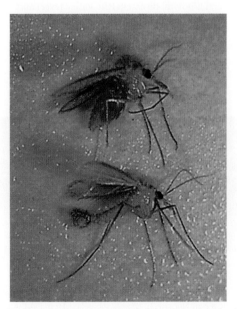

Fig. 2.5 Male and female *Phlebotomus papatasi,* vector for leishmaniasis in the Old World. (From Nabarro L, Morris-Jones S, Moore DAJ. Arthropod-borne diseases. In: Nabarro L, Morris-Jones S, Moore DAJ, eds. *Peters' Atlas of Tropical Medicine and Parasitology.* 7th ed. London, UK: Elsevier Ltd; 2019:1–108.)

species are vectors for human disease, whereas *Phlebotomus* species are of concern in the Old World. Although these insects inhabit a wide variety of environments (arid deserts to humid jungles), they prefer to rest in cool, dark, humid areas when possible. They normally only bite at night but will bite during the day if disturbed. Both sexes depend on nectar or other sources of sugar for sustenance; the female takes blood meals for her brood only.

2. Sandflies can transmit protozoans (*Leishmania*), bacteria (*Bartonella*), and viruses (Patapasi fever, Toscana virus, Punta Toro virus, Chagres virus) to humans. Additionally, the bite of *P. papatasi* and other species in the Middle East may cause an intense urticarial reaction in persons new to the region. Individual species in various areas demonstrate strong preferences for specific conditions. Additionally, sandflies in one area may transmit one disease (or more) but not another, whereas a different species in the area may transmit a different disease.

MOSQUITOES

1. *Anopheles*: only vector of malaria in man, feeds at night (Fig. 2.6). Over 200 species, only a handful are significantly anthropophilic instead of zoophilic; this is responsible for endemicity rates. For example, *A. gambiae* of Africa much more anthropophilic (and hence a greater threat) than any species in Latin America. Larvae lack air tube and are parallel to water surface. Adults females have palpi that are straight and nearly as long as the proboscis. Adults at rest are identifiable by stance; the proboscis and body are in a straight line at around a 45-degree angle to the surface.

2. *Aedes*: vector of several arboviral diseases (dengue, yellow fever, Zika virus) and filariasis, most species feed at day (Fig. 2.7). Larval stage has clear breathing tube and rest at an angle to surface of the water. Adult female has palpi that are straight but very small. Adult is identifiable by distinctive white patches on legs and body. When at rest, the adult's proboscis and body are at an angle to one another.

3. *Culex*: vector of several arboviral diseases (Rift Valley fever) and filariasis (Fig. 2.8).

4. Other
   a. *Armigeres*
   b. *Haemogogus*
   c. *Psorophora*

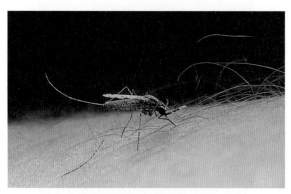

Fig. 2.6 *Anopheles gambiae*. (From Nabarro L, Morris-Jones S, Moore DAJ. Arthropod-borne diseases. In: Nabarro L, Morris-Jones S, Moore DAJ, eds. *Peters' Atlas of Tropical Medicine and Parasitology.* 7th ed. London, UK: Elsevier Ltd; 2019:1–108.)

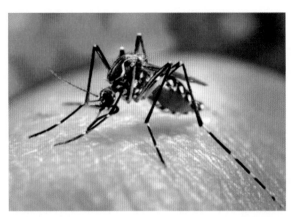

Fig. 2.7 *Aedes aegypti.* (From Nabarro L, Morris-Jones S, Moore DAJ. Arthropod-borne diseases. In: Nabarro L, Morris-Jones S, Moore DAJ, eds. *Peters' Atlas of Tropical Medicine and Parasitology.* 7th ed. London, UK: Elsevier Ltd; 2019:1–108.)

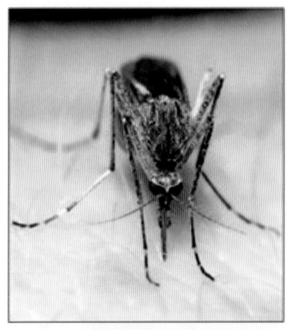

Fig. 2.8 *Culex pipiens.* (From Nabarro L, Morris-Jones S, Moore DAJ. Arthropod-borne diseases. In: Nabarro L, Morris-Jones S, Moore DAJ, eds. *Peters' Atlas of Tropical Medicine and Parasitology.* 7th ed. London, UK: Elsevier Ltd; 2019:1–108.)

MIDGES ("NO-SEE-UMS")

1. 1 to 4 mm long flies, the female of which imparts a painful bite, often attacking in large groups.
2. *Leptoconops*: day biters, shiny black with milky white wings, found in sandy beaches along the Indian Ocean, and the coast of the southeastern United States, eastern Central America, and the Caribbean. Some species also found with fine silt soils inland SE United States.

3. *Forcipomyia* serious pests in central Asia, Japan, China, and Asia.
4. *Culicoides*: widely found in temperate and tropical countries with extremely high (200–3000/h) biting rate. Lesions may cause significant swelling, and in some species, dermatitis. Species are significant vectors for *Mansonella ozzardi* in Latin America and *M. perstans* in Africa. *Culicoides* may also be a vector for several viruses, but none proven.

SIMULIUM FLIES (BLACKFLIES, BUFFALO GNATS, TURKEY GNATS)

1. 1 to 5 mm long flies with short antennae, the female can be a vicious biter. They are vectors for onchocerciasis, and more rarely, filariasis. Females lay eggs in running (oxygenated) water.
2. Africa: species can fly exceptionally long distances.
3. Latin America: in Central America, some species orange/yellow, not black. Many species breed in mere trickles of water. Some species in Brazil and Venezuela also transmit non-pathogenic *M. ozzzardi*.

TABANIDAE FLIES

1. *Chrysops* (deer flies, greenheads, mango flies, mangrove flies) 6 to 10 mm long, wings held over body like partly open scissors (Fig. 2.9). Day biters? Often in waterlogged scrub and marshy woodlands. Females feed on blood, have painful bite. Rarely enter homes. A mechanical vector of tularemia (*Francisella tularensis*), although ticks a more common vector. This genus is also the vector responsible for spread of loiasis (*Loa loa*) in sub-Saharan Africa.
2. *Tabanus* (horse flies, gad flies) and *Haematopota* (clegs, stouts) may be responsible for mechanical transmission of anthrax in some parts of the world, but if this occurs, it is rare.

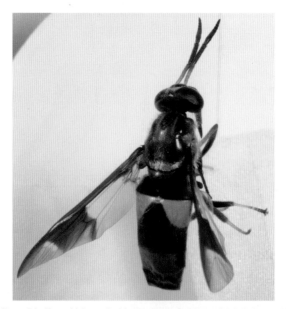

Fig. 2.9 *Chrysops* (Deer fly). (From Nabarro L, Morris-Jones S, Moore DAJ. Arthropod-borne diseases. In: Nabarro L, Morris-Jones S, Moore DAJ, eds. *Peters' Atlas of Tropical Medicine and Parasitology*. 7th ed. London, UK: Elsevier Ltd; 2019:1–108.)

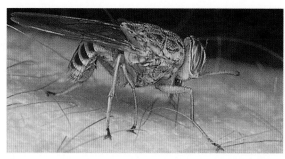

Fig. 2.10 Tsetse fly (*Glossina palpalis*). (From Nabarro L, Morris-Jones S, Moore DAJ. Arthropod-borne diseases. In: Nabarro L, Morris-Jones S, Moore DAJ, eds. *Peters' Atlas of Tropical Medicine and Parasitology.* 7th ed. London, UK: Elsevier Ltd; 2019:1–108.)

TSETSE FLIES

1. *Glossina* species are found in tropical Africa from 15 degrees N and 30 degrees S (Fig. 2.10). Various species have strong preferences for different ecological niches from jungle to arid regions. They are strongly attracted to large moving objects and are almost exclusively day biters—even overcast conditions retard their habits.

2. Typically, flies of the *palpalis* group are responsible for transmission of Gambian sleeping sickness and are fairly bound to terrain near water, whereas those of *morsitans* group usually transmit Rhodesian sleeping sickness and tend to be found in more arid regions. Further, *palpalis* feeds most often on domestic herds and has more contact with man. Consequently, Rhodesians sleeping sickness is far less common than Gambian disease and is found mainly in those who enter the bush (hunters, pole-cutters, etc.).

CIMICID AND TRIATOMINE BUGS

1. Cimicidae family, *Cimex*, (bed bugs) are globally distributed, all wingless, with a few parasitic to man. The species hide in crevices and feed at night exclusively on blood. Their feces can be found near small holes. Although sensitive to heat (a humid 37.8°C will kill), adults live for several months. Sulfur fumigation is an easy means to kill active stages but not all eggs. Otherwise, DDT, malathion, or pyrethroids can rid the house of bugs. Although some have speculated that they may transmit viral hepatitis, they are of import mainly because of their irritating bites.

2. Reduviidae family, subfamily triatominae, (triatomine bugs, "cone-nose bugs," "kissing bugs," "assassin bugs," *chinchas* [Mexico], *chipos* [Venezuela], *barbeiros* [Brazil], *vinchuchas* [Argentina])

   a. Triatomine bugs feed exclusively on vertebrate blood, but some reduviids have a painful bite but do not feed on blood (only a few triatomines have painful bite) (Fig. 2.11). Nonhematophagous reduviids have an inflexible, curved proboscis, whereas triatomines possess flexible, straight proboscis. Triatomine species vary from 5 mm to 4.5 cm.

   b. The majority of species are found in the Americas. Species can be found in epiphytic bromeliads, under logs, and in hollow trees. Many are fond of domestic animal housing (coops, sties, stables) and have adapted exceptionally well (*Rhodnius prolixus*, *Triatoma infestans*) to live in the crevices of simple mud/adobe housing with thatch roofs. Although all triatomines can harbor trypanosomes, only those that inhabit human dwellings transmit the disease. In some areas, when one dominant species keeps more timid and less numerous species from infecting humans, control of that species permits

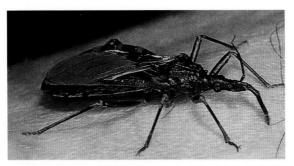

Fig. 2.11 *Triatoma infestans*, vector for Chagas disease. (From Nabarro L, Morris-Jones S, Moore DAJ. Arthropod-borne diseases. In: Nabarro L, Morris-Jones S, Moore DAJ, eds. *Peters' Atlas of Tropical Medicine and Parasitology.* 7th ed. London, UK: Elsevier Ltd; 2019:1–108.)

the establishment of others as significant vectors. Within homes, triatomines prefer dark places: crevices, boxes, bedding, clothing, frame-adorned mantles, and palm roofs have been used. Areas inhabited by hosts at nighttime/feeding time (i.e., bedroom) is where the insects tend to congregate.

   c. Eggs and nymphs may be carried long distances by migratory birds. Adults take up to 2 years to mature, and some stages can withstand up to several months of starvation.

   d. Transmission of trypanosomes occurs if vector defecates during/after feeding near wound. Hence only species that do this AND colonize houses to bite man are effective vectors. No vectors meet these criteria in the Amazonian basin, but *R. prolixus* is quite common from 3 degrees N (Colombia, Venezuela, Guyana) to 20 degrees N in Mexico, from sea level to 2000 m.

FLEAS

1. In general, fleas are associated with transmission of plague, murine typhus, tularemia, pseudotuberculosis, melioidosis, brucellosis, and lymphocytic choriomeningitis (Fig. 2.12). Fleas may also serve as intermediate hosts for dog and rat tapeworms. Regular cleaning and vacuuming are simple but effective means to control flea populations. To combat sand fleas, infested areas should be burned to the soil and livestock hooves inspected. Good shoes should be worn at all times.

2. Pulicidae
   a. *Pulex irritans*, the human flea, is a cosmopolitan nuisance in temperate and tropical areas. It may be responsible for outbreaks of bubonic plague, and definitely spreads vesicular and tonsillar plague in Ecuador.
   b. *Xenopsylla cheopis*, the oriental or black rat flea, normally affects rats in urban areas, although somewhat rare in northern temperate zones. Frequently attacking man in rat-infested buildings, it is the chief vector of epidemic plague (*Yersinia pestis*), and of murine typhus (*Rickettsia mooseri*), both among rats and from rat to man. The eggs of the rat tapeworm *Hymenolepis diminuta* may be ingested by *Xenopsylla* which may in turn be eaten by children; intestinal infection may result.
   c. *Ctenocephalides*, cat and dog fleas, may ingest eggs of dog tapeworm *Dipylidium caninum*. Individuals eating adult fleas with cysticercoids may develop intestinal infection.

3. Ceratophyllidae
   a. Includes the chicken fleas, medically unimportant except for a particularly painful bite, and the brown rat flea which may transmit dog tapeworm to man, as does *Ctenocephalides*.

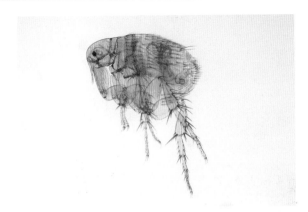

Fig. 2.12 *Xenopsylla cheopis*, rat flea, vector for plague. (From Nabarro L, Morris-Jones S, Moore DAJ. Arthropod-borne diseases. In: Nabarro L, Morris-Jones S, Moore DAJ, eds. *Peters' Atlas of Tropical Medicine and Parasitology.* 7th ed. London, UK: Elsevier Ltd; 2019:1–108.)

4. Tungidae (sand flea, jigger, chigoe, chique)
   a. *Tungae penetrans* has females adapted for intracutaneous permanent attachment on pigs, humans, poultry, and other animals in Central America, sub-Saharan Africa, and parts of the Indian subcontinent. Fertilized females crawl into exposed areas (usually on the feet) such as cracks, between toes, or at the base of toenails before growing pea-size over 8 to 12 days; only the posterior spiracles penetrate through the surface of the skin. This causes the host considerable irritation to the host, with inflammation, suppuration, and ulceration before the eggs are released. Surgical excision of the entire female, including the head is warranted, as chronic suppuration has resulted in cases of thrombophlebitis. (note: may be confused with cutaneous myiasis).

ZOONOSES AND OCCUPATION/EXPOSURE-RELATED GLOBAL

Diseases

1. Undercooked meat
   a. Salmonellosis (chicken), toxoplasmosis, trichinosis, cysticercosis
2. Drinking water/ice
   a. Salmonellosis, shigellosis, leptospirosis, amebiasis, giardiasis, dracunculiasis(?), hepatitis A/E, schistosomiasis, cryptosporidium
3. Unpasteurized milk products
   a. Brucellosis, salmonellosis, campylobacterosis, tuberculosis, listeriosis, toxoplasmosis, Q fever
4. Undercooked fish/shellfish
   a. Salmonellosis, hepatitis A, fish tapeworm, angiostrongyloidiasis, liver flukes, lung flukes, anisakiasis, paragonimiasis, gnathostomiasis, capillariasis, fish tapeworm (diphyllobothriasis)
5. Rodent contact
   a. Plague, leptospirosis, lymphocytic choriomeningitis, Venezuelan equine encephalitis, rickettsialpox, spotted fever, typhus, Hanta/Bolivian/other hemorrhagic fever
6. Farm animal contact
   a. Brucellosis, tuberculosis, salmonellosis, tularemia, glanders, anthrax, psittacosis, Q fever
7. Freshwater exposure
   a. Schistosomiasis (human and cercarial dermatitis), leptospirosis, melioidosis, neagleria/acanthamoeba

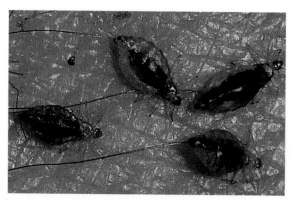

Fig. 2.13   *Pediculus humanus corporis* (body louse). (From Nabarro L, Morris-Jones S, Moore DAJ. Arthropod-borne diseases. In: Nabarro L, Morris-Jones S, Moore DAJ, eds. *Peters' Atlas of Tropical Medicine and Parasitology.* 7th ed. London, UK: Elsevier Ltd; 2019:1–108.)

   8. Contact with soil/sand
      a. Tungiasis, hookworm (human), cutaneous larvae migrans, strongyloidiasis, schistoso-miasis (*S. japonicum*), Hansen's disease
   9. Ingestion of fecally contaminated food or fomites, or person-to-person
      a. Ascariasis, enterobiasis, typhoid, echinococcosis, giardiasis, shigella, cryptosporidium
  10. Diseases potentially spread by contaminated clothing
      a. Tumbu fly, tinea capitis, pinworm, body louse (Fig. 2.13)
  11. Slaughtering animals
      a. Wildlife: ehrlichiosis (deer), tularemia (rabbits)
      b. Occupational (abbatoir): anthrax, brucellosis, leptospirosis, salmonella, Q fever
  12. Parturient animals
      a. Toxoplasmosis, brucellosis, Q fever, listeriosis

CHAPTER 3

Specific Infectious Diseases

Daniel S. Burns ▦ Lucy Lamb

Bacterial Infections

ANTHRAX

Anthrax is a zoonotic disease caused by the spore-forming bacteria, *Bacillus anthracis*. Humans acquire disease after contact with infected animals or animal products, with the route of exposure, cutaneous, gastrointestinal or inhalational, determining the clinical syndrome. *B. anthracis* is distributed throughout the globe, except where vaccination of livestock controls infection in the zoonotic host. Agricultural and industrial workers handling animal products are at greatest risk but inhalational anthrax from deliberate bioterrorism release is a potential threat.

Clinical Features

There are three main clinical syndromes.

Cutaneous. Typically, 2 to 7 days after exposure a painless pruritic papule develops which enlarges and ulcerates. A characteristic thick black eschar with surrounding edema covers the ulcer. Lesions will heal slowly over 2 to 6 weeks with minimal systemic symptoms although 10% to 20% of untreated patients will develop systemic disease with bacteremia. Injectional anthrax caused by injection of a contaminated agent, usually heroin in injecting drug users, can cause severe soft tissue infection, compartment syndrome, and necrotizing fasciitis, and progress to systemic disease with meningitis.

Respiratory. After a variable, dose-dependent incubation period, patients develop a prodrome of myalgia, fever, malaise, and cough. Some will transiently improve after 2 to 4 days before a fulminant stage with respiratory distress, high fever, and cyanosis. Mediastinal nodes undergo hemorrhagic necrosis, leading to septicemia, which may be accompanied by meningitis and/or pneumonia, almost invariably resulting in death within 1 day.

Gastrointestinal. Acquired from eating contaminated, undercooked meat, gastrointestinal (GI) anthrax occurs 2 to 5 days after exposure, not uncommonly in clusters (such as family units). Spores can be deposited in the oropharynx leading to neck swelling, sore throat, and dysphagia followed by a local lesion with a necrotic ulcer covered by pseudomembrane, or in the lower GI tract leading to nausea, vomiting, and bloody diarrhea. Fever occurs in both forms. Death may be from airway obstruction, or systemic bacteriaemia and shock.

Diagnosis

Culturing typical short chains of gram-positive rods from a lesion, blood, or stool is diagnostic, although frequently it is diagnosed on clinical grounds. Serology is generally unhelpful except for retrospective diagnosis.

Treatment

Cutaneous anthrax can be treated with penicillin. In mild cases, oral penicillin (250 mg qds for 5–7 days) and for more extensive lesions intravenous (IV) penicillin G (2 million units 4-hourly) should be given. For inhalational and GI anthrax, two IV agents should be used, penicillin G (4 million units) 4-hourly, plus ciprofloxacin or doxycycline. For bioterrorism-related infections, two agents are preferred, with fluoroquinolone and doxycycline usually advised.[1]

TETANUS

Clostridium tetani is a ubiquitous spore-forming anaerobic gram-positive soil bacterium that causes disease in humans via production of tetanospasmin toxin following inoculation, germination, and multiplication in a wound. Although present worldwide, most cases occur where vaccination is absent, or traditional birth practices result in inoculation of tetanus bacteria onto the umbilical stump. A total of 49,000 deaths from neonatal tetanus were estimated to occur in 2013.

Clinical Features

Symptoms start typically 7 to 14 days post inoculation with increasing muscle tone. Muscle tone increases over several days with spasms occurring 2 to 5 days after first symptoms. Trismus, opisthotonos, and risus sardonicus are characteristic findings. Autonomic instability, airway obstruction, and involvement of the respiratory muscles cause critical illness and death. Neonatal tetanus follows a similar clinical course. The World Health Organization (WHO) uses a clinical diagnosis: "an illness occurring in a child who has the normal ability to suck and cry in the first 2 days of life but who loses this ability between days 3 and 28 of life and becomes rigid and has spasms."

Diagnosis

Tetanus is a clinical diagnosis based on characteristic clinical features, and a portal of entry for the bacteria such as traumatic inoculation or peripartum. Where laboratory facilities allow, absence of protective antibodies, or positive wound cultures, may be helpful in reaching a diagnosis.

Management

Focus should be on prevention of tetanus. Immunization, effective wound management including debridement, and the use of prophylactic antibiotics, postexposure prophylaxis following tetanus prone wounds, and provision of safe, sterile midwifery practices are all effective. Management of clinical tetanus should include wound management, antibiotic therapy with penicillin or metronidazole and tetanus antitoxin when available. Supportive care is important but can be difficult in less-developed settings. Pharmacological reversal of the autonomic instability, sedation with benzodiazepines, intubation, and ventilation in the event of respiratory muscle involvement or airway compromise may be required. Nurse patients in a quiet, low-light atmosphere (to prevent spasms), and ensure nutrition, frequent turning, hydration, and awareness of the high rates of nosocomial infection.[2]

DIPHTHERIA

Diphtheria is a devastating disease, largely affecting under 5s where there is low vaccine coverage. It is caused by toxigenic strains of the gram-positive rods *Corynebacterium diphtheriae* or *ulcerans*. It is spread by respiratory droplets, or direct contact with cutaneous lesions. Outbreaks have occurred after natural disasters, including an outbreak in Haiti following the earthquake in 2010, likely because of prior low vaccine coverage and overcrowding, and amongst the displaced Rohingya population on the Bangladesh-Myanmar border in 2017/2018.

Clinical Features

After an incubation period of 2 to 6 days, diphtheria presents with malaise, sore throat, and fever. A gray-yellow pseudomembrane is present over the tonsils and enlarges to cover the oropharynx, soft palate, and associated structures. Marked fetor, cervical lymphadenopathy, nausea, and painful dysphagia accompany this. The pseudomembrane will become black and eventually slough off. Some patients will present with malignant diphtheria with a rapid-onset high fever and gross cervical lymphadenopathy with edema ("bullneck"). Local bleeding, cardiac involvement, and renal failure are common. Cardiovascular complications, including myocarditis and heart block, occur early, usually in the first week, and are commoner in malignant, or hypertoxic, diphtheria. Later, neurologic complications can occur, comprising typically of a segmental demyelinating neuropathy. Patients will recover if appropriate intensive care support is available, but unfortunately many die. Cutaneous diphtheria causes ulcerative punched-out lesions covered in a dark pseudomembrane. Although these are slow to heal and contribute to transmission of diphtheria, symptoms are usually mild and complications rare.

Diagnosis

As well as the typical clinical syndrome, *Corynebacteria* species can be cultured from swabs on appropriate selective media. Evidence of toxin production should be sought to confirm that a toxigenic strain of a *Corynebacteria* species has been produced. Elek's test, which depends on visualization of toxin-antitoxin precipitate in an agar plate cultured with suspected bacteria and filter paper containing antitoxin, is commonly used, although polymerase chain reaction (PCR)–based testing for the diphtheria toxin gene is of increasing importance.

Management

Intravenous penicillin (or erythromycin in allergic individuals) will eliminate the causative organism and prevent further toxin production. Diphtheria antitoxin is an effective treatment but needs to be given early, ideally within 48 hours of symptoms, so should be given on clinical suspicion rather than waiting for bacteriological confirmation. For diphtheria, 20,000 to 40,000 units should be given, or 40,000 to 80,000 when given more than 48 hours after onset of symptoms. For malignant disease, including rapid-onset disease, presence of a "bullneck," or renal or cardiac involvement, 80,000 to 10,0000 units should be given. Anaphylaxis may occur and facilities to treat this should be at hand. Good supportive care is required to treat cardiovascular and neurologic complications. Vaccination will prevent diphtheria infections, and should be instituted early in case of an outbreak.[3]

LISTERIOSIS

Listeria monocytogenes is a gram-positive soil bacterium that is widespread in nature. Consumption of contaminated food items, most commonly soft cheese, may cause clinical disease. Although listeria can cause disease in healthy individuals, most vulnerable are older patients, neonates, pregnant women, and those who are immunosuppressed or have underlying disease such as diabetes mellitus, renal, or liver disease, particularly alcohol-related liver disease.

Clinical Features

Meningoencephalitis and/or septicemia is the most common presentation. Onset of meningitis may be acute or follow an insidious course. Cerebritis is increasingly recognized, and brain abscess can occur. Rhombencephalitis (brainstem encephalitis) with cranial nerve palsies, cerebellar signs, and coma may develop. In maternal listeriosis, the mother presents with fever, headache, myalgia, and low backpain because of the bacteremic phase of the disease. The neonate is infected via the transplacental route resulting in placentitis, amnionitis, and spontaneous septic abortion or premature labor with delivery of a severely infected baby. Neonatal listeriosis has a high mortality. The neonate will be septic and jaundiced, with signs of purulent conjunctivitis, bronchopneumonia, meningitis, and/or encephalitis. Late-onset disease presenting days to weeks after birth with meningitis may occur. Immunocompetent patients may present with gastroenteritis, often as part of an outbreak.

Diagnosis

Culture of appropriate samples, such as cerebrospinal fluid (CSF), blood, amniotic fluid, placental tissue, or pus, in selective media will allow growth of gram-positive rods that can be biochemically identified. Lymphocytic meningitis in a vulnerable individual, or other compatible clinical syndrome such as maternal and fetal sepsis, should alert clinicians to the possibility of listeriosis.

Management

Listeria monocytogenes is intrinsically resistant to cephalosporins, the first-line treatment for meningitis in many countries. Where listeriosis is suspected as a cause of meningitis, high-dose IV amoxicillin (e.g., 2 g qds for adults; 200–300 mg/kg for children) should be added. Some advocate adjunctive gentamicin. Co-trimoxazole or chloramphenicol are alternatives.[4]

STAPHYLOCOCCAL SKIN AND SOFT TISSUE INFECTIONS

Staphylococcus aureus is a gram-positive bacteria commonly found to cause skin and soft tissue infections (SSTIs) as well as invasive disease (bacteremias, endocarditis, osteomyelitis). It is becoming more challenging to treat with the increasing presence of antibiotic resistant strains and virulence factors such as Panton Valentine leukocidin (PVL) toxin. *S. aureus* infections can arise endogenously from bacteria carried on the host skin surface or by exogenous acquisition from either carriers or other sources, including pets. In recent years there has been an increasing prevalence of community-acquired methicillin resistant *S. aureus* (CA-MRSA) worldwide, and particularly in the United States. The prevalence of MRSA varies worldwide. Asian countries have been shown to have very high rates (>50%), with a large proportion hospital acquired. A review of Latin American studies reports MRSA rates ranging from 29% in Brazil to 79% in Peru.

Clinical Features

S. aureus can cause a wide variety of SSTIs, from boils and furuncles to cellulitis and even necrotizing fasciitis. Invasive infection may follow a bacteremia from an SSTI and bacteremias, endocarditis, and osteomyelitis can all be challenging to manage. CA-MRSA, and especially the USA300 strain, which carries the PVL locus, has been associated with increased virulence. PVL *S. aureus* is commonly associated with recurrent skin abscesses, but can lead to necrotizing pneumonia and SSTIs.

Diagnosis

Diagnosis is usually dependent on laboratory culture and identification of typical colonies from samples such as pus, blood cultures, or skin swabs. Antibiotic disc testing can reveal resistant strains. PVL is often suspected clinically on grounds of recurrent abscesses or necrotizing pneumonia, but gene testing by PCR is available. The mortality of invasive *S. aureus* disease can be as high as 40% despite antibiotics and intensive care support, and even survivors may have significant morbidity.

Management

This will be dependent on the site of infection and whether there is an underlying bacteremia. Simple SSTIs can be treated with oral antibiotics for 7 to 10 days. If there is an underlying concern regarding a bacteremia, treatment should be extended to 14 days or longer depending on other sites involved. In cases with *S. aureus*–associated pneumonia, testing for other organisms (such as influenza) is extremely helpful. Treatment is tailored to the resistance profile and presence of PVL, with agents such as flucloxacillin, an antistaphylococcal penicillin, being used first line. Where PVL is suspected or confirmed, other antibiotics like clindamycin or linezolid may be required.[5,6]

STREPTOCOCCAL DISEASE

This is a gram-positive bacteria in which species are classified based on hemolytic properties, with alpha-hemolytic species causing partial hemolysis of red blood cells (greenish color on blood agar) and beta-hemolytic species leading to complete rupture of red blood cells. Beta-hemolytic streptococci are further classified by Lancefield grouping (a serotype classification describing specific carbohydrates present on bacterial cell wall). Several different streptococci cause human disease across the globe in different patterns including the alpha-hemolytic streptococci (such as *S. pneumoniae*), viridians group (*S. mitis*, *S. sanguinis*, *S. mutans*, *S. anginosus*, *S. intermedius*, and *S. constellatus*) and the beta-hemolytic streptococci of Lancefield group A (*S. pyogenes*) and group B (*S. agalactaie*). These will be discussed briefly.

Viridans Streptococci

These can be normal flora of the mouth and GI tract but can also cause bacteremia, endocarditis, and abscess (liver/brain) formation. Most are susceptible to penicillin or cephalosporins, with duration of treatment dependent on site of the disease. The *S. anginosus* group (*S. anginosus*,

S. intermedius, and *S. constellatus*; formerly the *S. milleri* group) are well known to cause abscess formation and are a not uncommon cause of brain and liver abscesses.

Group A Streptococci (*Streptococcus pyogenes*)

These cause a variety of clinical presentations from a mild pharyngitis or soft tissue infection through to invasive disease including necrotizing fasciitis, bacteremia, or pneumonia, associated with a high morbidity and mortality. Scarlet fever, which usually follows a streptococcal pharyngitis, causes a typical erythematous, symmetrical rash that may desquamate, along with the characteristic "strawberry tongue." Historically, Group A streptococcus was the leading cause of puerperal sepsis, bacterial infection of the mother peripartum, and caused significant mortality. Although easily preventable and much rarer in modern hospital settings, puerperal sepsis remains a risk for mothers, especially where access to good quality midwifery and obstetric care is difficult. Postinfectious sequelae of streptococcal disease, namely rheumatic fever and glomerulonephritis, are still common in parts of the developing world, causing significant mortality and morbidity.

Diagnosis of Group A streptococcal disease is usually made by clinical presentation and isolation of the organism from a sterile site (blood culture, sputum, aspirate, or tissue). Antistreptococcal antibody titers may aid diagnosis, especially when therapy has been commenced before taking appropriate samples, but sequential rising titers are more useful than a single measure.

Most strains are penicillin susceptible but clindamycin may be added in certain cases to inhibit strains producing exotoxins. Note there has been a rise in macrolide resistance recently, which may make it a less useful second-line agent.

Group B Streptococci (*Streptococcus agalactiae*)

These are frequently carried asymptomatically in the throat or perineum. Clinically, these are an important cause of neonatal infections, including meningitis and bacteremia, and postpartum infection of the mother. Risk factors include diabetes, liver disease and malignancy, and human immunodeficiency virus (HIV). Diagnosis is made by isolation of the organism from blood, CSF, sputum, urine, or other site. It is usually susceptible to penicillin, but other agents such as clindamycin may be used. Duration of therapy is 10 to 14 days, except for endocarditis or osteomyelitis (in which treatment is 4–6 weeks).

Streptococcus pneumoniae (Pneumococcus)

Pneumococcal infections including pneumonia, bacteremia, and meningitis are important causes of morbidity and mortality in young children, older adults, and those with chronic conditions across the globe. Smoking, chronic disease, and immunodeficiency, especially HIV, are important risk factors. HIV increases the risk of invasive pneumococcal disease by 50 times and drives much of the burden of disease where HIV is highly prevalent.

Streptococcus pneumoniae Respiratory Disease

Although relative rates of *Streptococcus pneumoniae* as a cause for pneumonia have fallen, it remains the commonest cause of community-acquired pneumonia in the developed and developing world and is responsible for a large number of hospital admissions at all age groups. Classically, patients present with fever, chills, cough productive of "rusty sputum," and pleuritic chest pain. Patients may show clinical signs of consolidation (dullness on percussion, bronchial breathing, and whispering pectoriloquy) with chest radiography showing classical lobar pneumonia. Complications include bacteremia, empyema, and lung abscess.

Diagnosis is frequently made from the history, physical examination, and chest radiograph changes without proving the bacteriological diagnosis. Sputum, blood culture, or the presence of a positive pneumococcal urinary antigen are helpful.

In most settings, pneumococci remain penicillin sensitive, and this forms the basis of most antibiotic regimes, with oral amoxicillin for mild cases or IV penicillin for severe cases effective. However, rising rates of penicillin resistance, largely because of variation among the penicillin binding proteins in some areas, has led to increasing use of cephalosporins or fluoroquinolones, particularly for severe disease. Vaccination using the polysaccharide or conjugate vaccine has reduced the number of invasive cases of pneumococcal disease.

Streptococcus pneumoniae Meningitis

S. pneumoniae can cause meningitis by hematogenous spread during a bacteremia or direct invasion of bacteria colonizing the nasopharynx. It is a common cause of meningitis in adults, particularly amongst the elderly. Cases have decreased since the introduction of the 7-valent pneumococcal conjugate vaccine, where it is available at least, although there has been concern over a rise in serotypes not in the vaccine.

The clinical features are those consistent with meningitis including fever, headache, photophobia, and neck stiffness. It is usually indistinguishable from other causes of meningitis at presentation, although risk factors such as concurrent pneumonia, middle ear infection, or trauma may point to the diagnosis.

Empiric treatment is with a cephalosporin such as ceftriaxone. In certain populations where there is concern over the rise of clinical failure because of cephalosporin resistance, other agents may be added such as vancomycin. Administration of dexamethasone has been shown to diminish the rate of hearing loss and neurologic complications. Duration of treatment is usually 10 to 14 days. Despite appropriate treatment, mortality can be high and recovery slow, and many patients are left with neurologic sequelae.

NONVENEREAL ENDEMIC TREPONEMATOSES (YAWS, ENDEMIC SYPHILIS/BEJEL, AND PINTA)

The endemic treponematoses are caused by subspecies of the spirochaete *Treponema pallidum*. Morphologically and serologically identical to the spirochaete causing venereal syphilis, *Treponema pallidum* subsp. *pallidum* (see Chapter 6), they are distinguishable by their epidemiology, pathogenic effects, and genome. They enter the body through abrasions and cuts and cause chronic, granulomatous infections, usually in the extremities.

YAWS

Yaws is caused by the spirochete *Treponema pallidum* subsp. *pertenue* and is spread person-person by direct contact with infective moist lesions to broken skin. Crowded, unhygienic conditions promote spread. Yaws is a disease predominantly of children, with a peak incidence of 6 to 10 years old. The WHO-led eradication program in the 1950s decreased cases by 95% from 50 million to 2.5 million. However, since the 1970s there has been a resurgence, and a new campaign to eradicate yaws was launched in 2012 using azithromycin. Yaws still persists in rural populations in West Africa, Ethiopia, Southeast (SE) Asia, and the Pacific Islands including Papua New Guinea, Solomon Islands, and Vanuatu.

Clinical Syndrome

Primary Yaws. After a few weeks' incubation period, a painless initial papule appears, typically on the extremities. This enlarges to form a raised, ulcerated raspberry-like papilloma 1 to 3 cm in size. The surface teems with spirochaetes and is highly contagious. Tender lymphadenopathy may also develop.

Secondary Yaws. As this lesion begins to heal, disseminated or satellite ulcerated papillomata appear in crops 2 to 6 months later. These may be accompanied by periostitis of the long bones and fingers. Papillomata and hyperkeratoses may occur as painful lesions on the palms and soles. Lesions heal spontaneously, but may relapse elsewhere.

Late Yaws. Up to 20% of patients go on to late-stage destruction of skin and bone, years after initial infection. Deep skin ulcers may cause disability, as may incapacitating hyperkeratotic lesions on the palms of the hand and soles of the feet. Bony destruction may cause deformity, especially of the palate and soft tissues of the nose.

Diagnosis

Diagnosis of endemic treponematoses is relatively simple in endemic areas where clinical assessment may reveal the typical features, supported by dark-ground microscopy demonstrating treponemes and/or positive treponemal serology. However, differentiating between syphilis and endemic treponematosis in this cohort (i.e., those who have lived in an endemic area) is difficult because in both the serology is positive. Therefore it is important that a thorough clinical history and assessment is performed, looking for evidence of old yaws (e.g., scars or periostitis). A history of treatment can be particularly helpful. If the decision is made to treat, this should be documented carefully to prevent unnecessary further treatments, as serology will remain positive life-long.

Treatment

A single intramuscular dose of benzathine penicillin at 0.6 million units (children aged under 10 years) and 1.2 million units (people aged >10 years) is the traditional treatment for all endemic treponematoses. The WHO now recommends a single dose of azithromycin at 30 mg/kg (maximum 2 g) for yaws as part of their eradication strategy (the Morges Strategy) because of the ease of administration in large-scale treatment campaigns and the reduction of yaws infection (2.4%–0.3% at 12 months) with no evidence of macrolide resistance.[7,8]

ENDEMIC SYPHILIS (BEJEL)

Caused by *T. pallidum* subsp. *endemicum*, it is transmitted via nonvenereal contact among children or in family groups. Transmission from contaminated drinking vessels is common. The form known as bejel is still prevalent among nomadic populations in North Africa (such as the Tuareg peoples living in the Sahara in Mali, Niger, Mauritania, and Burkino Faso) and the Arabian Peninsula.

Clinical Syndrome

Clinical features are similar to yaws although primary lesions are often found around the mouth or in the mucus membranes, reflecting transmission via contaminated drinking vessels. Cardiovascular and neurologic complications are rare but bone lesions and ulcerative nodules do occur as late complications.

Diagnosis and treatment are as per yaws.

PINTA

The spirochete *Treponema pallidum* subsp. *carateum* is spread person to person from skin lesions, especially if skin is trauma present. Tribal rituals involving skin scratches may play a part. Various arthropods bites (e.g., blackflies) have also been implicated. It is found in rural, isolated, warm areas of the American tropics including foci in southern Mexico, Columbia, Peru, Ecuador, and Venezuela.

Clinical Syndrome

Lesions from pinta are limited to the skin. Several weeks after exposure (which is typically prolonged), a painless, itchy scaling papule develops, typically on the extremities. This may enlarge and sometimes regional lymphadenopathy develops. Satellite lesions may form and coalesce before healing to leave depigmented atrophic scars. Months to years later a disseminated secondary rash may develop, typically on the scalp or nails, which may change into dyschromic skin splotches (blue, violet, and brown) before becoming an achromic and treponema-free scar.

Diagnosis and treatment are as per yaws.

LEPTOSPIROSIS

Leptospirosis is a zoonotic disease with multisystem manifestations caused by the spirochete *Leptospira interrogans*. Leptospira are found in urine of domestic and wild animals: livestock, dogs, and small rodents. The spirochete enters the host through skin, mucous membrane, or conjunctiva. Globally widespread, rates are particularly high in SE Asia. Occupation exposure is common, including sewage and rubber plantation workers, and is well described in adventure travelers. Outbreaks commonly occur after flooding, such as an outbreak in Guyana after flooding in 2005 for which doxycycline chemoprophylaxis may have prevented more deaths.

Clinical Features

The vast majority of cases are mild or asymptomatic, with only around 10% of symptomatic cases resulting in severe icteric disease. After an incubation period of 2 to 20 days, typically 10, the acute phase begins abruptly with high fever and chills, intense headaches, severe myalgia, and malaise. Distinguishing between this and dengue, malaria, or typhoid is clinically challenging. Conjunctival suffusion appearing after 2 to 3 days is useful diagnostically but is not universal. In some patients, jaundice will develop around day 5 to 9 of illness. This may progress with renal failure, hemorrhage (including pulmonary hemorrhage), and liver dysfunction, potentially leading to death. A biphasic disease is commonly described in textbooks, but in reality this has been overemphasized as a clinical indicator of leptospirosis.

Diagnosis

Biochemical abnormalities include a neutrophilia, biochemical jaundice, a raised alkaline phosphatase, and acute kidney injury. Definitive diagnosis can be by PCR early in the disease, with serologic methods such as microscopic agglutination test (MAT) becoming positive from the second week onwards. Culture of urine or blood on specialized media is possible early in disease but frequently results will not be known until after recovery or death. Where PCR is not available, timely diagnosis of leptospirosis can be difficult. Suspecting leptospirosis in patients with exposure and an undifferentiated febrile illness, especially if they have renal or liver impairment, and treating on suspicion, is key.

Management

Intravenous penicillin G (1.5 million units qds) is indicated for severe disease, oral doxycycline for mild disease. Where leptospirosis is being treated on clinical suspicion, a cephalosporin such as ceftriaxone maybe appropriate to ensure coverage of other causes of febrile illness such as typhoid. Doxycycline 200 mg once weekly is an effective prophylactic agent but defining who is at sufficient risk to benefit is challenging.[9,10]

LYME DISEASE

Lyme disease is a spirochaete infection caused by *Borrelia burgdorferi*, and a few other related spirochaetes, transmitted by hard-bodied ticks of the *Ixodes ricinus* group, usually in woodland and heathland areas of the temperate Northern Hemisphere, including in the United States, Europe, and Russia. Most cases occur between June and September, and rates in individuals with exposure to backcountry areas can be high with, for example, 54% of asymptomatic hunters seropositive for Lyme in one area of Austria.

Clinical Features

Erythema migrans, an expanding red patch, usually greater than 5 cm and with a distinct edge and central clearing, is the commonest skin manifestation. It typically develops 1 to 4 weeks after a tick bite, usually at the site of the bite, although distant erythema migrans and multiple lesions occur. Systemic symptoms such as fever, myalgia, and fatigue may occasionally occur. Neurologic manifestations include meningitis, radiculitis, and cranial nerve palsies, especially facial nerve palsies. Encephalitis is rare. Lyme carditis, usually presenting as atrioventricular conduction problems developing weeks to months after exposure, with myocarditis or pericarditis, is rare. Arthritis is well described and may be recurrent, and is typically of the large joints, with the knee most commonly reported. "Late" disease is poorly defined, rare, and not universally accepted to occur, except in neurologic infection. Thus persistent Lyme-related symptoms may be a result of tissue damage and do not necessarily imply persistent infection.

Diagnosis

Erythema migrans can be diagnosed clinically and treatment started empirically. Extracutaneous manifestations are usually diagnosed serologically via a two-step approach, with a sensitive immunoglobulin (Ig)M and IgG enzyme-linked immunosorbent assay (ELISA; usually to the C6 peptide) performed first and confirmed by immunoblot testing if positive. Testing may need to be repeated at 4 weeks if initially negative in early disease. Both serologic tests should be positive to diagnose Lyme, as overreading of weakly positive IgM ELISA leads to false positives. Laboratories offering single-step testing or that are not accredited/validated should be avoided. In Lyme meningitis there is a lymphocytic picture, and CSF serology may be helpful.

Management

A number of national and regional guidelines are available with, at the time of writing, the UK and US guidelines currently being written/updated. Treatment is generally dependent on the clinical manifestation, with erythema migrans, cardiac, neurologic, and late Lyme having different recommended treatments. Readers are advised to consult up-to-date national guidance but, broadly, erythema migrans should be treated with an oral regime (doxycycline 100 mg bd preferred; amoxicillin 500 mg tds alternative; azithromycin third line) for 14 days; neurologic Lyme where there is meningitis or radiculitis treated parentally with 14 days of ceftriaxone (2 g od) or an oral regime for 14 to 21 days where there is isolated cranial nerve features (some guidelines suggest that meningitis without complicating encephalitis or radiculitis can also be treated orally); cardiac disease with parental therapy for 14 to 21 days (with oral therapy potentially used to complete the course once stable); Lyme arthritis with a 3- to 4-week oral treatment; and late disease a 14-day parental course for neurologic disease, or 28 days of oral therapy. Chronic sequalae of treated Lyme such as persistent arthralgia, fatigue, or neurologic symptoms do not necessarily imply ongoing bacterial replication and there is little to no evidence to support an extended course of antibiotics, "pulsed" antibiotic regimes, combination therapy, or antibiotic agents beyond those discussed earlier. Supporting patients, symptomatic treatment, advice that Lyme sequalae may take time to resolve, and/or investigating for alternative diagnoses is likely to be more helpful in those with persistent symptoms who have completed adequate therapy. Nonevidence-based treatments (and diagnostic approaches) are strongly advocated by some patient groups, and a few physicians. Generally, these should be avoided and referral to an expert for a second opinion may be helpful to try to reassure the individual patient.[11]

RELAPSING FEVERS

Louse-borne relapsing fever (LBRF) and tick-borne relapsing fever (TBRF) are caused by spirochaete organisms of the *Borrelia* genus transmitted by an arthropod vector, human-human by the body louse *Pediculus humanus corporis* for LBRF and zoonotic transmission via soft ticks (genus *Ornithodoros*) from various mammal and bird species for TBRF. In the wake of war and famine LBRF can cause devastating epidemics, with 10 million cases between 1943 and 1946, although it is now confined largely to small foci, typically in mountainous regions. The potential for epidemic disease, especially after complex emergencies or in refugee settings, remains. At least 15 different species of TBRF exist and are geographically widespread across temperate and tropical zones. Relapsing fevers are an important medical problem in parts of Africa, including Tanzania and Rwanda. Antigenic variation allows escape from immunogenic control and underlies the relapse phenomenon.

Clinical Features

Louse-Borne Relapsing Fever. After a 4- to 18-day incubation period there is a sudden onset of high fever and rigors. Headache, myalgia, nausea, vomiting, and diarrhea follow. Patients are commonly confused and prostrate. A tender, enlarged liver is often palpable. Jaundice, petechial rash, and spontaneous hemorrhage are common. Meningitis, myocarditis, and multiorgan failure can all occur, with an untreated case fatality rate of up to 40% dropping to 5% with treatment. After resolution, multiple relapses with declining severity can occur after 5 to 9 days.

Tick-Borne Relapsing Fever. After an average incubation period of 1 week, disease presents similarly to LBRF with fever, headache, myalgia, and extreme fatigue. The initial episode may only last for 3 to 4 days before recurring 1 to 2 weeks later. Although generally less severe than LBRF, with death unusual, similar complications do occur. Additionally, neurologic complications similar to Lyme disease, such as cranial nerve palsies, lymphocytic meningitis, and radiculitis, are commoner. Untreated patients may relapse multiple times with decreasing severity, with ocular complications including optic neuritis, uveitis, and keratitis often occurring during the third and fourth relapse.

Diagnosis

Diagnosis is typically by demonstration of spirochaetes by staining (e.g., Giemsa's, or Wright's) on thick and thin blood films, or on clinical suspicion. PCR and serology can also provide the diagnosis, when available.

Management

For LBRF, stat doses of tetracycline (500 mg), erythromycin (500 mg), or doxycycline (100 mg) are effective, or for patients who cannot tolerate oral medication IV tetracycline (250 mg), erythromycin (300 mg), or a penicillin (such as benzylpenicillin 300,000 units) can all be used. However, penicillin may fail to prevent relapse. Milder TBRF requires multiple dose regimens such as tetracycline 500 mg qds for 10 days, or erythromycin 500 mg qds for 10 days to prevent relapse. Clinicians should be aware that treatment may precipitate a Jarisch-Herxheimer reaction (JHR) with endotoxin release causing worsening fevers, tachycardia, hypotension, and myalgia. Use of penicillins is associated with a less severe, if more prolonged JHR, and 100 mg of meptazinol given IV or hydrocortisone given preantibiotics may ameliorate the reaction.

Control

Delousing to prevent onward transmission is essential to control epidemics of LBRF and measures to prevent tick infestation or tick bite in TBRF are effective. Doxycycline 200 mg as a postexposure dose can prevent TBRF.[12,13]

TYPHOID AND PARATYPHOID (ENTERIC FEVER)

Enteric fever, typhoid, and paratyphoid is caused by *Salmonella enterica* serovar *typhi* and serovars *paratyphi A, B,* and *C.* Transmission is via fecooral contamination of food or water, with chronic carriage from previously infected patients contributing to ongoing transmission. There are an estimated 27 million cases per year, with 100,000 deaths. South and SE Asia, and sub-Saharan Africa are hotspots. Outbreaks of typhoid have been seen in disaster medicine settings, especially in overcrowded refugee camps with overwhelmed sanitary facilities or postflood.

Clinical Syndrome

Enteric fever presents as a febrile illness, often without clear focus, after an incubation period of typically 1 to 2 weeks. There is an insidious onset of fever accompanied by malaise and headache with diffuse abdominal pain. Constipation is commoner than diarrhea earlier in the illness. Rose spots, sparse macular lesions typically on the trunk, a dry cough, and relative bradycardia, where the pulse is below 100 beats per minute despite a fever of over 40°C, may also all occur (although clinicians should be aware other infections may cause "Faget's sign"). Typically, 2 weeks into the illness a host of complications occur caused by disseminated disease. These include intestinal perforation and hemorrhage, myocarditis, lobar pneumonia, meningitis, and typhoid abscess. Severe toxemia, shock, and confusion are more common in Papua New Guinea and Indonesia, with a higher associated mortality rate. Generally, 10% of cases are fatal, and up to 10% relapse without proper antibiotic therapy.

Diagnosis

Diagnosis of typhoid ideally rests on successfully culturing the organism from appropriate samples. Repeated sampling of an adequate volume of blood increases yield. Bacteria may be isolated from blood (especially early in disease); bone marrow; CSF; aspirates of rose spots; urine; and stool, typically after the first week of illness, with bone marrow giving the highest yield. Care must be taken when interpreting stool cultures because they may represent carriage rather than infection. Serology, largely the Widal test, is usually unhelpful but still widely used. A four-fold rise in titer is considered diagnostic, but may occur too late to aid clinical decision-making. Unpaired serologic tests are unhelpful, with vaccination or past exposure leading to false positives. These should generally be disregarded.

Treatment

Effective antimicrobial treatment is key to treating typhoid. Amoxicillin, chloramphenicol, and co-trimoxazole are the traditional agents, with chloramphenicol the drug of choice, but their use is now limited by growing antimicrobial resistance, particularly in SE Asia. Cephalosporins such as ceftriaxone, fluroquinolones, and azithromycin remain effective in most parts of the world (with some fluroquinolone resistance in South Asia). Treatment should be guided by local resistance patterns, and culture results where available. Vaccination is available for typhoid but does not protect against paratyphoid; protection declines over time and can be overwhelmed by, for example, a large infective dose. As a result, uptake is poor except in travelers, and a history of vaccination should not rule out typhoid infection.[14,15]

CHOLERA

Cholera is caused by the gram-negative bacterium *Vibrio cholerae*, transmitted via the fecooral route, particularly where sanitation and water supplies are inadequate. Cholera is thus a disease of poverty, endemic in many of the poorest places of the world, but with the potential to cause devasting outbreaks and epidemics. Recent outbreaks in Haiti in 2010 (700,000 cases; 9000 deaths) and Yemen 2016 to 2017 (771,945 cases and counting) have occurred after earthquake, hurricane, and civil war, and have been challenging to control even with a global humanitarian response.

Clinical Features

Most patients (90%–95%) will develop mild, self-limiting diarrhea. However, 5% to 10% of patients will suffer from severe, painless diarrhea. In the severe form, 500 to 1000 mL diarrhea can be produced per hour, rapidly leading to severe dehydration, electrolyte disturbance, and death.

Diagnosis

The mild diarrhea is clinically indistinguishable from other causes of diarrhea such as the diarrheagenic *E. coli*, but generally the severe form is a distinct enough entity to allow identification on clinical grounds alone and the use of case definitions for diagnosis in outbreaks. Confirmation can be by culture of the organism on specialist media (TCBS), PCR, or, increasingly in field settings, immune-diagnostic dipsticks.

Treatment

The key to treatment is fluid resusitation. Oral rehydration therapy has saved millions of lives and relies on the coupling of sodium transport to glucose in the gut enterocyte to drive water absorbtion. Commercial preparations are available but home-made recipes containing the requisite concentrations of glucose and salts are widely available and are cheaper to produce at scale during an epidemic. IV rehydration is used in severe dehydration (10%+) where rapid rehydration is required, typically with lactated Ringers' or similar crystalloid solutions. Antibiotics including tetracyclines, fluoroquinoles, and azithromycin will all shorten the duration of illness and reduce the volume of diarrhea produced. With good case management and careful attention to fluid status the case fatality rate is less than 1%, but can be much higher, particularly in the early stages of an epidemic when case numbers may outstrip resources required to treat.

Control

Controlling a cholera outbreak requires a coordinated public health response. Isolation and case management of large numbers of infected individuals provides a substantial logistic challenge, with family or peer nursing care often required. Improving sanitation, providing adequate clean water supplies, improving hygiene at household level by, for example, provision of soap and containers, and health education messaging are important in preventing further cases. Vaccination has now been shown to help bring an epidemic under control with useful data on the real-life efficacy of a single dose of the oral cholera vaccine coming from the recent South Sudan outbreak in 2016.[16,17]

MELIOIDOSIS

Melioidosis is caused by the soil-dwelling bacteria *Burkholderia pseudomallei*, with most infections originating in SE Asia, especially NE Thailand, and northern Australia, although sporadic cases have been reported from Brazil, India, and China. Transmission is most often through contact with contaminated soil or water through wounds but may occur after aspiration or ingestion of contaminated water, or by inhalation of dust from the soil. Age, occupational exposure such as in rice farmers without protective footwear, environmental conditions, especially heavy rain, chronic illness including diabetes and renal failure, and use of steroids are all risk factors.

Clinical Features

Incubation can be from 2 days to several years. Although asymptomatic infection is common, clinical presentations include septicemic disease with bacteria seeding to distant sites, and local disease. Pneumonia is the most common localized infection occurring in 50% of cases, either secondary from septicemia or from inhalation. Cavitation is common. Skin pustules and abscesses are also common.

Diagnosis

Any chronic, suppurative disease (especially with pulmonary cavitation) in one who has traveled to or been resident in an endemic area should provoke suspicion of melioidosis. Presence of risk factors such as diabetes mellitus will also increase suspicion. Isolation of causative agent from culture of blood, pus, urine or wound, or throat swabs sputum, clinches the diagnosis. Yield can be low so multiple clinical samples are encouraged. *Burkholderia pseudomallei* is a group 3 biological agent requiring containment laboratory handling, so inform the lab of the suspected diagnosis. Where culture is negative but suspicion remains, serology can be helpful, especially a four-fold rise in titers taken two or more weeks apart, but the high background seropositivity in endemic areas limits their use and warrants caution, especially when interpreting single titer results.

Treatment

Treatment requires an IV phase, usually with ceftazidime or meropenem (or when unavailable, amoxicillin-clavulanate as an alternative) for at least 10 days (or clinical improvement) followed by an oral eradication phase of co-trimoxazole for 12 to 20 weeks. Deep-seated abscesses may need drainage ± a longer IV phase.

GLANDERS

Burkholderia mallei causes glanders in horses, with occasional transmission to humans. Equine outbreaks do occur still in the Middle East, with potential for human infection. Glanders is similar to melioid in clinical features and diagnostic tests. Treatment regimens for *B. pseudomallei* will also treat *B. mallei.*[18]

MENINGOCOCCAL DISEASE

Neisseria meningitidis is asymptomatically carried in the nasopharynx in up to 10% of people, higher in the 19- to 25-years age range. It can be spread from person to person in droplets. Virulent strains invade through the nasopharynx causing severe disease. The disease is present globally, with young children most commonly affected and a second incidence peak in juveniles and young adults. Vaccination has led to reducing incidence in developed countries and outbreaks are now rarely reported. Across the meningitis belt (sub-Saharan Africa from Gambia to Ethiopia) rates are still high and large epidemics occur.

Clinical Features

Neisseria meningitidis may cause meningococcal meningitis with or without septicemia, or more rarely, may cause septicemia alone. The features of the meningitis are typical with fever, headache, photophobia, and neck stiffness. The onset of meningitis may be insidious, but untreated mortality is high as rising intracranial pressure causes brainstem herniation. Where septicemia is present the distinctive nonblanching rash occurs, caused by bleeding into the skin, often with petechiae. Circulatory collapse, often with a severe coagulopathy, may cause rapid deterioration in a patient's condition. Despite heroic measures in the intensive treatment unit (ITU), patients may die, or be permanently disabled with neurologic sequelae or loss of limbs and/or digits.

Diagnosis

Rapid identification and administration of treatment saves lives, so antibiotics are often given on clinical suspicion for patients with a presentation compatible with bacterial meningitis. Lumbar puncture shows a neutrophilic meningitis with a high opening pressure and low glucose. *Neisseria* can usually be cultured (gold standard of diagnosis) from blood or CSF with characteristic gram-negative diplococci seen, although when antibiotics are given before sampling, PCR of CSF or blood may be useful.

Treatment

The treatment of choice is usually with a third-generation cephalosporin such as ceftriaxone (2 g twice daily). Often intramuscular benzylpenicillin is administered in a prehospital setting to prevent early dissemination, and is currently used across the globe for first-line hospital therapy. However, it is generally not recommended in most Western hospital guidelines because of concern regarding penicillin-resistant strains, although these are generally rare and high doses are still likely to be effective. Chloramphenicol 25 mg/kg qds is an alternative, although there is increasing worldwide resistance. Good nursing and medical care including ITU-level care and ionotropic support may be required. Steroids are probably not effective in meningococcal meningitis, but UK guidelines recommend 10 mg dexamethasone IV qds is commenced at presentation in case of pneumococcal meningitis but discontinued if this is not confirmed. Some patients will be left with significant morbidity and follow-up care and rehabilitation are often required. There are a number of effective vaccines against meningococcal meningitis.[19]

LEGIONELLOSIS

Legionellosis is caused by several species of *Legionella*, of which *L. pneumophila* causes most human disease. It is a gram-negative rod that multiplies in warm water, often in man-made sources. Humans are infected when aerosolized bacteria from whirlpools, showers, air-conditioning equipment, etc. is inhaled. It is most reported in developed settings where it makes up 2% to 9% of community-acquired pneumonia.

Clinical Features

Between 2 and 10 days after infection, patients develop fever, headache, and myalgia. A lobar pneumonia with accompanying signs and symptoms develops, although respiratory symptoms, including cough, can be minimal. Diarrhea and confusion are often present. Abnormal liver function tests and hyponatremia occur in around half of patients. *Legionella* can also cause Pontiac fever, a nonpneumonic form where the main symptoms are of an undifferentiated febrile illness.

Diagnosis

Travel, exposure to contaminated water sources, hyponatremia, or deranged liver function tests may all lead to a suspicion of Legionnaire's disease. Risk factors include chronic lung disease, smoking, and solid organ transplant. The mainstay of diagnosis is urinary antigen detection, which is sensitive and specific but only detects serotype 1, although that is the main cause of disease. Culture requires specialist media and is rarely performed. Serologic diagnosis relies on a four-fold increase between acute and convalescent titers, so is often positive too late to be of use. PCR of sputum or a nasal swab is increasingly used, and is sensitive and specific when available.

Treatment

Penicillins, which are the mainstay of treatment for community-acquired pneumonias, are not effective. A macrolide such as clarithromycin is effective and is commonly used, although a recent meta-analysis suggests fluoroquinolones are more effective. Longer courses may need to be considered in immunocompromised patients with severe illness.[20]

NONTYPHOIDAL SALMONELLOSIS

Nontyphoidal salmonella are gram-negative bacteria with an animal reservoir, which typically cause enteric infection. Human infection is usually from contaminated food, particularly chickens and eggs, although direct contact with chickens, reptiles, or other animals also causes disease. When safe food preparation techniques are neglected, large outbreaks may occur. After a short incubation period of 4 to 48 hours the disease usually presents with fever, abdominal pain, and diarrhea. The disease is usually self-limiting in 2 to 3 days but some, especially those at the extremes of age, may suffer from severe disease. Invasive salmonellosis is increasingly recognized as a health problem in sub-Saharan Africa. Bacteremia may lead to metastatic infection, with osteomyelitis in children with sickle-cell anemia well described. HIV infection is associated with recurrent disease. Diagnosis is generally by culture of feces on selective media and slide agglutination testing, although multiplex PCR methods are increasingly used. Oral rehydration solution and general supportive care are important, and antibiotics reduce length of illness and are important for treating metastatic disease. Ciprofloxacin is the treatment of choice but rising antibiotic resistance in some areas means azithromycin is increasingly used. Also of note, antibiotic therapy may prolong fecal excretion of salmonella after acute salmonellosis.[21]

CAMPYLOBACTER INFECTIONS

Campylobacter spp. are gram-negative zoonotic bacteria that cause bacterial gastroenteritis when accidentally consumed, usually in chicken, eggs, or other meat products that are undercooked. It is a common cause of an acute diarrheal illness with an incubation period of 3 days. There may be bloody stools, and occasionally a bacteremia. The disease may self-resolve, although an immune-mediated reactive arthritis or Guillain-Barré will occur in some patients weeks after infection. Diagnosis is by culture on selective media. Supportive management with fluid and electrolyte replacement is the mainstay of treatment. Where antibiotics are required, macrolides such as azithromycin are first line because of the high rates of resistance to fluoroquinolones. For severe life-threatening infection consider using an aminoglycoside or carbapenem.

SHIGELLOSIS

Shigellosis is an enteric illness caused by *Shigella dysenteriae*, *S. flexneri*, *S. sonnei*, and *S. boydii*, gram-negative bacteria closely related to *E. coli*. Transmission is via the fecooral route and is human to human with no significant animal reservoir. Epidemics and outbreaks occur, especially where many people are gathered with limited water-sanitation infrastructure, and have been reported from festivals, summer camps, and most devastatingly in refugee camps, including in the aftermath of the Rwandan genocide. Outbreaks of bloody diarrhea and fever in such settings should prompt diagnostic testing, syndromic management, and robust outbreak control measures. Infection may cause watery diarrhea and abdominal pain but severe infections with bloody diarrhea and fever are common, especially with *S. dysenteriae*. More recently there is an increased risk of antibiotic resistance to ceftriaxone, azithromycin, or fluoroquinolones, especially for *Shigella* infections in men who have sex with men. Outbreaks linked to international travel have been caused by ciprofloxacin-resistant *S. sonnei*. Diagnosis is by culture on appropriate selective media or PCR. Antibiotic treatment is recommended for those with severe illness or to prevent outbreaks, with local antibiotic sensitivity data guiding treatment where available.[22,23]

ESCHERICHIA COLI INFECTIONS

Escherichia coli are gram-negative bacteria inhabiting the human gut. They cause disease in several ways depending on location and virulence determinants and are often characterized by their serotypes.

Gut *E. coli* organisms in normally sterile sites cause infection, typically in the urine or bile duct, causing urinary tract infections and cholangitis, respectively, but also in the CSF, joints, or soft tissue causing meningitis, septic arthritis, or wound abscess, and can be identified by growing *E. coli* on appropriate agar from a sterile site. Resistance testing should guide therapy, especially given growing worldwide antibiotic resistance, with some *E. coli* producing enzymes that break down antibiotics including carbapenamases and extended-spectrum B-lactamases, making therapy challenging. Duration of therapy and need for surgical intervention will depend on site and response.

A number of pathogenic serotypes can cause gastroenteritis. Enteropathogenic *E. coli* (EPEC), enterotoxigenic *E. coli* (ETEC), enteroinvasive *E. coli* (EIEC), enterohemorrhagic *E. coli* (EHEC), and enteroaggregative *E. coli* (EAEC) are divided according to their pathogenic mechanism and serotype. All apart from EHEC are zoonoses. Several cause self-limiting diarrhea, but EIEC causes a disease indistinguishable from shigellosis, and EHEC, of which the most important is serotype O157, can cause bloody diarrhea and a hemolytic-uremic syndrome, especially at extremes of age. Antibiotic treatment, usually ciprofloxacin or azithromycin, shortens treatment, but should be avoided in EHEC as it may worsen illness. Management is supportive here. Growth on culture and identification by antisera will identify particular pathogenic strains but is laborious and not particularly sensitive. PCR-based approaches including multiplex PCR are replacing this.[24]

PLAGUE

The bacillus *Yersinia pestis* is responsible for this zoonotic disease, spread by fleas, most commonly the oriental rat flea, *Xenopsylla cheopis,* from mammals to man, with the black rat, *Rattus* as the most famous reservoir host. Epidemics have caused devasting economic and social consequences including the plague of Justinian, the Black Death, and epidemics causing millions of deaths in India and China in the 19th and early 20th century. Endemic disease continues to occur in various countries across the globe including Madagascar, where there was a recent large outbreak in 2017, Tanzania, Democratic Republic of Congo (DRC), Vietnam, India, Burma, Peru, and the United States (Fig. 3.1). Plague has been developed, and used, as a bioweapon.

Clinical Syndrome

The disease presents with sudden-onset fever, chills, and headache. In bubonic plague, the vast majority of cases, painful, swollen lymphadenitis (buboes) develops in the groin, axilla, or neck around the time of disease onset or shortly after. Buboes enlarge and suppurate. Hematogenous dissemination (secondary septicemic plague) and seeding to the lung (secondary pneumonic plague) or meninges may follow. Sepsis and disseminated intravascular coagulation (DIC) result in a mortality of 50% to 90% in untreated cases. Some cases may present as sepsis without buboes (septicemic plague; 10%–20%) or primary pneumonic plague from aerosol transmission or deliberate bioterrorism release. Mortality rates from primary pneumonic plague approach 50% even in those treated.

Diagnosis

The organism may be identified from bubo aspiration, sputum, blood or CSF where microscopy reveals bipolar-staining small gram-negative rods. Culture will allow a definitive diagnosis but should be done in specialist containment laboratories. Given that prognosis is much better when treatment is started early, presumptive treatment based on clinical features, especially in an outbreak situation, is encouraged, although the validated dipstick test for F1 antigen also allows for rapid diagnosis.

Treatment

Historically, streptomycin is the drug of choice at 1 g intramuscular (IM) bd for 10 days, but good quality evidence suggests gentamycin, which is often easier to get hold of, is as effective. Doxycycline at standard 100 mg bd doses is also effective, although most people prefer using

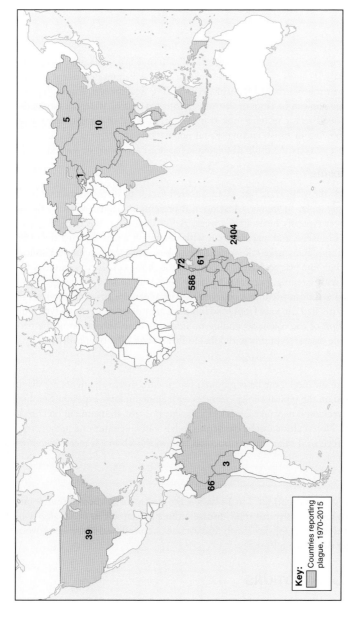

Fig. 3.1 Map of distribution of plague. (From Nabarro L, Morris-Jones S, Moore DAJ. Arthropod-borne diseases. In: Nabarro L, Morris-Jones S, Moore DAJ, eds. *Peters' Atlas of Tropical Medicine and Parasitology*. 7th ed. London, UK: Elsevier Ltd; 2019:1–108.)

Key:

Countries reporting plague, 1970-2015

IV drugs. Fluoroquinolones are effective in mouse models and are widely recommended as an alternative treatment where aminoglycoside therapy is not appropriate. Postexposure prophylaxis in cases of known exposure, such as close contact with a pneumonic plague patient, laboratory or bioterrorism exposure, is recommended. Doxycycline 100 mg bd or ciprofloxacin 500 mg bd for 7 days are the current recommended regimes.[25,26]

TULAREMIA

Francisella tularensis is a gram-negative coccobacillus found in rabbits, hares, small rodents, and other small animals. It causes a zoonotic disease with clinical features dependent on mode of infection. It is found in the Northern Hemisphere, including Scandinavia, Russia, Japan, and North America. Transmission can be from meat from an infected animal, water contamination, inoculation via an arthropod vector, or inhalation from airborne spread of contaminated material by, for example, lawn mowing or brush cutting. Rural populations are more at risk, especially hunters, walkers, and forest workers. Aerosolized tularemia has been previously developed as a bioweapon.

Clinical Syndrome

Infection through the skin, via a bite of an infected vector or direct contact with animal flesh, results in ulceroglandular tularemia. Most often it presents as papule, often on the hand, which ulcerates. The ulcer typically heals after a week. A few days after infection, systemic symptoms including chills, headache, and malaise occur with the lymph nodes draining the ulcer becoming enlarged and painful. They make take some time to heal, and may suppurate. Clinically this can be mistaken for bubonic plague. Rarely, infection through the conjunctiva can lead to oculoglandular tularemia with swelling, purulent discharge, and lymphadenopathy. Ingestion of bacteria via contaminated meat can produce a pharyngitis with ulceration, swollen cervical lymph nodes, and a gastroenteritis that can vary from mild but persistent diarrhea to a fatal syndrome involving extensive ulceration of the colon, depending on infecting dose. Inhalation of the pathogen may lead to pneumonic disease, typically with lobal infiltrates and hilar lymphadenopathy.

Diagnosis

Prolonged culture on special media is required for growth, so most patients are diagnosed serologically, or based on the typical clinical features with epidemiologic exposure. Serologic response peaks at 4 to 6 weeks and may take 2 weeks to become positive, so treatment on clinical suspicion may be required. Note, culture can be dangerous to lab staff and requires a suitably equipped containment laboratory, so if tularemia is suspected, inform the lab in advance of submitting clinical specimens.

Treatment

Gentamicin (or streptomycin) for 7 to 14 days is the treatment of choice. Fluoroquinolones and tetracyclines are also effective for mild disease although relapse can occur after withdrawal of treatment. Postexposure prophylaxis with doxycycline or ciprofloxacin has been advocated in case of exposure after deliberate release.[27]

BARTONELLA INFECTIONS

Bartonella species are slow-growing fastidious gram-negative bacteria that causes a variety of human infections including cat scratch disease, endocarditis, trench fever, and bartonellosis, which is also termed Carrion's disease, Oroya fever, and Verruga peruana (Peruvian wart). The three most important Bartonella species are: *Bartonella bacilliformis* (Bartonellosis), *B. henselae* (cat scratch disease), and *B. quintana* (trench fever).

BARTONELLOSIS

B. bacilliformis multiples in erythrocytes and endothelial cells and is transmitted to humans by the bites of various *Lutzomyia* sandfly (active at twilight). Cases are seen in Andean and high jungle areas of Peru and adjacent countries, with transmission greatest toward the end of the rainy season. Its many synonyms attest to its long history in South America, being present since pre-Columbian times.

Clinical Features

The disease is biphasic. After an incubation period typically of 60 days patients develop a febrile illness with malaise, headache, backache, and lethargy. Approximately 1 in 6 patients will develop the classical clinical picture with a severe hemolytic anemia, which may be accompanied by jaundice, hepatosplenomegaly, lymphadenopathy, myocarditis, and purpura. This typically lasts 2 to 4 weeks, and has a high fatality rate in pregnant women. Patients that recover are then well for weeks-months before multiple, red, or purple hemangioma-like lesions erupt over the body. These persist for 3 to 4 months, and can become secondarily infected.

Diagnosis

In the acute phase, blood smear and staining (e.g., Giemsa's) may be positive in up to 90% with intraerythrocytic bacteria visible. PCR and antibody detection are useful but not widely available, with most cases diagnosed based on the typical clinical features; hemolysis with a febrile illness in the acute phase, or the classic skin lesions in the eruptive phase.

Treatment

A wide range of antibiotics are effective including co-trimoxazole, penicillin, the macrolides, and cephalosporins. Ciprofloxacin 500 mg bd for 14 days is usually preferred because of the frequent association with salmonellosis, or ceftriaxone plus ciprofloxacin for severe disease.

CAT SCRATCH FEVER

B. henselae can cause cat scratch disease and is found throughout the globe. The bacterium is typically inoculated after a cat scratch, with kittens most often responsible, and a few weeks later a lymphadenopathy in the draining lymph nodes develops which can last weeks, or even years. Systemic symptoms including fever, fatigue, and headache may also occur. Diagnosis can be tricky, with PCR or antibody testing not widely available. Often lymph node biopsy and Warthin-Starry staining can confirm the diagnosis, and are often done to exclude tuberculosis (TB) or lymphoma as a cause. Treatment is not usually required as in the immunocompetent the disease will be self-limiting. Antibiotic response is often minimal, but excision or drainage of lymph nodes and azithromycin can be used where disease is persistent or associated with systemic symptoms. Note that the JHR can occur after the first few doses of antibiotic.

TRENCH FEVER

Trench fever, also known as "quintan fever," "Wolhynia fever," or "5-day fever," is caused by *B. quintana*, a small gram-negative rod spread person-person by the body louse, *Pediculus humanus*. Often seen in homeless persons and those in poverty, it caused a million cases of trench fever during World War I and II. Some 15 to 25 days after exposure an acute febrile illness develops with severe headache, malaise, splenomegaly, pain in the long bones of the leg, and occasionally a rash. Fever episodes last 1 to 5 days, and then an asymptomatic period of 4 to 6 days is followed by further episodes of fever. Debility is common, but mortality rare. *B. quintana* may also cause culture-negative endocarditis. Definitive diagnosis usually requires reference laboratory techniques; PCR assays are useful, but serology is more widely used although cross-reactions with other *Bartonella* species can make interpretation difficult. The recommended treatment regime is with doxycycline 200 mg od for 4 weeks (6 weeks in culture-negative endocarditis) and 14 days of gentamicin 3 mg/kg.[28]

BRUCELLOSIS

Brucellosis is a zoonosis caused by four species of small gram-negative coccobacilli, *Brucella melitensis*, found in sheep goats and camels in the Mediterranean, Middle East, and Central and South America; *B. abortus*, in cattle in Africa, India, and some temperate areas; *B. suis* from pigs; and *B. canis*, which rarely causes human infection. Transmission is predominantly through consumption of unpasteurized dairy products, although consumption of raw liver, bone marrow, or meat also causes disease. Occupational exposure of abattoir workers, veterinarians, or farmers, including through aerosolization of the products of abortion and/or placenta, is not uncommon. There are around 500,000 cases a year, although pasteurization of milks and control in herds with vaccination has eradicated the problem of brucellosis in many parts of the world.

Clinical Features

Brucellosis has a long incubation period, typically 1 to 3 weeks but it can be several months. The main clinical feature is recurrent bouts of fever, which have an insidious onset. The fever pattern is described as undulating, with fever, usually associated with sweating, worse in the evening or at night. Patients look well, although depression, malaise, and fatigue are common. Musculoskeletal pain, especially lumbar backache, is common, affecting more than 80%. A septic arthritis or osteomyelitis is a frequent localizing feature. Vascular infection, including infective endocarditis, a meningoencephalitis, and genitourinary involvement, are all well reported. A quarter will have splenomegaly. Often the fevers will continue for several months if undiagnosed, with debility common but mortality rare.

Diagnosis

Blood cultures are often positive, but may require extended incubation, up to 6 weeks for solid systems. Multiple cultures improves the yield, as will sampling a range of fluids, including urine, synovial fluid, and bone marrow (highest yield). Often patients have a mild hepatitis, leukopenia, and relative lymphocytosis. Serologic tests can be very helpful but caution must be used. They may cross react with other gram-negative bacteria (e.g., *Yersinia*), the patient may have had previous exposure giving a false positive, or the "prozone" effect (a false negative at low dilutions of serum) may give a false negative if not diluted to 1/320 or 1/640. A four-fold rise in titer between acute and convalescent samples is helpful, but clearly takes some time. Increasing use of PCR-based testing will help. It is important to exclude TB as a cause, which presents in a similar fashion. When sending samples to the laboratory, adequate clinical information and warning is key: brucellosis will aerosolize readily, and should be handled in a category 3 biosafety laboratory.

Treatment

Two major combination regimes are used: doxycycline (200 mg daily) plus rifampicin (600–900 mg daily) is an effective oral combination, although traditionally an aminoglycoside (streptomycin 1 g/day for 2–3 weeks or gentamicin 5 mg/kg per day for 10–14 days) plus doxycycline was used, and probably has a lower relapse rate. The oral agent should be given for 6 weeks, or 3 months in chronic or focal disease. Triple therapy (doxycycline, rifampicin, and an aminoglycoside) is used for endocarditis or meningitis. Co-trimoxazole may replace doxycycline when tetracyclines are contraindicated. Inadvertent exposure to brucellosis in the laboratory should be followed by a risk assessment, and then serology and/or prophylaxis (e.g., doxycycline 100 mg bd for 21 days) as appropriate. The UK guidelines are freely available and easy to use.[29,30]

WHOOPING COUGH

Bordetella pertussis (and six other less important bordetella species) cause whooping cough and occasionally pneumonia in humans and are transmitted person-person by respiratory droplet spread. Whooping cough was historically an important cause of mortality in Western nations but rates have dropped because of widespread vaccination. However, in areas of low vaccine coverage, often in the aftermath of civil war and famine, whooping cough can cause devastating outbreaks of disease with mortality particularly significant in those under 5 years of age and malnourished.

Clinical Features

There are generally three stages of illness, with a catarrhal stage in the first 1 to 2 weeks (treatment is effective at this stage but the disease is rarely recognized), then paroxysmal coughing for 2 to 4 weeks (treatment not beneficial after 2 weeks of cough), with the last stage 1 to 2 weeks of convalescence (where treatment is used to eradicate carriage of the organism to prevent transmission). During the middle stage, the coughing is often worse at night and may prevent feeding, or lead to vomiting, dehydration, and even malnutrition. Apnea and cyanosis may also occur.

Diagnosis

Bacterial culture is difficult as specialized media are required, and the organism will not be present once the patient has had 3 weeks of cough, so can be negative for much of the illness. Serology can be very useful, especially in the unimmunized, with oral fluid assay sensitive, specific, and easy to use. PCR is also very useful. In an outbreak setting a clinical diagnosis can usually be made but other causes of chronic cough including TB, asthma, and respiratory infections should be considered.

Treatment

Macrolides, such as azithromycin, will reduce the duration of illness (when given within 2 weeks) and the infectivity of the patient. They are less effective in late illness but are often used to reduce transmission. Supportive care, especially in young, malnourished children, including careful observation, fluid and nutritional supplementation, and treatment of any secondary bacterial infections, is vital.[31]

RICKETTSIAL INFECTIONS

Rickettsia are obligate intracellular pathogens that are taken up by macrophages and replicate in endothelial tissues, causing vasculitis. They are generally zoonoses with mammalian reservoirs and an arthropod vector, the bite from which may leave an eschar. There are a great many rickettsia, covering a large portion of the globe, although individual species may have a fairly localized distribution. Clinical symptoms include fever, headache, and myalgia, often with an associated rash that may be vasculitic or maculopapular. Diagnosis can be difficult, with treatment often initiated on clinical suspicion. PCR of blood, or better of the eschar, is sensitive and specific but not widely available. Serology, including the Weil-Felix test, is commonly used, but may only become positive in the second week of illness, and there are commonly cross-reactions between the rickettsia. The rickettsia can be clinically grouped into the spotted fever group, the typhus group, scrub typhus, and ehrlicosis and anaplasmosis. Each will be briefly described below.

SPOTTED FEVER GROUP

This is a group of around 20 rickettsioses, of which Rocky Mountain spotted fever (RMSF) is the best known, and most severe. Together they have a wide geographical range with RMSF, caused by *Rickettsia rickettsii*, present in the United States (mostly significantly to the east of the Rocky Mountains), Mediterranean spotted fever, *R. conorii,* in Europe and North Africa, particularly in urban areas, and African tick-bite fever, *R. africae,* often seen in agricultural workers, hunters, and tourists on safari in Africa. The other rickettsioses have their own geographical range covering Australasia, South America, Africa, and Asia including Siberia. Transmission is from a variety of zoonotic hosts to humans by the bite of a variety of infected ticks, *Dermacentor andersoni* in the case of RMSF.

Clinical Features

Between 4 and 10 days after an infected tick bite, patients develop high fever, retroorbital headache, and myalgia. An eschar, a thick black lesion at the site of tick attachment, develops in many species of rickettsia. The rash that gives the group its name is a macular "spotted" rash which starts in the hands and feet and moves inwards toward the trunk. The severity varies according to species with case fatality rates (untreated) varying from 2.5% in Mediterranean spotted fever to 50% in RMSF. Vasculitis with gangrene, and other vascular complications, mediate severe disease.

Diagnosis

Treatment is often empiric based on exposure and clinical features. PCR assays are available for many rickettsia with PCR of an eschar or blood sensitive and specific. Serology can be helpful but may be negative early in disease, and cannot necessarily distinguish between species.

Treatment

Doxycycline 200 mg od is the treatment of choice, with short courses (even as short as 3 days) often effective and producing a rapid response. Chloramphenicol is an alternative but there is evidence of poorer outcome in RMSF.

EPIDEMIC TYPHUS

Caused by *R. prowazekii*, this is spread from person to person by the body louse, *Pediculus humanus*. Outbreaks have accompanied conflict and natural disasters, with large outbreaks during World War II, and Napoleon's retreat from Russia. Recent outbreaks are rarer but occurred, for example, in Burundi during the civil war in the 1990s.

Clinical Features

Headache, fever, myalgia, and a macular-papular or petechial rash develop some 10 to 14 days after exposure. The disease can be severe, especially among the malnourished (e.g., in Bergen-Belsen concentration camp in 1945) with vasculitis leading to many complications including gangrene. The disease may reappear years after the initial infection, termed Brill-Zinsser disease.

Diagnosis

Serology is frequently used, although the old Weil-Felix test, although still used widely, lacks sensitivity and specificity. PCR is useful and is positive early in the disease, when available.

Treatment

Doxycycline is highly effective, given 100 mg bd for several days with an excellent, rapid clinical response, or where resources are limited, 200 mg as a stat dose. Chloramphenicol may be used second line, but a stat dose of doxycycline is likely to be safe, even in children. Delousing clothes, blankets, etc. is crucial during an epidemic to avoid spread, and was used successfully many times during World War II.

MURINE (ENDEMIC) TYPHUS

R. typhi is spread from rats to humans by the rat flea, *Xenopsylla cheopis*. It has a worldwide distribution, which is probably underappreciated. Anywhere with a significant population of rats may harbor the disease, although it seems to be more common in coastal areas. The disease presents with fever, headache, and myalgia, but is generally mild. There may be a maculopapular rash. Diagnosis is often missed or made retrospectively on serology, after the patient has improved. The illness will generally resolve after 7 to 14 days, but a course of doxycycline will bring more rapid resolution.

SCRUB TYPHUS

Orientia tsutsugamushi is a zoonotic disease transmitted from a wild rodent reservoir host to humans by the bite of the chigger mite when humans encroach on their grassy scrubland habitat. The disease is distributed widely in SE Asia, from northern Australia to Japan, and across to Pakistan, with disease usually focally distributed in "mite islands" in rural areas (Fig. 3.2).

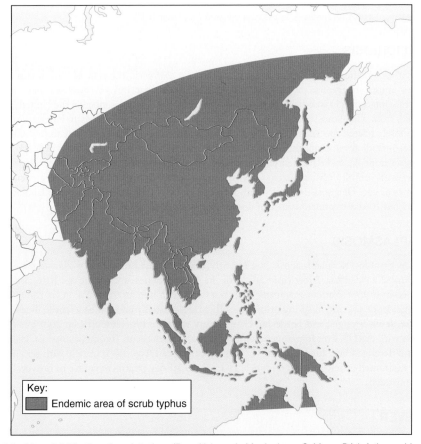

Fig. 3.2 Map of distribution of scrub typhus. (From Nabarro L, Morris-Jones S, Moore DAJ. Arthropod-borne diseases. In: Nabarro L, Morris-Jones S, Moore DAJ, eds. *Peters' Atlas of Tropical Medicine and Parasitology.* 7th ed. London, UK: Elsevier Ltd; 2019:1–108.)

Clinical Features

Bites are usually painless, but an eschar will typically develop at the site of the bite during the 10 or so days' incubation period, forming a thick, blackened, necrosed scab, often with regional lymphadenopathy. Fever, headache, and myalgia are common, with hearing loss, conjunctival suffusion, and a faint macular rash useful specific diagnostic signs. The disease may self-resolve or increase in severity with pulmonary infiltrates worsening as acute respiratory distress syndrome (ARDS) or meningoencephalitis develops.

Diagnosis

A thorough search for an eschar when presented with a patient with compatible symptoms in an endemic area is often the most useful diagnostic test, although one is not always apparent. The Weil-Felix serology test lacks sensitivity, and other more sensitive serologic tests are not always available. Empiric therapy is often required.

Treatment

Prompt antibiotic therapy, usually with 100 mg doxycycline bd (or chloramphenicol as second line) reduces mortality, and usually produces a prompt clinical response. Weekly doxycycline 200 mg is an effective prophylactic, and should be considered in high-risk groups such as construction workers clearing scrubland, trekkers, or soldiers on exercise (Table 3.1).

EHRLICHIOSIS

Human monocytic ehrlichiosis is caused by *Ehrlichia chafeensis*, transmitted to humans from various animal reservoirs, most commonly by the Lone Star tick, *Ambylomma americanum*. Transmission occurs in woodland or meadows. The disease was first described in the United States in 1986, from where most cases have been reported, although there are likely to be cases (at least from closely related species) in Brazil and elsewhere. Incidence peaks from May to July. Clinical features include fever, headache, myalgia, malaise, and rash, usually accompanied by leukopenia, thrombocytopenia, and deranged liver function. Most patients can remember a tick bite. Severe disease with central nervous system (CNS) features and multiorgan failure occurs, especially at extremes of age. Diagnosis is usually with serology or PCR performed at reference laboratories, and a 7- to 10-day treatment course of doxycycline is recommended.

ANAPLASMOSIS

Human granulocytic anaplasmosis is a recently described disease caused by *Anaplasma phagocytophilium*, a rickettsia. Most cases are from the United States, although cases have also been reported in Europe. Various mammals act as reservoirs with human transmission via ixodes ticks, with incidence peaking in spring or summer. The disease usually presents as a febrile illness with malaise, fever, myalgia, and headache. Case fatality rates are low (around 1 in 200) but severe disease with ARDS, liver impairment, or CNS features does occur. Thrombocytopenia, leukopenia, and deranged liver function tests (LFTs) are common. Diagnosis is usually with serology or PCR performed at reference laboratories, and a 7- to 10-day treatment course of doxycycline is recommended.

Q FEVER

Humans develop Q fever, a zoonosis, after inhaling aerosols contaminated with the small gram-negative bacteria, *Coxiella burnetti*. The usual source of bacteria is from sheep or goats, typically from dried birth products on windy days. Transmission from ticks or from ingesting infected meat

TABLE 3.1 ■ Selected Rickettsioses

Pathogen	Disease	Vector (Tick Unless Otherwise Indicated)	Distribution	Notes
Rickettsia rickettsii	Rocky Mountain spotted fever	*Dermacentor andersoni* (and others)	United States (esp. South Atlantic region); occasionally South and Central America	Historically most severe although severity appears to be declining
Rickettsia siberica siberica	Siberian tick typhus	*Dermacentor* spp.	Former USSR and China	Rural disease in spring/summer
Rickettsia conorii conorii	Mediterranean spotted fever	*Rhipicephalus sanguineus*	Southern Europe; North Africa	Reported severity increasing
Rickettsia africae	African tick-bite fever	*Amblyomma* spp.	Sub-Saharan Africa; West Indies	Eschars almost universal; often reported in travelers on Safari
Rickettsia australis	Queensland tick typhus	*Ixodes holocylus* and *tasmani*	East coast of Australia and Thursday Islands	Rural disease; not typically severe
Rickettsia japonica	Japanese spotted fever	Various ticks	Japan	Often associated with agriculture, e.g., bamboo cutting
Rickettsia conorii caspia	Astrakhan fever	*Rhipicephalus* spp.	Caspian and Balkan regions. Recently detected in Africa	Rash very common, eschar less so
Rickettsia prowazekii	Epidemic typhus	*Pediculus humanus humanus* (human body louse)	Historically, globally, but especially during war in Europe; mountainous areas of Asia, Africa and America currently.	Outbreaks associated with war and famine. Often severe, especially in malnourished
Rickettsia typhi	Endemic typhus	*Xenopsylla cheopis* (rat flea)	Global where rats and fleas are present	Generally mild
Orientia tsutsugamushi	Scrub typhus	*Leptotrombidium* spp. (trombiculid mites)	Southeast Asia	Rural areas in "mite islands"

From Ericsson CD, Jensenius M, Fournier P-E, et al. Rickettsioses and the international traveler. *Clin Infect Dis.* 2004;39(10):1493–1499.

or milk products is possible but less common. The disease has a global range; it was discovered in Australia, there has been a large recent outbreak in the Netherlands, and members of the UK Armed Forces acquired Q fever in Afghanistan. Transmission is most important where there are infected ruminants, and dry windy conditions facilitate aerosolized spread.

Clinical Features

Acute Q fever develops after an incubation period of 2 weeks. Q fever causes one of two clinical entities. It may cause an undifferentiated febrile illness, with fatigue, fever, and headache common. The differential diagnosis is broad here, especially in travelers. Q fever also presents as a pneumonia, which is usually mild but can be severe. Both are accompanied by a hepatitis which may give a clue as to the diagnosis. Chronic Q fever develops in 1% to 5% of those infected. Symptoms may include fever and fatigue but are often nonspecific. Infections are usually vascular, with a culture-negative endocarditis the commonest manifestation, but vasculitis, including of prosthetic tissue, hepatitis, and osteomyelitis, are all reported.

Diagnosis

The nonspecific features, apart from hepatitis, and different manifestations mean a low threshold to considering Q fever a patient may have been exposed is key to diagnosis. Q fever is fastidious and cultures are generally not used, not least because its high infectivity means that as well as making it a potential biowarfare agent, it requires biosafety level 3 laboratory conditions to grow safely. A new PCR assay is very useful, and is positive early in disease with good sensitivity, although access to this assay is limited. Serology is more widely used, with the phase II antibody response, somewhat perversely, higher in acute disease than phase I, and phase I titers very high in chronic Q fever. Interpretation can be tricky, and expert help may be required. In particular, antibody assays may not be positive at the onset of acute disease but will diagnose chronic Q fever.

Treatment

Tetracyclines are the treatment of choice with 14 days of doxycycline 100 mg bd a commonly recommended regimen. Quinolones are an alternative where tetracyclines are contraindicated. Chronic Q fever requires prolonged treatment with dual therapy, hydroxychloroquine, and doxycycline for 1 to 2 years. Antibody titers can be used to measure response. Monitoring for side effects, especially retinal toxicity, is important. A fatigue syndrome after Q fever has been well described. If there is no evidence of chronic Q fever (for example PCR is negative and phase I antibody titers are reducing) then antimicrobial therapy is not required.[32]

TUBERCULOSIS

TB is a disease of worldwide importance and is the second-leading cause of death from infection after HIV. Mycobacteria from the *Mycobacterium tuberculosis* (MTB) complex: *M. tuberculosis*, *M. africanum*, and *M. bovis*, are transmitted from person to person via aerosolized transmission. In some agricultural areas, zoonotic TB from *M. bovis* is important. Globally TB is widespread, with one-third of the world's population having been infected at some point, and around 9 million cases and a million deaths per year. Risk factors for disease include increased transmissibility by aerosolized droplets, such as overcrowding, and poor-quality housing and working conditions, especially poorly ventilated areas with little natural light, including prisons and mines, or the tendency to develop disease after exposure, usually by affecting cell-mediated immunity, such as HIV. In a complex emergency setting, particularly a protracted one, overcrowding in refugee or IDP camps and malnutrition can lead to a large increase in TB cases in a population. The requirement for prolonged, complex drug treatment makes treating cases in these settings difficult. Globally, TB rates are highest in sub-Saharan Africa, but with moderate-high rates and large populations, Asia has numerically more cases. Rates of TB have recently increased in Eastern Europe, and rates in certain populations, including people living with HIV, prisoners, miners, and the homeless, can be high, even in countries with low overall rates.

Risk of Infection and Clinical Disease

Whether someone exposed to TB will develop an infection depends on the duration of the exposure (with hours of face-face exposure being required usually); the infectivity of the index case, with cavitatory disease very infectious; and the environmental conditions. Some 5% to 10% of people with an infection will fail to control it and will develop early progression with clinical TB within 2 years. For the remaining 90% to 95% of people exposed, their immune system will control the infection, but with a subsequent risk of reactivation leading to clinical disease. The lifetime risk of reactivation is 10%, although host factors include malnutrition, chronic illness (including renal disease, and immunosuppressive drugs including corticosteroids and TNF-alpha inhibitors), and most importantly HIV, affect this.

Clinical Syndrome

The cardinal clinical features of TB are fever, night sweats, and weight loss, although they are not always present, especially in immunosuppressed patients, or those with extrapulmonary TB. The presentation is usually fairly indolent, with symptoms present for weeks before diagnosis. Additional features depend on the site of infection. Most TB is pulmonary, with productive, often bloodstained, sputum the commonest manifestation. Radiology classically demonstrates cavitary disease in the upper zones with associated hilar lymphadenopathy, although a wide range of appearances, including noncavitary, nonapical, and pleural disease, occur. Extrapulmonary TB can occur anywhere in the body with lymphatic, genitourinary, bone and joint (especially spine), CNS, abdominal, and disseminated TB all relatively common (in that order). Presentations can vary depending on the location, and diagnosis of extrapulmonary TB can be challenging. In areas of high TB incidence or where risk factors are present, clinicians should have a low threshold for suspecting TB in any chronic illness, especially in patients with weight loss, fever, and night sweats. CNS TB can have devastating consequences, so lymphocytic meningitis with a raised protein or ring-enhancing mass lesions without other cause should always prompt suspicion of TB.

Diagnosis

Diagnosis will depend on what is available to you. Tuberculin skin testing, looking for a cell-mediated delayed-type hypersensitivity reaction to an intracutaneous injection of purified proteins of MTB, or interferon gamma release assays will demonstrate if someone has been exposed to TB, although sensitivity is worse in the immunosupressed. These cannot distinguish between active and latent infection although, limiting their usefulness. To determine if active TB is present, demonstating presence of the bacillus is key. Microscopic staining using the Ziehl-Neelsen method (for example) is cheap, rapid, and simple. However, sensitivity is poor as many bacilli are needed to visualize the acid- and alcohol-fast mycobacteria, with up to 50% of proven pulmonary cases being smear negative. Repeated testing, typically three samples, fluorescent microscopy (with an auramine stain), or adjunctive methods in those not coughing (such as bronchoscopy or induced sputum, or gastric washings in children) can improve diagnostic yield. Culture of MTB is more sensitive than microscopy (up to 90%), allows definitive diagnosis differentiating from the nontuberculous mycobacteria, and allows for sensitivity testing, which is of importance given the rise of multidrug resistant (MDR) and extensively drug resistant (XDR) TB. However, growth is slow, with 3 to 6 (or more) weeks required; specialist media and expertise is needed, and it should be performed where containment laboratories are available to prevent laboratory transmission. This limits its use, especially in the less-developed world, to reference laboratories. Nucleic acid amplification tests can circumvent many of these issues. The GeneXpert system, for example, which uses a simple cartridge system requiring little training or lab support, approaches the sensitivity of culture, gives information on rifampicin sensitivity, and is rapid, with a result in 2 hours. These advantages mean it has been rolled out to many centers across the world with WHO support. Despite these many diagnostic tools, there will be occasions when TB needs to be treated empirically based on clinical features, epidemiology, and radiological features, either because of the difficulty of making a diagnosis, the patients condition requiring urgent treatment before definitive laboratory results, or in settings where these tests are unavailable. However, persuing a definitive diagnosis, and ideally drug sensitivity, is encouraged when possible.

Treatment

Treatment for TB requires the use of combination antimicrobials for many months. The current WHO-approved standard regime uses a 2-month intensive phase with isoniazid, pyrazinimide, ethambutol, and rifampicin, followed by 4 months of rifampicin and isoniazid. Treatment is 95% effective, although some patients will suffer side effects, including hepatotoxicity. Daily dosing is recommended, although intermittant treatment during the continuation phase (three times per week) can be effective where this is the only feasible option. Smear-positive patients, especially those with cavitatory disease, present an infection control risk, although their infectivity falls rapidly after a few days of treatment. Given the length of current treatment, retaining patients in care, and thus preventing development of MDR TB, is important. This may include health education and counseling, which should always be offered, and directly observed (or video-observed) therapy (DOT or VOT), which can be useful. Samples should be tested for drug resistance when possible, and tailored therapies used. Treatment for MDR TB is currently 18 to 24 months long and should be provided under specialist care. HIV testing is recommended for people with TB; checking hepatitis B and C status and for vitamin D deficiency is prudent given the risk of hepatotoxicity of drugs and the role of vitamin D deficiency in pathogenesis. Immune reconstitution inflammatory syndrome (IRIS) in patients with HIV and active TB remains a concern, so TB therapy should be initiated before starting antiretrovirals (ARVs). Current guidelines recommend not delaying starting ARVs past 8 weeks, or 2 weeks for those whose CD4 count is below 50 cells/mm^3.

Control

Early identification and effective treatment of cases, screening of contacts of cases, and treatment of individuals with latent TB, for example, with isoniazid for 6 months, all play a role in controlling TB.[33,34]

LEPROSY

Leprosy is caused by the acid-fast bacillus *Mycobacterium leprae*. It is transmitted via the respiratory route before being distributed around the body by a brief bacteremia, with reproduction largely in cooler areas of the body (e.g., skin) intracellularly in macrophages. The incubation period is long, with years or even decades elapsing between exposure and clinical features. Historically, the disease was globally distributed, and well described in medieval Europe. Today, most cases are in Brazil, India, the DRC, Indonesia, and Bangladesh, but with foci of disease in other countries. There were over 200,000 new cases in 2016.

Spectrum of Disease and Classification System

The clinical features of leprosy depend on the host immune response. In those with a brisk cell-mediated immune response, replication of bacilli is controlled by granuloma formation, and there will be only a few lesions, with features of tuberculoid leprosy. Where there is a poor cell-mediated immune response, bacilli will be abundant in affected tissues, lesions multiple, and lepromatous leprosy seen. This immune response underlies the two classification systems. The

Ridley-Jopling system classifies disease according to microbiological and clinical features on a scale from tuberculoid to lepromatous leprosy, with borderline states in between, and correlates well to the immune response, as well as helping to predict the likelihood of reactions to therapy. The simpler WHO classification is based purely on the number of lepromatous skin lesions with 1 in solitary lesion paucibacillary leprosy, 2 to 5 in paucibacillary leprosy, and >5 in multibacillary leprosy. Roughly, this correlates with the immune response, with paucibacillary lying at the tuberculoid end of the spectrum although it lacks some of the clinical subtlety of the Ridley-Jopling system. However, it is easy to train people to use, and correlates with current WHO treatment guidelines.

Clinical Features

The cardinal features of leprosy are anesthetic skin lesions, peripheral nerve damage and thickening, and the presence of acid-fast bacilli in the skin. Skin lesions are few in tuberculoid leprosy, numerous in lepromatous. They are often hypopigmented macules with a slightly raised edge, but may be papules, or even nodular in lepromatous leprosy. They feel dry owing to loss of the autonomic nerve supply and thus sweating, and are insensate. Damage to peripheral nerves causes muscle weakness and loss of sensation in the distribution of the nerve, or sometimes a glove and stocking distribution with lepromatous leprosy. Nerves are typically thickened and are often palpable. Median, ulnar, common peroneal, posterior tibial, sural, and facial nerves are commonly affected. In lepromatous leprosy, loss of the outer third of the eyebrow may occur "madarosis", and eye complications including iritis and cataract can lead to blindness. The effects of nerve damage, including foot ulcers, charcot joint, burns to the hand, deformity, and subsequent infection, should be carefully elicited.

Diagnosis

Leprosy is usually made as a clinical diagnosis with identification of the cardinal features. Lack of experience with the disease often delays the diagnosis in settings where leprosy is nonendemic. Supportive evidence can be sought with skin biopsy showing characteristic granulomatous pathology with neural inflammation, plus acid-fast bacilli. Split-skin smears are often used in addition where, after an epidermal incision, dermal material is scraped onto a slide. Several sites are sampled and the presence of acid-fast bacilli can confirm the diagnosis, indicate a high bacillary burden (thus toward the lepromatous end of the Ridley-Jopling classification), and help demonstrate response to therapy. This is often negative in tuberculoid leprosy/paucibacillary disease. Serology is not helpful.

Treatment

WHO treatment guidelines are based on the number of lepromatous skin lesions, and use multidrug therapy. Single drug regimens should not be used. For single skin lesion paucibacillary leprosy, rifampicin 600 mg, ofloxacin 400 mg, and minocycline 100 mg given together as a single stat dose is recommended. Paucibacillary leprosy requires dapsone 100 mg daily, and monthly (supervised) rifampicin 600 mg for 6 months. Multibacillary leprosy is treated with rifampicin (600 mg monthly), dapsone (100 mg daily), and clofazimine (50 mg daily and 300 mg monthly). During treatment, it is important to monitor the patient for reactions, which are common, especially in borderline disease. These include immune-mediated new or worsening skin or nerve lesions (type 1 reactions) and erythema nodosum leprosum—immune complex deposition-driven erythematous skin lesions often accompanied by fever and malaise. Multidrug therapy should be continued but steroids are often required to manage reactions, with thalidomide increasingly used, with caution. Prevention of disability, for example, foot care in those with neuropathic foot ulcers, reconstructive surgery, and awareness of stigma and social isolation in treating patients with leprosy, should not be neglected.[35]

BURULI ULCER

Mycobacterium ulcerans is a fastidious nontuberculous mycobacterium that causes a disabling skin infection, Buruli ulcer. It was originally named after the Buruli district in Uganda, where many of the first cases were described. It is the third most common mycobacterial infection after TB and leprosy. It is endemic in the tropical rainforests of Africa, SE Asia, South and Central America, and Australia.

Clinical Features

Buruli ulcer usually begins as a painless nodule less than 5 cm in diameter, with the limbs most commonly affected. The initial lesion usually breaks down after days to weeks, forming an ulcer with characteristic undermined edges. Superficial *M. ulcerans* infection can progress to involve deeper tissues including tendons, joints, and bones. Contiguous or hematogenous spread leads to osteomyelitis in up to 15% of cases. Interestingly, up to 25% patients with osteomyelitis have no history of Buruli ulcer skin lesions. Disseminated disease in association with HIV has been described. The natural history of Buruli ulcer includes slow spontaneous healing in up to one-third of cases.

Diagnosis

The diagnosis of Buruli ulcer is frequently based upon clinical manifestations and is often not confirmed because of limited access to laboratory services. Laboratory diagnostic tools include staining for acid-fast bacilli, histopathology, mycobacterial culture, and PCR.

Treatment

Antimicrobial therapy is the cornerstone of treatment, with a high cure and low recurrence rate. Antimicrobial treatment alone is highly efficacious in small, relatively new Buruli ulcer lesions. Primary regimens consist of rifampicin with a macrolide (e.g., clarithromycin) or a quinolone (e.g., moxifloxacin). Streptomycin was used but the requirement for injection therapy makes it less attractive. Normal treatment duration is 8 weeks. Often, antibiotic therapy alone is effective and surgery is reserved for those with large defects or intolerant of antibiotics. New evidence has suggested that application of local heat for 5 to 14 hours per day may be effective.[36]

Protozoa

MALARIA

Malaria is the most important parasitic infection globally, with an estimated 216 million cases across 91 countries in 2016, causing 445,000 deaths (Fig. 3.3). Some 90% of cases and 91% of deaths occur in the WHO Africa region. There are five species of the protozoa parasite *Plasmodium* that cause human disease. All are transmitted by the female *Anopheles* mosquito. Of the five species, *P. falciparum* is the most important, responsible for the most deaths and able to cause cerebral malaria. Of the "benign" malarias (a poor term as infection with a benign malaria may still be fatal: "nonfalciparum" is a better term), *P. vivax* and *ovale* can cause recurrent malaria, via a dormant liver stage, the hypnozoite; *malariae* has a "quartan fever" pattern rather than tertian; and *knowlesi* is a zoonosis, a monkey malaria that may infect humans, limited to the island of Borneo, and the only zoonosis of the five human species.

Epidemiology

Malaria is widely distributed across the tropics. In 1900, malaria was distributed even more widely, and into subtropical areas including foci in the UK and United States. Control efforts have halved the area of the world where the population is at risk of malaria from 53% to 27%. However, over

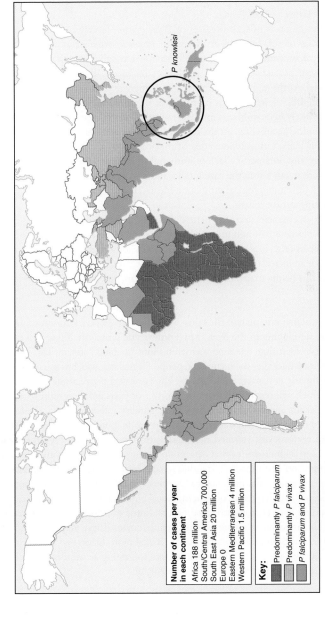

**Number of cases per year
in each continent**

Africa 188 million
South/Central America 700,000
South East Asia 20 million
Europe 0
Eastern Mediterranean 4 million
Western Pacific 1.5 million

Key:

Predominantly *P falciparum*

Predominantly *P vivax*

P falciparum and *P vivax*

P knowlesi

Fig. 3.3 Map of distribution of malaria. (From Nabarro L, Morris-Jones S, Moore DAJ. Arthropod-borne diseases. In: Nabarro L, Morris-Jones S, Moore DAJ, eds. *Peters' Atlas of Tropical Medicine and Parasitology.* 7th ed. London, UK: Elsevier Ltd; 2019:1–108.)

the same period, population growth has meant that the number of people exposed to malaria risk has increased from 1 billion to 3 billion people. *Vivax* has the widest geographic range including India, Central America, and China, accounting for around half of malaria outside Africa, and 10% inside. *Ovale* is largely limited to West Africa (where it occupies the same niche as *vivax* elsewhere, because of widespread indigenous resistance to *vivax* there) and *knowlesi* to Borneo. *Malariae* has a patchy distribution. *Falciparum* is present in many countries in the tropics, especially sub-Saharan Africa and SE Asia.

There are several patterns of transmission of *P. falciparum* largely based on the intensity of transmission. In areas of sub-Saharan Africa with *Anopheles gambiae* as the predominant and highly effective vector, transmission is intense. Children will usually develop malaria a few months after birth, often with protective maternal antibodies on board. They will have repeated, often severe, attacks of malaria throughout childhood, and many will die of the disease. However, those that survive into adulthood will have a high degree of immunological protection and further attacks as adults are likely to be mild and unlikely to lead to death, except in pregnant women. This is termed holoendemic transmission. At the other extreme, in areas of hypoendemic transmission, such as much of SE Asia, transmission rates of malaria are low, clinical disease will be spread across all age groups, and because of a lack of immunological protection, although overall rates of malaria and death are much lower, the case fatality rate for an individual infection will be higher. In addition, the lack of immunological protection means that after rains or floods, epidemics may occur with devastating consequences.

During complex emergencies and after natural disasters, malaria rates may increase substantially, either because of displacement of nonimmune individuals into a malaria endemic zone, lack of protection from the vector (e.g., loss of housing or bed nets), comorbid illness such as malnutrition, lack of health care, or an increase in vector populations (e.g., after flooding). Humanitarian workers should be aware of this before malaria rates increase and plan, prevent, and mitigate accordingly.

Lifecycle

Sporozoites are inoculated into man in the saliva of the female *Anopheles* mosquito. These circulate in the blood before developing in the liver as preerythrocytic schizonts. These will take a variable time to mature before rupturing, releasing merozoites into the blood stream. This liver maturation before merozoite release underlies the incubation period for malaria, which is usually 7 to 30 days for *falciparum*, longer for the non-*falciparum* species. For *ovale* and *vivax*, some sporozoites develop into hypnozoites which will remain dormant for months or years before resuming replication and causing a relapse, despite successful treatment of the primary infection. Once the liver schizonts rupture, the released merozoites will undergo asexual reproduction in erythrocytes. After 48 to 72 hours, the infected erythrocytes (termed merozoites, trophozoites, then erythrocytic schizonts) rupture releasing 12 to 24 merozoites that can set up further rounds of erythrocytic reproduction. This progressive infection and rupture of red blood cells with release of cell contents and subsequent inflammation mediates the pathological effects of malaria. *P. falciparum* has an additional ability to sequester into capillary beds, obstructing local blood flow causing complications such as cerebral malaria, pulmonary edema, and renal failure. Some merozoites entering red blood cells develop not into schizonts but into male or female gametocytes. These may be taken up by a passing female *Anopheles* mosquitoes before undergoing sexual reproduction within the mosquito gut to complete the lifecycle over a total of around 20 days, migrating as sporozoites to the mosquito saliva gland, where the mosquito remains infectious for life.

Clinical Features

Malaria presents with fever and a range of other symptoms, and may do so months (or even occasionally years) after a bite from an infected mosquito, although 7 to 14 days is more typical in *P. falciparum*. Thus malaria should always be considered, and ruled out, in any febrile traveler returning from an endemic zone (even up to 2 years after) or person living in an area of transmission. Fever is the cardinal symptom, which will start at the onset of the erythrocytic stage. The fever is often periodic but the historical described tertian or quartan periodicity is rarely seen unless treatment is delayed. The fever is accompanied by a range of symptoms including most commonly headache, myalgia, and malaise, and less commonly dry cough, abdominal pain, and backache. Paroxysmal attacks of fever with rigors, severe headache, tachypnea, and palpitations lasting 8 to 12 hours and terminated by drenching sweats leaving the patient exhausted are common. GI symptoms including diarrhea can occur, especially in children, and may cause a clinician to overlook malaria as a cause. Splenomegaly and anemia are frequent, both more commonly with repeated infections, and anemia can be severe in children. Mild jaundice occurs typically owing to hemolysis during the erythrocytic stages.

Severe disease is seen most with *P. falciparum* but can occur with *vivax* and *knowlesi*. The nonimmune, children, and pregnant women are all at higher risk of severe malaria. Cerebral malaria, a global encephalopathy caused by *P. falciparum* (and present even after correcting for anemia and hypoglycemia) is a significant cause of death. Coma, seizure, raised intracranial pressure, and white matter hemorrhage may all occur. Other severe manifestations include severe anemia, especially in children and pregnant women, hypoglycemia, which is correctable but only if identified, acidosis because of tissue hypoxia, and pulmonary edema/ARDS. "Algid malaria," that is, malaria with hypotension and shock, may be a result of the above complications or from complicating gram-negative bacteremia. Renal failure is present in one-third of adults and intravascular hemolysis and hemoglobinuria (termed "blackwater fever") also occur, more commonly in patients who are glucose-6-phosphate dehydrogenase (G6PD) deficient.

Diagnosis

Malaria is most frequently diagnosed by repeated examination of appropriately stained blood films by a trained individual. Thick film, a film with 10 to 20 red blood cells (RBCs) hemolyzed on top of each other, is extremely sensitive at the hands of a skilled, experienced practitioner with a parasite count as low as 0.0001% detectable. Thin films, one rbc thick, are useful for speciation and estimating a parasite count. Three thick and thin films should be examined over 72 hours before malaria is excluded. Because of the skill and time required for microscopy, many labs now use antigen-based or rapid diagnostic tests (RDTs). These are highly sensitive and specific, generally easy to use, and can be performed at the bedside. However, they can be expensive, need to be stored correctly, do not give information on a parasite count, and may be less sensitive in non-*falciparum* species, so they must be used with caution. PCR-based tests are highly sensitive and are increasingly used at national reference laboratories but are not yet usable in field or small lab settings. Biochemically, thrombocytopenia is almost universal and should prompt consideration of malaria (if not already considered) in a febrile patient. Patients also typically have a mildly raised bilirubin from hemolysis.

Assessment of Severity

While treating malaria clinicians should attempt to identify the species as at least *falciparum* or non-*falciparum* and make an assessment of the severity of disease. Treating as *falciparum* if species information is not available or treating as severe malaria if an accurate assessment of severity cannot be performed is safer than undertreating. Impaired consciousness, prostration, multiple convulsions, acidosis, hypoglycemia, severe malarial anemia, significant jaundice, renal impairment, pulmonary edema, and significant bleeding are all used to define severe malaria according to the WHO (see table) as well as a high parasite count (>10%). However, not all the information required (including a lactate, parasite count, and renal function) may be available when treating without laboratory support. A careful clinical assessment including looking for cerebral dysfunction, assessing for shock, tachypnea (which may indicate ARDS or an acidosis), bedside glucose

---

BOX 3.1 ■ Features of Severe Malaria

Clinical
- Impaired consciousness
- Multiple convulsions (>1 in 24 h)
- Acute pulmonary edema
- Evidence of acidosis (e.g., tachypnea)
- Shock (systolic blood pressure <80 mmHg)
- Clinically evident jaundice with other organ dysfunction
- Clinical evidence of coagulopathy (e.g., abnormal bleeding)
- Hemoglobinuria

Laboratory
- Hypoglycemia (<2.2 mmol/L)
- Metabolic acidosis (bicarb <15 mmol/L; lactate >5 mmol/L)
- Severe (malaria-related) anemia (Hb <5 g/dL [children]; <7 g/dL [adults])
- Acute kidney injury (oliguria <0.4 mL/kg per hour; creatinine >256 mcg/L)
- Hyperparasitemia (>10% parasitemia; especially in malaria naïve)

Adapted from World Health Organization and BIA guidelines.

---

measurement, urine output, anemia, bleeding, and risk factors for severe malaria (such as pregnancy, or travel from nonendemic area) should be performed (Box 3.1).

Treatment

Severe *P. falciparum*. Patients with severe malaria should be given IV (or IM) artesunate for at least 24 hours (Table 3.2). The AQUAMAT and SEAQUAMAT trials established the superiority of artemisinin treatments in severe malaria, showing reduced mortality in children in Africa, and adults

TABLE 3.2 ■ Treatment of Malaria

Condition	First line	Alternative	Pregnant women
Severe falciparum malaria	Intravenous (IV) artesunate for at least 24 hours; Artemisinin combination therapy (ACT) follow-on therapy once stable	IV quinine plus oral clindamycin or doxycycline for at least 24 hours; ACT follow-on therapy once stable	IV artesunate for at least 24 hours; ACT follow-on therapy once stable
Nonsevere falciparum malaria	ACT	Quinine plus doxycycline/clindamycin OR malarone	1st trimester quinine plus clindamycin; alternative and 2nd/3rd trimester ACT
Nonfalciparum malaria (no chloroquine resistance)[a]	Chloroquine or ACT	Chloroquine or ACT	Chloroquine
Nonfalciparum malaria (chloroquine resistance)[a]	ACT		Oral quinine

[a]Consider 14-day primaquine course in those not glucose-6-phosphate dehydrogenase (G6PD) deficient to eradicate in vivax/ovale except infants <6 months old, pregnant women, and women breastfeeding infants <6 months old.
If unsure of species or mixed infection treat as falciparum; if unsure of severity treat as severe.
Modified from World Health Organization recommendations.

in SE Asia. It is the WHO recommended treatment of choice in adults, children (dose adjusted) and pregnant women at all trimesters. Where artesunate is not available, IV quinine should be given. Patients will require follow-on oral therapy once improving and able to tolerate. Artemisinin combination therapy (ACT) is recommended, but if unavailable, oral quinine + clindamycin or doxycycline can be used. Patients should ideally be nursed on an intensive care unit or similar, with regular observations, including coma score, urine output, and blood glucose, with an eye for the complications outlined above. Management of complications, and in particular, fluid management can be difficult and reference should be made to appropriate guidance or expert advice, including the WHO Management of Severe Malaria handbook. Patients treated with artesunate may have a delayed anemia, and a Hb check 1 to 2 weeks after recovery or if symptomatic is advised.

Nonsevere *P. falciparum*. Current WHO recommendations are to treat with an ACT, a combination of a rapidly acting artemisinin-related drug with a longer-acting partner. This is effective and safe. Using drug combinations prevents development of drug resistance. Examples include artemether-lumefantrine (Riamet) dosed bd for 3 days in fixed dose combinations or artesunate-amodiaquine (fixed dose, once daily for 3 days). If ACTs are not available, quinine plus doxycycline or clindamycin, or malarone (atovaquone-proguanil) would be suitable alternatives. For pregnant females in the first trimester, a lack of data means the safety of artesunate is not established. Here quinine plus clindamycin for 7 days is recommended but if not available promptly then an ACT should be used.

Nonfalciparum Malaria. Chloroquine has been the treatment of choice for the nonfalciparum malarias for some time and is still widely used, although ACTs are a safe alternative. Resistance to chloroquine is increasing and is present in Indonesia and Oceania. Where there is established chloroquine resistance, ACTs should be used first line. As discussed, vivax and ovale may recur because of the presence of hypnozoite stages in the liver. To prevent relapse, in G6PD-negative patients, a 14-day course of primaquine should be given, except to infants younger than 6 months, pregnant women, and breastfeeding mothers.

Control

Malaria control efforts including early identification and treatment of cases, provision of long-lasting insecticide-treated bed nets, and indoor residual spraying to prevent bites have resulted in 37% fewer malaria cases and 60% fewer malaria deaths between 2000 and 2015, with several new countries, including Sri Lanka, now certified malaria free. However, continued progress in the face of potential donor fatigue, rising resistance to artemisinins, and areas with stubbornly high transmission will require intensification of current efforts and new tools such as the malaria vaccine RTS,S pilot program in three sub-Saharan African countries starting in 2018.[37–40]

LEISHMANIASIS

Leishmaniasis is caused by a number of species of protozoan parasites of the genus *Leishmania* and is spread from human to human or from animals to humans by the bite of the sandfly. Three major clinical forms of leishmaniasis exist—cutaneous, mucosal (Espundia), and visceral (kala-azar). The various species of *Leishmania* are microscopically identical so speciation, which can be useful for determining treatment, relies on knowledge of local epidemiology and laboratory testing.

CUTANEOUS LEISHMANIASIS

Cutaneous leishmaniasis is an important cause of chronic ulcerating skin conditions. Old World leishmaniasis is caused by a variety of species of *Leishmania* including *L. tropica* and *L. major* and is present across North Africa, the Middle East, South Asia, and the Horn of Africa where it is

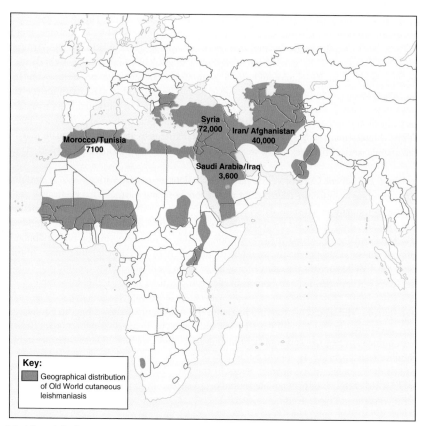

Fig. 3.4 Map of distribution of Old World cutaneous leishmaniasis. (From Nabarro L, Morris-Jones S, Moore DAJ. Arthropod-borne diseases. In: Nabarro L, Morris-Jones S, Moore DAJ, eds. *Peters' Atlas of Tropical Medicine and Parasitology.* 7th ed. London, UK: Elsevier Ltd; 2019:1–108.)

spread by sandflies of the genus *Phlebotomus* (Fig. 3.4). New World leishmaniasis is caused by *L. mexicana* complex, *L. Viannia* subgenus, and *L. chagasi*, in Central and South America, spread by sandflies of the genus *Lutzomyia* (Fig. 3.5). New World leishmaniasis can also cause mucocutaneous leishmaniasis. Transmission may be rural or, increasingly, urban or periurban. Outbreaks have been seen in areas of political instability, including a recent upswing in cases in the Middle East following the large displacement of people because of the Syrian conflict.

Clinical Features

After a bite from an infected sandfly an erythematous nodule will develop weeks to months later that enlarges and ulcerates over several weeks, resulting in a central depressed ulcer with a raised indurated edge. Satellite lesions are common, and a nodular lymphangitis may occur. There are many variations of this classical presentation, with *Leishmania* species and host immunity playing a part. *L. major* lesions tend to form and heal more rapidly (3–5 months) but with inflammation and exudation—a wet sore. *L. tropica* lesions are less inflamed and exudative, forming and healing more slowly (10–12 months)—a dry sore. *L. braziliensis* (and the whole *Viannia* subgenus) often cause deep, spreading ulcers that can take up to 2 years to heal, with an appreciable (15%) recurrence rate. Appearances can be atypical in HIV infection, with delayed healing and poor response

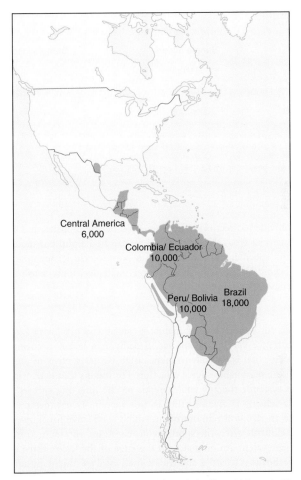

Fig. 3.5 Map of distribution of New World cutaneous leishmaniasis. (From Nabarro L, Morris-Jones S, Moore DAJ. Arthropod-borne diseases. In: Nabarro L, Morris-Jones S, Moore DAJ, eds. *Peters' Atlas of Tropical Medicine and Parasitology.* 7th ed. London, UK: Elsevier Ltd; 2019:1–108.)

to treatment. In the immunosuppressed, visceral leishmaniasis can even occur with infection from a species that normally causes cutaneous leishmaniasis. Given species tend to be confined geographically; knowing the pattern of local presentations and species present is very helpful.

Mucocutaneous leishmaniasis, espundia, is only found in the New World, typically from the *Viannia* subgenus. A variable time after infection with the original skin lesion (up to years) amastigotes spread to the nasooropharyngeal mucosa. The resultant nodule, typically in the nasal mucosa, causes nasal obstruction then enlarges slowly and destructively over years, causing septal perforation and deformity of the entire mouth and nose if untreated.

Diagnosis

Diagnosis is usually by demonstration of the parasite. A punch biopsy can be used to make an impression smear which is stained and examined for parasites. Histologic examination is also useful as although amastigotes may not be seen, presence of granulomas and foamy

TABLE 3.3 ■

Species	Simple lesion	Complex lesion[a]
Old world species	Local therapy	Systemic therapy
Leishmania mexicana complex	Local therapy	Systemic therapy
L. Viannia subgenus	Systemic therapy	Systemic therapy

[a]Complex lesions are usually defined as ones that are multiple, with cosmetic or functional issues, are large (>40 mm), and that fail to respond to simple therapy or lymphatic spread.
From Blum J, Buffet P, Visser L, et al. LeishMan recommendations for treatment of cutaneous and mucosal leishmaniasis in travelers, 2014. J Travel Med. 2013;21(2):116–129.

macrophages can provide indirect evidence. Aspirates, needle biopsies, and slit skin smears are also used to gain material from the lesion. Culture can be helpful but requires special media. PCR is sensitive and specific, and can be used in New World leishmaniasis to speciate into *Viannia* or non-*Viannia*, which is helpful for treatment decisions. Serology is not useful in cutaneous leishmaniasis.

Treatment

Treatment decisions for cutaneous leishmaniasis can be complex, with rates of spontaneous resolution and recurrence varying by species. Broadly, if a lesion is cosmetically unimportant, and from a species that is unlikely to metastasize, be destructive, or recur, then leaving to spontaneously heal is a reasonable course of action. For lesions that need treatment, the choice is between local or systemic therapy and depends on the infecting species and complexity of infection. A simple schema is given further in this section. Local therapy includes heat and cryotherapy, as well as paromomycin ointment, which is effective for *L. major*. Estimating the efficacy of these is difficult given the spontaneous cure rate. Intradermal injection of sodium stibogluconate, a pentavalent antimonial, into the edge of the lesion three times per week for 3 weeks is probably the most effective and widely used local treatment. Systemic therapy agents include sodium stibogluconate 10 to 20 mg/kg IV or IM for 21 days (28 days for visceral), which is effective for all species (except *L. aethiopica*) including for mucocutaneous leishmaniasis, although side effects are common. Amphotericin is effective but expensive. Oral systemic agents include fluconazole or ketoconazole, but these only have specific efficacy (e.g., *L. major*). Miltefosine is a promising oral agent with good efficacy across species, including for mucosal leishmaniasis, although it can be difficult to get hold of and expensive, and data for some species is limited (Table 3.3).

VISCERAL LEISHMANIASIS

Visceral leishmaniasis is caused by three species, *Leishmania donovani* (causing disease in India and East Africa), *L. infantum* (Mediterranean basin, Middle East, and parts of China), and *L. chagasi* (South and Central America) (Fig. 3.6). Transmission is often confined to local hot spots, and 90% of the 500,000 cases yearly are in Bangladesh, India, Nepal, Sudan, and northeastern Brazil. The reservoir is humans and various species of canines and rodents with sandflies as the vector. Amastigotes are taken up during a blood meal and multiply in the sandflies developing into promastigotes, which migrate to the mouthparts and are injected during feeding. Transfusion and sharing needles also transmit disease, the latter particularly relevant in IV drug users where HIV coinfection makes treatment problematic.

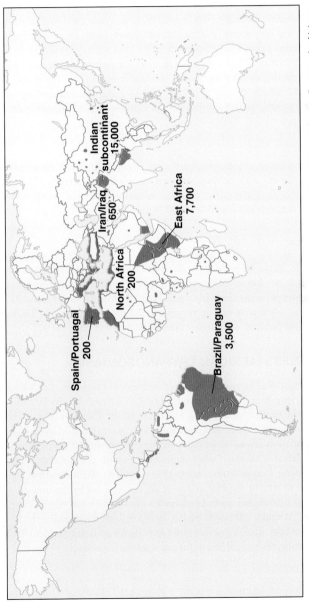

Fig. 3.6 Map of visceral leishmaniasis (kala-azar). (From Nabarro L, Morris-Jones S, Moore DAJ. Arthropod-borne diseases. In: Nabarro L, Morris-Jones S, Moore DAJ, eds. *Peters' Atlas of Tropical Medicine and Parasitology*. 7th ed. London, UK: Elsevier Ltd; 2019:1–108.)

Labels on map:

Spain/Portuagal 200

North Africa 200

Iran/Iraq 650

Indian subcontinant 15,000

East Africa 7,700

Brazil/Paraguay 3,500

Clinical Features

The incubation period may be as short as 2 weeks, but is usually 2 to 10 months. A dormant state may persist for years, only for disease to be activated by a drop in host immunity. Most cases are asymptomatic or subclinical, but host factors including HIV infection and malnutrition make clinical disease much more likely. Onset is usually insidious with low-grade fever. As the disease progresses, lymphadenopathy, wasting, and anemia become common. On examination hepato-splenomegaly, which may be massive, is apparent, and hyperpigmentation (leading to the name kala-azar or black disease) may be seen. Splenomegaly causes a dragging sensation or abdominal pain because of splenic infarcts. Intercurrent infections are common with pneumonia, measles, dysentery, and TB often the reason patients seek medical attention, and the mode of death. Post kala-azar dermal leishmaniasis causing a rash on the face and trunk may develop after treatment, usually in Sudan (50%) or India (10%). This is a parasitological phenomenon and requires extended treatment.

Diagnosis

Anemia, thrombocytopenia, and leucopenia are seen, usually with a low albumin (20 g/L) and high globulins. Amastigotes may be demonstrated in splenic aspirates (>95%), bone marrow (53%–86%), or lymph nodes (50%–60%). Serology is useful with good sensitivity and specificity with rk39 antigen dipstick kits useful in "field" settings. However, serology is less sensitive in HIV-positive patients.

Treatment

Sodium stibogluconate, 20 mg/kg per day for 20 to 40 days is effective but nausea, arthralgia, and pancreatitis can limit its use. Liposomal amphotericin B is an attractive but expensive option and is becoming the treatment of choice in many areas: 3 mg/kg on days 1 to 5, 14, and 21 is a standard regimen. Miltefosine is an effective oral agent given at 2.5 mg/kg for 28 days. Treatment is more difficult in HIV-positive patients, with higher rates of relapse and side effects.[41]

SLEEPING SICKNESS (AFRICAN TRYPANOSOMIASIS)

African trypanosomiasis, also known as sleeping sickness, is caused by two subspecies of the protozoan parasite *Trypansoma brucei*. It is transmitted to humans by the bite of the tsetse fly (*Glossina* spp.) generally south of the Sahara and north of the Zambezi (Fig. 3.7). Broadly, the majority (90%) of cases occur west of the Great Rift Valley and are caused by *T. b. gambiense* with human-human transmission following an indolent clinical course. *T. b. rhodesiense* occurring east of the Great Rift Valley is a zoonosis with an animal reservoir predominantly in the antelope family. The clinical course is much more acute than *gambiense*. Vector control, mass screening programs, and patient treatment resulted in a large decline of cases by the mid-1960s. However, war and civil strife have interrupted control programs and caused a resurgence of sleeping sickness, especially in the DRC, Angola, and South Sudan. Refocused efforts, including by Médecins Sans Frontières (MSF), have begun to reverse this but it remains a significant problem in the DRC and Central African Republic, with small loci of disease remaining elsewhere.

Clinical Features

The earliest sign of sleeping sickness is usually a chancre developing after a painful tsetse bite. These are red, inflamed, and ulcerated but not usually painful and resolve in 2 to 4 weeks. A chancre is less common in *T. b. gambiense*. Trypanosomes will invade the hemolymphatic system and multiply causing fever, chills, headache, and joint pain, which may be mistaken for malaria. Winterbottom's sign, lymphadenopathy in the posterior triangle of the neck, may give a clue to the diagnosis. *T. b. rhodesiense* causes more severe illness, and patients may even die at this stage,

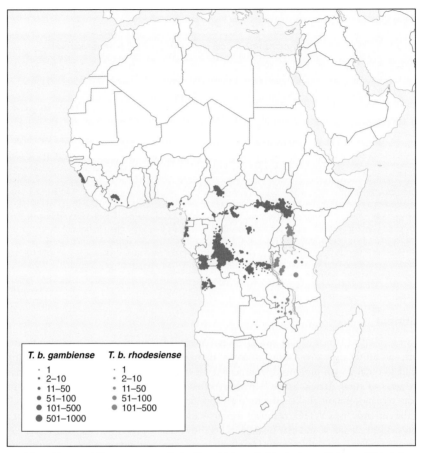

Fig. 3.7 Map of human African trypanosomiasis. (From Nabarro L, Morris-Jones S, Moore DAJ. Arthropod-borne diseases. In: Nabarro L, Morris-Jones S, Moore DAJ, eds. *Peters' Atlas of Tropical Medicine and Parasitology*. 7th ed. London, UK: Elsevier Ltd; 2019:1–108.)

usually of cardiac involvement. Weeks (*rhodesiense*) to months (*gambiense*) later the trypanosomes invade the CNS causing headache, behavioral change, and, progressively, convulsions, somnolence, and coma. The sleep-wake cycle may be disturbed. Onset is usually insidious, but if untreated the disease is fatal, frequently by wasting and dehydration caused by an inability to eat or drink.

Diagnosis

Diagnosis is usually by demonstration of trypanosomes or serology. Trypanosomes may be visible on lymph node aspirates, blood, or CSF, depending on the stage. Thick films, concentration methods (e.g., by centrifuging and examining the buffy coat layer) and repeated examination increase sensitivity as blood parasite levels, especially in *gambiense,* are often low. Serology methods, including ELISA, and the field-screening card agglutination test for trypanosomiasis (CATT), are very useful but ideally the diagnosis should be confirmed parasitologically. All positive cases require staging, which means looking for CNS invasion. A lumbar puncture demonstrating a lymphocytosis, high protein, trypanosomes, or the morular cells of Mott indicates stage II disease.

TABLE 3.4 ■

	Trypansoma brucei gambiense	*T. b. rhodesiense*
Stage I	Pentamidine	Suramin
	4 mg/kg intramuscular (IM) or intra-venous (IV) daily for 7–10 days	Day 1: Test dose 4–5 mg/kg IV
		Days 3, 10, 17, 24, 31: 20 mg/kg (max. 1 g) IV
Stage II (central nervous system involvement)	Eflornithine[a]	Melarsoprol[b]
	100 mg/kg qds for 14 days (IV usually preferred)	2.2 mg/kg daily for 10 days, slow IV injection

[a]Nifurtimox-eflornithine combination therapy is increasingly used, requiring reduced doses of eflornithine while maintaining the efficacy of the treatment. Médecins Sans Frontières use oral nifurtimox 15 mg/kg per day in three divided doses for 10 days plus eflornithine infusions 400 mg/kg per day in two divided doses for 7 days
[b]Daily prophylactic steroids (1 mg/kg prednisolone up to 40 mg) are frequently given to prevent the immune-mediated acute encephalopathy that occurs in 5%–14% patients typically between days 5 and 8.
From Büscher P, Cecchi G, Jamonneau V, et al. Human African trypanosomiasis. *Lancet.* 2017;390(10110):2397–2409; Médecins Sans Frontières. Chapter 6: Parasitic diseases. In: *Clinical Guidelines—Diagnosis and Treatment Manual.* Geneva: MSF; 2016:148–150.

Treatment

The drugs used to treat sleeping sickness were developed some time ago, have significant side effects, and can be expensive (although cost is now covered by a WHO donation program) and difficult to obtain, with prolonged treatment regimes. In addition, most cases occur in hard to reach areas of rural Africa. Stage II patients often have complex medical needs. This makes African trypanosomiasis challenging to treat. Specific drug treatment depends on stage and species. The currently used WHO treatment regimens and dosages are laid out in Table 3.4, but good quality evidence is sparse and new treatments urgently needed. Prevention includes vector control, case management (preventing onward human transmission), and bite avoidance. *Glossina* spp. are attracted by blue-colored clothing, and avoiding wearing this in endemic areas can prevent disease (Table 3.4).

CHAGAS' DISEASE (AMERICAN TRYPANOSOMIASIS)

American trypanosomiasis is caused by the kinetoplastid protozoan *Trypanosoma cruzi*, closely related to the causative agent of sleeping sickness, *T. brucei*. It is a zoonosis with mammalian hosts (including opossums, guinea pigs, dogs, and cats) with autochthonous transmission in Central and South America (Fig. 3.8). There is evidence of some ongoing transmission in the southern states of the United States. Transmission is predominantly vector borne with triatomine bugs (also known as assassin bugs, reduviids, or kissing bugs) taking a blood meal from an infected host and then, after gut replication of trypanosomes, excretion in the feces. Infection occurs when these feces are rubbed into a wound or the conjunctiva. Additionally, transmission can occur via blood transfusion, organ transplantation, and orally, particularly in the Amazon where drinking fruit juices contaminated with crushed reduviid bugs causes around 1000 cases per year. Chagas' disease is commonest in rural areas, where the presence of the mammal hosts and poor-quality housing providing a habitat for the vector leads to high rates of infection, with seroprevalence of up to 50% in some areas. Migration from South America and the chronicity of the illness means cases are seen outside of South and Central America, and transmission from blood transfusion has occurred.

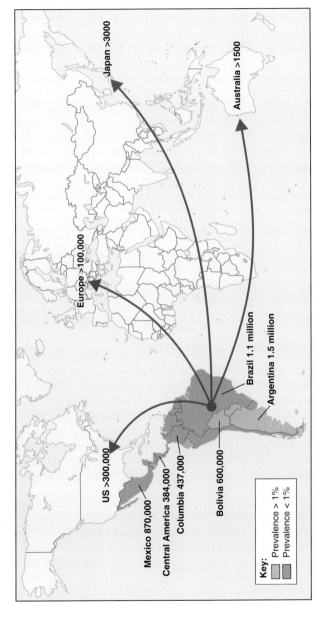

Fig. 3.8 Map of distribution of American trypanosomiasis. (From Nabarro L, Morris-Jones S, Moore DAJ. Arthropod-borne diseases. In: Nabarro L, Morris-Jones S, Moore DAJ, eds. *Peters' Atlas of Tropical Medicine and Parasitology.* 7th ed. London, UK: Elsevier Ltd; 2019:1–108.)

Clinical Features

Infection can be asymptomatic initially but up to one-third develop acute symptoms, particularly children. Local parasite multiplication causes edema at the site of entry known as a chagoma, or orbital edema if infection is via the conjunctiva, termed Romaña's sign. A few weeks later fever, myalgia, lymphadenopathy, and hepatosplenomegaly may occur. Most will control the infection in 1 to 3 months but will have a low level parasitemia and remain at risk of chronic sequalae. Some, especially younger children or those with HIV, may acutely develop meningoencephalitis or cardiac complications, which carry a poor prognosis. Some 10 to 20 years after initial infection, chronic sequelae become apparent in around 30%. Heart disease, especially conduction abnormalities, and destruction of the parasympathetic nerve plexus leading to megaesophagus and megacolon cause morbidity and mortality.

Diagnosis

Acute infection may be diagnosed with identification of organism in peripheral blood smears especially when aided by hemoconcentration techniques, or by PCR. Culture, xenodiagnosis (triatomine bugs unexposed to Chagas feed on patient, allowing demonstration of the parasite in insect feces after a few weeks) or serology can be helpful in diagnosing chronic infection, although culture and xenodiagnoses are technically challenging and serology requires careful interpretation. Presence of amastigotes on biopsy specimens is diagnostic but requires development of pathology and appropriate sampling.

Treatment

Acute presentations should be treated promptly with nifurtimox or benznidazole. Antiparasitic treatment of chronic disease is more problematic. Although the BENEFIT trial showed reduced parasite detection with treatment in the chronic phase, no improvement in clinical outcomes was seen with 5 years of follow-up, and supportive management is the only current evidence-based strategy for chronic infection.[42]

TOXOPLASMOSIS (SEE ALSO CHAPTER 6)

Toxoplasma gondii is an intracellular protozoan whose definitive host is the cat. Cats shed oocysts in their feces and intermediate hosts such as rodents and birds become inadvertently infected after ingesting food or water contaminated with oocysts. Oocysts develop in the intermediate host in muscles and neural tissue, before completing the cycle when intermediate hosts are eaten by cats. Humans may become infected by accidental ingestion of oocytes from cat feces through food or water contamination, or eating undercooked meat from an intermediate host, including beef and lamb. Transmission transplacentally or by blood transfusion or organ transplant from an infected donor can occur. The disease is globally widespread with seroprevalence up to 40% in France.

Clinical Features

In immunocompetent adults and children, infection is usually asymptomatic or causes lymphadenopathy (cervical or generalized) that self-resolves. Congenital infection, where parasites are transmitted from mother to child via the placenta during maternal parasitemia, can lead to hearing loss, learning difficulties, chorioretinitis (which may reactive later in life), and stillbirth or miscarriage. The earlier it is acquired in gestation the more severe the illness. The commonest manifestation in the immunodeficient, especially patients with advanced HIV, is CNS space-occupying lesions, which are often multiple. This is covered is Chapter 6.

Diagnosis

Serology with or without histologic evidence of toxoplasmosis is usually required for diagnosis although in HIV-infected patients with CNS lesion(s) treatment is often started presumptively.

Treatment

Immunocompetent, nongravid individuals need no specific treatment. Spiramycin is used in pregnant women if diagnosed with acute infection at less than 16 to 18 weeks of gestation, to prevent congenital transmission. Later in pregnancy pyrimethamine and sulfadiazine may be used. For patients with chorioretinitis, congenitally acquired infection or those with toxoplasmic encephalitis, pyrimethamine and sulfadiazine in combination are used most, with folinic acid. In active chorioretinitis, patients require prednisolone 1 mg/kg per day in two divided doses until CSF protein concentration falls or inflammation subsides.[43]

INTESTINAL AMEBIASIS

Entamoeba histolytica is an intestinal protozoan that causes GI infection including dysentery (bloody diarrhea) and extrahepatic abscess, most commonly in the liver. The cystic form is excreted from the gut and can survive in the environment for months before being ingested in food or water contaminated with feces. Widespread across the globe, there are an estimated 40 to 50 million cases per year and 40,000 to 100,000 deaths. It is particularly prevalent where poor hygiene or sanitation are present, with Central and South America, SE Asia, and West Africa all hotspots.

Clinical Features

There is a wide spectrum of clinical presentations from asymptomatic infections or minor changes in bowel habit to fulminant colitis. Colitis is caused by invasion of the trophozoites through the gut wall causing flask-shaped ulcers in the colon. Diarrhea is usually bloody, and abdominal pain common, although fever and systemic symptoms are rare even in those with severe disease. A fulminant colitis may develop, especially in those given steroid treatment, so care should be taken to exclude intestinal amebiasis in patients being investigated for inflammatory bowel disease.

Amebic abscess may occur anywhere throughout the body, with the liver as the most common site. Multiple abscesses are present in one-third of cases, and right lobe abscesses are four times commoner than left. Less than half the patients with an amebic liver abscess have a history of amebic colitis or even recent diarrhea. Patients usually present with fever and right upper quadrant pain (and tenderness). Abscesses may rupture into the pleura, pericardium, or externally.

Diagnosis

Wet microscopy of stool may reveal *Entamoeba* cysts but as these are clinically indistinguishable from *E. dispar*, a nonpathogenic protozoon, stool antigen detection for *histolytica* should be performed to confirm the diagnosis. When "hot stool" can be obtained and examined, ideally within 15 minutes, visualization of trophozoites containing red blood cells is diagnostic. More practically, stool antigen tests and PCR-based assays are sensitive and specific. Amoebic liver abscesses may be seen on ultrasound or computed tomography (CT) scan, or identified indirectly by noticing a raised hemidiaphragm or small pleural effusion on chest x-ray. Antibodies can be detected in 95% of patients (70% with intestinal disease). This becomes negative within 6 to 12 months, so if positive is not usually because of past disease.

Treatment

High-dose metronidazole (800 mg tds for 5–10 days) or tinidazole (2 g for 3–6 days) is the treatment of choice for intestinal amebiasis and amebic abscess (with abscess at the longer end of the treatment duration). These will not eradicate cysts in the lumen of the gut, so a luminal amebicide such as diloxanide or paromomycin should be used to prevent reinfection. Surgery is generally best avoided in amebic colitis as the gut is often friable, but may be required when there is intestinal perforation or toxic megacolon. Most abscesses will respond to medical therapy but where they do not, secondary bacterial infection is suspected or there is diagnostic doubt, aspiration is helpful. Pus is typically "anchovy sauce"-like, and trophozoites may be seen on microscopy.[44]

GIARDIASIS

Giardia lamblia (also known as *G. intestinalis*), a flagellate protozoon causing disease by adherence to the small bowel lumen, is globally widespread. The cystic form is environmentally hardy. Infection usually arises from drinking contaminated water, especially untreated water from lakes and rivers.

Clinical Features

Most cases are asymptomatic. Those that develop symptoms get a predominantly upper GI picture with abdominal pain, cramps, bloating, and flatulence. Nausea and malaise are common, with watery diarrhea. Although the infection self-resolves for some, infection may persist leading to weight loss and malabsorption. Even after clearing the infection, postinfectious irritable bowel syndrome or lactose intolerance means for some bowel habit takes months to normalize afterwards.

Diagnosis

Stool microscopy, ideally of three samples, will reveal presence of giardia cysts (up to 90% sensitivity with three samples, in expert hands). Multiplex PCR methods and point-of-care stool antigen testing is now widely available.

Treatment

Metronidazole or tinidazole are the treatments of choice and show good efficacy. When symptoms are persistent other infectious and noninfectious causes of diarrhea, immunodeficiency (especially HIV and IgA deficiency), evidence of reinfection, noncompliance with treatment, and postgiardia lactose intolerance should be considered. Antimicrobial resistance is increasingly reported and combination metronidazole/albendazole treatment, nitazoxanide, and quinacrine have all been used as second-line therapies.[45]

OTHER GUT PROTOZOAN INFECTIONS

There are a variety of other intestinal protozoa that cause disease including *Cryptosporidium parvum*, *C. hominis*, *Cyclospora* species, *Cystoisospora belli*, *Balantidium coli*, and the numerous microsporidia species (now thought to be intracellular fungi). These have variable worldwide distributions. All are transmitted fecoorally, with *C. hominis* by human-human transmission but the others mostly zoonoses. Apart from *B. coli*, which causes a spectrum of disease similar to amebiasis, most cause self-limiting watery diarrhea in immunocompetent individuals. Persistent diarrhea and weight loss can occur in immunosuppressed patients and are well described in patients with advanced HIV. Diagnosis is usually by microscopy (±) special stains (e.g., modified ZN for cyclospora). PCR approaches are increasingly used.

In the immunosuppressed, symptoms may be prolonged, with ARVs a key treatment in patients with advanced HIV. Nitazoxanide can be effective in cryptosporidiosis in the immunosuppressed; *Cystoisospora* and *Cyclospora* will respond to oral co-trimoxazole; *B. coli* responds to tetracycline (500 mg qds) as well as metronidazole and paromomycin, and the microsporidia often clinically respond to albendazole.

FREE-LIVING AMOEBAE INFECTIONS

The free-living species of amoebae survive encysted in dry environments and reproduce as trophozoites in moist environments. *Naegleria*, *Acanthamoeba*, and *Balamuthia* species can all cause human disease, albeit rarely.

Naegleria fowleri causes a primary amebic meningoencephalitis in immunocompetent children and young adults, typically 2 to 14 days after swimming in warm fresh or spa water. Amebic meningitis is rarely suspected as clinically appearances are typical for bacterial meningitis. Most patients will die. When epidemiologic exposure suggests the diagnosis, wet specimens should be examined for amoebae, and culture attempted on a bacterial lawn. Amphotericin B is the treatment of choice but data on efficacy is limited.

Granulomatous amebic encephalitis may be caused by *Acanthamoeba* species and *Balamuthia madrillaris*. Most patients are immunosuppressed, often transplant patients, apart from a few cases of *Balamuthia* from Peru. Amoeba enter the respiratory system (or occasionally the skin), often with a primary lesion from soil contamination before spreading to the CNS and causing either headache and meningism or a focal brain lesion. Microscopy of wet specimens of CSF, or special stains are required for diagnosis. Treatment is not clearly defined but usually includes fluconazole for *Balamuthia* or co-trimoxazole for *Acanthamoeba*. Most patients do not survive.

Helminths: Nematodes

ASCARIASIS

Ascaris lumbricoides infects 819 million people worldwide, particularly in areas of poor sanitation and high humidity or where human feces are used as fertilizer. Children are most commonly infected. It is acquired by ingestion of ascaris eggs, and then follows a rather complex lifecycle in humans, involving migration through the lungs before settling in the small intestine. There it has a life span of 1 to 2 years, producing 200,000 eggs per day, which require 2 to 6 weeks development in the soil before becoming infective.

Clinical Features

Migration through the lung, especially second and subsequent infections, may cause pneumonia. When associated with fever, bronchospasm, eosinophilia, and lung infiltrates it is termed Loeffler's syndrome. Infection is usually subclinical, although children may suffer from malnutrition and delayed development in proportion to worm burden. Very heavy infestation can cause a bolus of worms leading to acute intestinal obstruction.

Diagnosis

Diagnosis is by demonstration of the presence of oval, fertilized eggs with a typical appearance on stool microscopy. Occasionally, adult worms may be visualized, either in situ during surgery or endoscopy, or migrating out of the mouth, nose, or anus precipitated by fever, acute, drugs, or anesthesia.

Treatment

Mebendazole (100 mg bd for 3 days) or albendazole (400 mg stat) are effective treatments. Piperazine salt (75 mg/kg to maximum of 3.5 g, once daily for 2 days) causes a flaccid paralysis of the worms and is used when there is intestinal obstruction, along with decompression of the gut with a nasogastric tube and IV rehydration.[46,47]

HOOKWORM INFECTION

Hookworm infection is caused by the nematodes *Ancyclostoma duodenale* and *Necator americanus*. Over 500 million people are infected, with the heaviest burden in sub-Saharan Africa and SE Asia but with a global distribution including temperate areas, such as the southern states of the United States. Hookworm has a fascinating lifecycle. Larvae in moist soil penetrate through the skin and then into the circulation before migrating to the lungs, then up to the pharynx where they are swallowed. From there, they move down the gut until attachment to the small bowel wall. Females will produce 10,000s of eggs per day, which are excreted in the feces. These will larvate in moist soil after 48 hours and can then complete the lifecycle by invading the next host.

Clinical Features

Hookworm may cause clinical features throughout the lifecycle in humans. "Ground itch" may arise at the site of penetration, causing a pruritic rash. Migration through the lungs is generally asymptomatic but may cause a pneumonitis with cough, eosinophilia, and wheeze. The commonest, and most important, symptom is an iron deficiency anemia caused by chronic blood loss at the site of hookworm attachment in the small bowel. Anemia is proportional to worm burden and can be severe leading to significant morbidity.

Diagnosis

Acute infection causing ground itch or a pneumonitis can usually be diagnosed clinically, along with the presence of eosinophilia. Intestinal infection is usually diagnosed by microscopy of stool demonstrating an ovoid egg with multiple nuclei. Concentration techniques or microscopy of multiple samples (three is ideal) increases the yield in light infections.

Treatment

Albendazole 400 mg stat will eliminate approximately 80% of worms, which is usually sufficient for clinical cure, although dosing can be repeated to completely eradicate the helminths. Mass treatment campaigns, better sanitation, and provision of footwear have all been used in control, although promising steps are also being taken to produce an effective hookworm vaccine.

TRICHURIASIS

Trichuris trichiuria is acquired by ingesting food or water contaminated with human feces containing *Trichuris* eggs. It has a worldwide distribution, especially in areas of poor sanitation, or where human feces are used as fertilizer.

Clinical Features

Light infections are usually asymptomatic but heavy infections, especially in children, can cause bloody diarrhea because of colitis. Rectal prolapse may occur. Developmental delay and iron deficiency anemia also occur with heavy infections.

Diagnosis

Typical barrel-shaped eggs with mucoid polar plugs can be visualized on wet film stool microscopy. Individual worms may be visualized attached to the mucosa during endoscopy, or after prolapse.

Treatment

A single oral dose of mebendazole (500 mg) is effective, as is albendazole (400 mg). Severe infections may need repeated dosing (e.g., albendazole 400 mg od or mebendazole 100 mg bd for 3 days). Ivermectin is also effective.[48]

CUTANEOUS LARVA MIGRANS

Infection with a nonhuman hookworm (e.g., *Ancylostoma braziliense*, a dog hookworm) can cause cutaneous larva migrans. Here the larva cannot complete migration through tissues and thus track along the skin leaving a characteristic itchy, inflamed, serpiginous rash which slowly migrates. Infection is usually acquired by exposure to sandy soils or beaches contaminated with dog excrement. The hookworms will eventually die, and the rash resolves, although albendazole or ivermectin will speed this process up.

STRONGYLOIDIASIS

Strongyloides stercoralis is found mostly in tropical and subtropical regions and infects 30–100 million people worldwide. It has a free-living soil lifecycle that can maintain an environmental reservoir, as well as a parasitic lifecycle in humans which produces disease. Larvae in the soil penetrate directly through skin. From there they have a similar lifecycle to hookworm, migrating through the bloodstream to the lungs before being coughed up and swallowed to mature in the upper intestine. Helminth eggs germinate into larvae inside the gut, and may be excreted to complete a free-living lifecycle, or reinvade the host via the perianal skin, causing autoinfection. This can maintain life-long infection even after the host has left an endemic area. The ability to cause life-long infection has led to discovery of the parasite many years after travel to tropical areas, including in a significant number of British Far East Prisoners of War.

Clinical Features

Skin eruption at the site of penetration, larva currens, produces a typical migratory serpiginous, pruritic, erythematous rash. It migrates more quickly and is more diffuse than the cutaneous larva migrans rash. While migrating through the lungs, cough, wheeze, and an eosinophilic pneumonia may be seen. Intestinal symptoms are generally mild, but diarrhea, which may be bloody, along with epigastric pain and malabsorption, occur.

Strongyloides Hyperinfection. In immunosuppressed patients, including those given corticosteroids, chemotherapy, or immunosuppressants, as well as those with hematologic malignancies, human T-lymphotropic virus 1 (HTLV-1), or HIV, Strongyloides hyperinfection can occur with loss of immune control of the helminth, resulting in multiplication and migration through tissues. Severe bloody diarrhea, gram-negative sepsis, bowel perforation and bacterial peritonitis, pulmonary disease, and bacterial meningitis (often gram-negative) are common features. Mortality is high, and although eosinophilia is often absent, Strongyloides larvae are usually easy to demonstrate in multiple body fluids. Strongyloides hyperinfection many years after leaving the tropics in a host with previously asymptomatic infection can be a surprising finding, requiring an alert clinician and a good history to diagnose.

Diagnosis

Stool microscopy (saline smear) for motile larvae is a useful test but often larvae are only present in small numbers and produced intermittently in chronic infection, so multiple stool samples should be examined. Concentration and charcoal culture methods improve yield, as does examining duodenal contents, which have a high larval concentration, either from duodenal aspirated taken during endoscopic examination or using the famous "string test." Serology is highly sensitive and specific and is very useful, especially in screening patients who may be at risk of hyperinfection. Empiric therapy is occasionally required, especially when Strongyloides hyperinfection is suspected.

Treatment

Ivermectin at 200 mcg/kg given for 2 days is the treatment of choice. Albendazole 400 mg once or twice daily for 3 days is an alternative treatment. Patients with hyperinfection will need supportive care, and anthelminthic treatment may need to be repeated. For patients who have recently traveled to an endemic area or reside in one and require corticosteroids, immunosuppressive therapy, or are likely to become immunosuppressed, screening (usually by serology) is advocated.[49]

TRICHINELLOSIS

Trichinella spiralis and related species are nematodes found in the intestines of a wide variety of wild and domestic mammals, especially domestic and wild pigs, around the world. Ingestion of viable encysted larvae in undercooked contaminated meat leads to maturation in the host small intestine. Female worms release larvae for a few weeks before being expelled. The larvae disseminate throughout the body via the bloodstream and encyst in skeletal muscle. Global burden usually depends on local practices with regard to consumption of domestically raised meat and wild animals.

Clinical Features

GI symptoms can appear within days of ingestion, including diarrhea. Typically 1 to 2 weeks post ingestion, but occasionally longer, systemic symptoms may appear. These include fever, myalgia, and muscle tenderness across a range of muscle groups, often starting in the extraocular muscles. Periorbital edema, a petechial rash, subconjunctival hemorrhage, and cough may all occur. These usually subside over a few weeks although occasionally a fulminant infection with myocarditis or meningoencephalitis can occur.

Diagnosis

The diagnosis is made by a relevant exposure history in combination with clinical features, supported by laboratory findings including eosinophilia and an elevated creatinine kinase. Serology can confirm the diagnosis, but results often take several weeks. Muscle biopsy, although demonstrating characteristic spiral encysted larvae within muscle tissue, is rarely required.

Treatment

Prevention, by elimination in the animal reservoir, proper cooking of meat, or, less reliably, freezing below −18° C for more than 1 week, is preferable to treatment. Mebendazole or albendazole therapy may reduce parasite burden if given early, and corticosteroids may help with symptom relief or in critically ill patients but evidence of benefit for either is scant.[50]

PARASTRONGYLUS (ANGIOSTRONGYLUS) COSTARICENSIS

The reservoir for this disease is various rat species including the cotton rat *Sigmodon hispidus* in Costa Rica. Slugs are the intermediate host, and human disease is caused usually by accidental ingestion of the slug or its slime trail on salad. As the name suggests, it is found largely in Central America. The nematodes cause a granulomatous inflammation in the colon, known as abdominal angiostrongyliasis. The disease presents similarly to appendicitis, with right iliac fossa and flank pain, fever, and diarrhea. The eosinophilia may help differentiate it from appendicitis. Surgery is the commonest modality of treatment, often because of understandable confusion with appendicitis or other surgical abdominal problem, and the disease is often diagnosed retrospectively on visualization of the adult nematode, or characteristic histology on examination of pathology specimens. Antihelminthics such as mebendazole are often used for treatment but the evidence base is weak.

PARASTRONGYLUS (ANGIOSTRONGYLUS) CANTONENSIS

Parastrongylus cantonensis, previously *Angiostrongylus cantonensis* and more commonly known as the rat lungworm, is a nematode which normally parasitizes rodents and has a mollusk intermediate host. Accidental ingestion of infective larvae while consuming raw or undercooked snails causes epidemics of disease, particularly in Asia, including China, Taiwan, and Japan recently, as well as the Caribbean and Pacific regions. One to four weeks following ingestion of raw or undercooked snails meningism occurs, often with cranial nerve lesions, but less frequently encephalitis. CSF from a lumbar puncture shows an eosinophilic meningitis, with larvae visible in 25% of cases. Prednisolone is the treatment of choice, with anthelminthics showing no additional benefit in a clinical trial, although albendazole is still widely used. Recovery is usually gradual over a few weeks.

DRACUNCULIASIS

Dracunculiasis, or Guinea worm, is set to be the second disease eradicated after smallpox. The disease is endemic in four countries with only 25 human cases found in 2016. Transmitted by drinking water containing copepods infected with third-stage larva, it produces a distinctive clinical entity, with a blister forming, typically in the lower limbs, which ruptures, and a gravid worm emerges. Local complications including pain, deformity, and secondary bacterial infection can occur. Surgical removal or gradual light traction can remove the worms. Antibiotics may be needed for secondary infection.

GNATHOSTOMIASIS

The third-stage larvae of *Gnathostoma* are infectious to humans. The nematode is transmitted to the human host by ingestion of uncooked fish, shrimp, or frogs (intermediate hosts). Within 1 to 2 weeks the patient may present with fever, abdominal pain, cough, and eosinophilia although most acute infections are asymptomatic. The most common clinical manifestation is migratory swellings, which develop rapidly and persist for 1 to 2 weeks. If the nematode migrates through the CNS then neurologic deficit, including Brown-Sequard syndrome, hemiplegia, coma, and even death, may occur. However, there is CNS involvement in less than 1% of patients with cutaneous migratory swellings. The disease is usually diagnosed based on clinical features and an accompanying eosinophilia. A confirmatory serology test is available in some specialist laboratories. Albendazole 400 mg bd for 2 to 3 weeks causes migration of the parasite to the skin where it may be removed. However, success is not guaranteed. Ivermectin can be useful when albendazole has failed, but despite treatment some patients are left with ongoing symptoms, and must wait nervously for the helminth to expire, while hoping it does not migrate fatally through their CNS.

TOXOCARIASIS

Toxocara cani and *T. cati* are cosmopolitan roundworms that infect dogs and cats. Humans (mainly children) ingest embryonated eggs from soil. Larvae hatch in the intestine, then migrate through various tissues. They will not develop into adults in humans, instead becoming walled off in granulomas. Two clinical entities exist, visceral larva migrans and ocular larva migrans. In visceral larva migrans, although most infections are asymptomatic, patients may present with myalgia, urticarial rashes, anorexia, cough, and wheeze. Marked eosinophilia is usually present, often with hepatomegaly. Serology and/or visualization of the larva or granulomas on biopsy leads to diagnosis. In ocular larva migrans, granuloma formation in the critical structures in the eye, especially the macula, can cause blindness. Eosinophilia is often absent but fundoscopic features and positive serology help make the diagnosis. In terms of treatment, albendazole is often used for both but is not of proven efficacy. Corticosteroids reduce inflammation from the migratory larva and may help. Vitrectomy and laser ablation of visible larvae have been tried in ocular larva migrans.

FILARIASIS

Filariasis is disease caused by nematode infections where microfilaria (filarial larvae) are transmitted to humans by insects, various mosquito species for lymphatic filariasis, and simulum flies for cutaneous filariasis, which includes onchocerciasis and loa loa (Table 3.5). The microfilaria mature into adult worms in humans, producing more microfilaria, which are able to infect the insect vectors.

TABLE 3.5 ■ Summary of Filarial Diseases

Species	Clinical Disease	Location of MF (Periodicity)	Sheath	Main Characteristics	Distribution
Wuchereria bancrofti	LF	Blood (nocturnal[a])	+	Tail—pointed tail, nuclei not to tip. Body—275–300 × 9 μm, smooth curves. Sheath—stains pale mauve with Giemsa.	All tropics
Brugia malayi	LF	Blood (nocturnal[b])	+	Tail—tapers irregularly, two nuclei at tip. Body—200–275 × 6 μm, kinked. Sheath—stains bright pink with Giemsa.	Southeast Asia
Brugia timori	LF	Blood (nocturnal)	+	Tail—tapers irregularly, two nuclei at tip. Body—290–325 × 6 μm, kinked. Sheath—stains poorly with Giemsa.	Timor-Leste
Loa	Eye worm	Blood (diurnal)	+	Tail—rounded tip, nuclei to tip. Body—250–300 × 9 μm, kinked. Sheath—does not stain with Giemsa.	West Africa, forested areas
Onchocerca volvulus	River blindness	Skin (no periodicity)	−	Tail—long and pointed, nuclei not to tip, crooked. Body—240–360 × 8 μm. Head—spatulate. No sheath.	Africa, Central and South America, Yemen

TABLE 3.5 ■ Summary of Filarial Diseases—cont.

Species	Clinical Disease	Location of MF (Periodicity)	Sheath	Main Characteristics	Distribution
Mansonella perstans	Most asymptomatic	Blood (no periodicity)	–	Tail—nuclei extended to tip of rounded tail, large nucleus at tip. Body—190–240 × 5 µm. No sheath.	Sub-Saharan Africa, Central and South America
Mansonella azzardi	Most asymptomatic	Blood/skin (no periodicity)	–	Tail—long pointed tail with no nuclei. Body—150–200 × 5 µm, anterior nuclei positioned side by side. No sheath.	Central and South America, Caribbean
Mansonella strepto-cerca	Asymptomatic dermatitis	Skin (no periodicity)	–	Tail—nuclei extended to tip of rounded, hooked tail. Body—180–240 × 5 µm. Single file anterior nuclei. No sheath.	Central and West Africa

[a]In the South Pacific, microfilariae may be diurnally subperiodic.
[b]In the Philippines, microfilariae may be nocturnally subperiodic.
LF, Lymphatic filariasis.
From Nabarro L, Morris-Jones S, Moore DAJ. Arthropod-borne diseases. In: Nabarro L, Morris-Jones S, Moore DAJ, eds. *Peters' Atlas of Tropical Medicine and Parasitology.* 7th ed. London, UK: Elsevier Ltd; 2019:1–108.

LYMPHATIC FILARIASIS

Lymphatic filariasis is a globally widespread filarial disease caused by the nematodes *Wucheria bancrofti*, *Brugia malayi*, and *B. timori*, which are all transmitted by mosquitoes (Fig. 3.9). The species of transmitting mosquito varies according to the filarial species and location. Transmission can be day or night depending on mosquito species, but night is generally commoner, except in Polynesia. Bancroftian filariasis (caused by *W. bancrofti*) causes 90% of lymphatic filariasis and is present in the Indian subcontinent, Oceania, Central and South America, and parts of Africa. *B. malayi* and *B. timori* are responsible for substantially fewer cases and are limited to India and SE Asia, and Timor-Leste and Indonesia, respectively. In total, around 120 million people are affected by lymphatic filariasis, with 60% of those in SE Asia. Adult worms reside in the lymphatics, most commonly of the groin, and that drives the major pathological consequences.

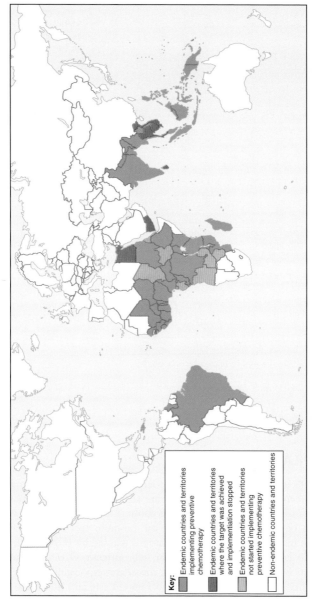

Fig. 3.9 Map of distribution of lymphatic filariasis. (From Nabarro L, Morris-Jones S, Moore DAJ. Arthropod-borne diseases. In: Nabarro L, Morris-Jones S, Moore DAJ, eds. *Peters' Atlas of Tropical Medicine and Parasitology*. 7th ed. London, UK: Elsevier Ltd; 2019:1–108.)

Key:

- Endemic countries and territories implementing preventive chemotherapy
- Endemic countries and territories where the target was achieved and implementation stopped
- Endemic countries and territories not started implementing preventive chemotherapy
- Non-endemic countries and territories

Clinical Features

Acute infections may cause no symptoms, or merely fatigue or malaise. Death of an adult worm may result in tender lymphadenopathy with retrograde lymphangitis. This may be accompanied by localized skin inflammation, ulceration, and bacterial infection. However, most pathology is chronic in nature with repeated infection, inflammation, filarial death, and scarring leading to lymphatic obstruction. This leads to lymphedema of the affected limb, progressing to elephantiasis with thickened, firm skin and permanent brawny edema. Sites include the legs and arms, but also scrotum and breasts. Secondary bacterial infection is common. Other manifestations include chyluria, chylous diarrhea, and chylous ascites because of lymphatic disruption, glomerulonephritis, and a monoarthritis.

Diagnosis

Acute filariasis is usually accompanied by an eosinophilia. A parasitological diagnosis relies on taking a blood sample when microfilariae are present in blood, which varies according to species (2200-0200 for *W. bancrofti*), and is dependent on a sufficiently high microfilariae burden. Concentration methods help. Antibody tests are useful diagnostically, especially in visitors to endemic areas, and live adult worms may be demonstrated by ultrasound. In endemic areas, clinical features are usually sufficient to make a diagnosis.

Treatment

On an individual basis, a single dose of diethylcarbamazine (DEC; 6 mg/kg) is the treatment of choice. It is as effective as the traditional 12-day course. Coinfection with loa loa or onchocerciasis requires care because of the chance of adverse reactions with DEC, and thus doxycycline ± ivermectin is preferred. Most patients globally are managed in community settings with mass drug administration of combination therapy (albendazole + ivermectin or DEC), alongside programmatic efforts to eliminate filariasis including vector control. Management of lymphedema, including skin care, exercise, massage, early treatment of secondary bacterial infection, and surgical intervention, is required alongside parasitological treatment.

ONCHOCERCIASIS

Onchocerciasis, or river blindness, is a tissue filarial disease caused by *Oncocerca volvulus* transmitted by blackflies of the genus *Simulium*. The vector typically breeds near freshwater, and 95% of cases are in Africa, but foci of disease are found in Central and South America, and Yemen (Fig. 3.10). Around 18 million people are infected, with blindness or visual impairment in three-quarters of a million. However, efforts at control, including vector control and mass administration of ivermectin, are reducing the burden globally.

Clinical Features

Clinical features are caused by the immunological response to dead and dying microfilariae and typically manifest 15 to 18 months after exposure.

Skin and subcutaneous tissue. Skin disease may vary from a localized maculopapular rash with mild itching to a more severe, generalized chronic rash with intense itching. Edema, excoriations, and hyperpigmentation occur in severe disease. The skin may lichenify and atrophy, and in chronic infection degenerates producing typical pathology including "hanging groin," apron-like folds of saggy atrophic skin in the groin area, or "leopard skin," with depigmentation of the pretibial area.

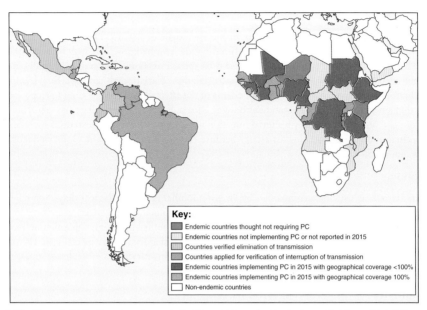

Fig. 3.10 Map of distribution of onchocerciasis. (From Nabarro L, Morris-Jones S, Moore DAJ. Arthropod-borne diseases. In: Nabarro L, Morris-Jones S, Moore DAJ, eds. *Peters' Atlas of Tropical Medicine and Parasitology*. 7th ed. London, UK: Elsevier Ltd; 2019:1–108.)

Eye. Onchocerciasis can cause anterior and posterior eye disease with geography and intensity of filarial burden driving risk of blindness. More intense infections and those in the West African savannah are most likely to result in blindness. A keratitis in response to death of microfilariae in the cornea results in a "snow flake" opacity that may be reversible in the early stages. However, an irreversible sclerosing keratitis can develop, leading to blindness. In the posterior eye, chorioretinitis is the most common pathology, resulting in tunnel vision. Optic atrophy can also occur. Vision is generally lost progressively.

Diagnosis

Eosinophilia is often present acutely, but is not specific, and may not be present in chronic disease. Microfilaria are best demonstrated via skin snips. Between four and six skin snips can be taken from a range of locations in a sterile fashion, immersed in saline, and the fluid examined for microfilariae some 30 minutes or so later. PCR, antibody, and antigen-based tests are all either available or in development and are increasingly used. The Mazzotti test, where 50 mg of DEC is given and the patient observed for development of itching and rash, has been well described. However, this can be dangerous in patients with a heavy microfilarial load, leading to fever, edema, and hypotension, and is now infrequently used. It should only be used when the skin snips and eye examination are normal.

Treatment

Ivermectin has replaced DEC as the treatment of choice as it effectively kills microfilariae with a much lower risk of a severe Mazzotti reaction. The standard treatment is 150 to 200 µg/kg po once but as adult worms are not affected this needs to be repeated each year until adult worms die naturally. Heavy infections may require dosing every 6 months.[51]

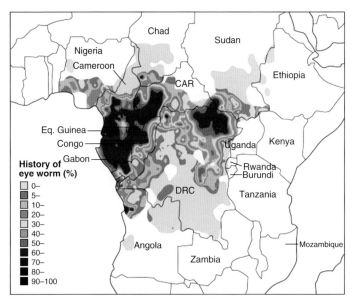

Fig. 3.11 Map of distribution of loiasis. *CAR,* Central African Republic; *DRC,* Democratic Republic of Congo; *Eq. Guinea,* Equatorial Guinea. (From Nabarro L, Morris-Jones S, Moore DAJ. Arthropod-borne diseases. In: Nabarro L, Morris-Jones S, Moore DAJ, eds. *Peters' Atlas of Tropical Medicine and Parasitology.* 7th ed. London, UK: Elsevier Ltd; 2019:1–108.)

LOIASIS

Loa loa is transmitted by the day-biting *Chrysops* flies in the tropical rainforests of Central and West Africa (Fig. 3.11). Microfilaria mature into adult worms and cause disease as they migrate through fascial planes.

Clinical Features

Months or even years after infection abrupt erythematous, itchy swellings occur. These are termed Calabar swellings, and may occur after heavy exercise or exposure to heat. Migrating worms might also be seen, either in the skin, or most dramatically when an adult worm migrates across the eye. Loa loa is often called "the eye worm." As with other filarial infection, endomyocardial fibrosis may occur, but the most feared complication is a meningoencephalitis, precipitated by treatment (often for another helminth infection) with DEC or ivermectin.

Diagnosis

Clinical findings of a visualized migratory worm or Calabar swelling combined with an eosinophilia are usually enough for a diagnosis but confirmation can be sought be examining a daytime peripheral blood smear for microfilaria.

Treatment

The standard treatment is DEC 2 mg/kg tds for 7 to 10 days. Single-dose ivermectin pretreatment can reduce the chances of a Mazzotti reaction in those who have concomitant onchocerciasis. For patients with very high microfilaria counts (>2500 Mf/mL), pretreatment with albendazole 200 mg bd for 21 days reduces the microfilarial burden, and the risk of precipitating encephalitis.

Helminths: Cestodes

TAENIA SAGINATA INFECTION

Taenia saginata, the beef tapeworm, is acquired by eating uncooked beef. Cattle are the intermediate host, whose flesh contains cysticerci, the larval stages. In the human small intestine, after ingestion, these develop into long, flat, segmented adult worms. The head, or scolex, is attached by suckers, with the worm growing by developing new segments. Eggs develop inside the tail segments or proglottids, which break off and are excreted in the stool. Highest rates of infection are found in East Africa, and the major human impact is economic because of spoiling of "measly" beef. Symptoms are usually minimal, but can include nausea, anorexia, or abdominal pain. Often asymptomatic patients may notice a proglottid segment passed in the stool. Diagnosis is usually by identification of proglottids macroscopically or the typical appearance of the eggs on microscopy of a wet preparation of stool. Beef and pork tapeworm eggs are morphologically identical but proglottids can be distinguished by examination of the lateral uterine branches. Single-dose praziquantel (10 mg/kg) or niclosamide (2 g for adults) are effective but given the lack of symptoms in most patients they usually given because of the distress of having tapeworm rather than the direct clinical effects.

TAENIA SOLIUM INFECTION AND NEUROCYSTICERCOSIS

The pork tapeworm, when acquired by eating undercooked pork, has a similar lifecycle, symptoms (minimal), diagnosis, and treatment as the beef tapeworm, except it is rare in those who do not consume pork (including amongst Muslims, Jews, and vegetarians). However, ingestion of eggs of *T. solium*, because of fecooral contamination, may lead to cysticercosis. On ingestion of eggs the oncospheres are released by the action of gastric acid in the stomach, penetrate the bowel wall, and are carried throughout the body by the bloodstream where they develop into larval cysts. Cysticercosis is an important cause of epilepsy in the less economically developed world and is prevalent in Latin America, Africa, and Asia, including India.

Clinical Features

Intestinal *T. solium* as per *saginata*.

Cysticercosis may present in a number of ways depending on the number, size, and location of cysts. Neurologic consequences, neurocysticercosis, are commonest, with epilepsy affecting 50% to 80% of people with parenchymal brain cysts. Focal signs are less common but may include pyramidal tract signs and movement disorders. Hydrocephalus and increased intracranial pressure, which usually develops slowly, may be the first presentation. Although most presentations follow a chronic or subacute course, in younger patients brisk host immune response to cysts may provoke encephalitis. Neurocysticercosis should be suspected in chronic and subacute neurologic deficits in an endemic area, or after potential exposure. Extra-CNS disease is rare; disease in the eye and muscles is reported.

Diagnosis

Intestinal *T. solium* as per *saginata*.

Diagnosing on clinical grounds alone is difficult given the protean manifestations. Presence of cysterici in subcutaneous tissue, skin, or the eye (seen clinically or on x-rays) is helpful but typical CNS CT or magnetic resonance imaging (MRI) appearances such as focal enhancing lesions with surrounding edema, or calcifications, are the most useful diagnostic clues. Serology is also very helpful, and where a biopsy has been performed, histologic appearances will be diagnostic.

Treatment

Intestinal *T. solium* as per *saginata*.

Treatment with antiparasitic agents will destroy active cysts and reduce seizure activity long-term. Albendazole 15 mg/kg per day in two divided doses for 8 to 15 days is recommended, or a prolonged praziquantel course as second line. Death of cysts and resulting inflammatory reaction can cause a worsening of symptoms on days 2 to 5, so coadministration of 0.1 to 0.2 mg/kg per day of dexamethasone during treatment is usually given. Repeated course of steroids and/or antiparasitic agents may be required. For those with inactive, calcified cysts, treatment is not generally recommended. Anticonvulsant therapy, holistic epilepsy care, neurorehabilitation, and/or surgery for hydrocephalus should not be neglected.[52]

FISH TAPEWORM INFECTION

The cestodes *Diphyllobothrium latum* and a few other recently discovered *Diphyllobothria* species are found in freshwater lakes and ponds in subarctic, temperate, and tropical zones, and cause tapeworm infections in humans. Persons acquire the tapeworms via ingestion of inadequately cooked (or raw) fish. Many individuals are asymptomatic or only mildly symptomatic, remaining infected for long periods. Heavy infections in the jejunum may lead to vitamin B12–deficient anemia. Diagnosis is by identification of eggs or proglottids in the stool. Praziquantel at 10 mg/kg is usually effective but can be repeated at 25 mg/kg if not cleared. Prevention is by thorough cooking of fish, or freezing.

HYDATID DISEASE

The cestodes *Echinococcus granulosis* and *E. multilocularis* cause hydatid disease in humans. *E. granulosis*, the commonest cause of human infections, maintains a lifecycle between dogs and sheep, with *E. multilocularis* having a wild cycle involving rodents and canines. Humans are infected by accidental ingestion of eggs excreted by dogs, which develop into larval oncospheres that in turn penetrate the GI tract to be disseminated throughout the body by blood and lymphatics. The disease is largely a rural one, and especially present in sheep-rearing areas, where dogs are used for flock control. It is globally distributed, but particularly in South America, parts of Europe, northern Africa, and Asia Minor.

Clinical Features

Both species cause cysts to grow over years in various organs. Symptoms are caused by mass effect, secondary bacterial infection, or cyst rupture. Rupture, spontaneously or from trauma or surgery, causes leakage of cyst fluid into organ cavities provoking a hypersensitivity reaction that may cause wheeze, urticaria, and fever, or even a life-threatening anaphylactoid reaction with hypotension and shock. The cyst fluid will seed body cavities, typically the peritoneal or pleural cavity, and the very many daughter cysts are difficult to treat. In *E. granulosis*, 70% of cysts develop in the liver, 20% in the lungs, and 10% elsewhere. Occasionally patients will present with cough productive of salty water and eosinophilia, where a cyst has ruptured into a bronchus. *E. multilocularis* is more likely to cause disease by invasion, decades after initial exposure, and may be mistaken for a tumor or cause erosive bony disease.

Diagnosis

Eosinophilia is usually present after a cyst has ruptured. Plain x-ray, ultrasound, and CT/MRI appearance may be suggestive or diagnostic. Ultrasound allows hydatid disease to be classified according to the WHO 2001 classification, which guides treatment. MRI probably gives most information, but is least available. Serology is useful, but false negatives in extrahepatic cysts or false positives with cross-reactions with other cestodes occur. Serology titers often increase after rupture, and reduce with treatment, allowing monitoring.

Treatment

Stable asymptomatic, calcified cysts may be monitored over several years. For active cysts, surgery to remove the cysts whole, where feasible, is commonly used and is effective. Percutaneous aspiration, injection, aspiration (PAIR) under ultrasound guidance is increasingly used, with cyst fluid aspirated and then hypertonic saline injected to kill viable cestodes. It is less invasive, but is not suitable for all lesions. Albendazole treatment, usually 400 mg bd, to suppress replication or prevent seeding, is important. It should be given for 1 to 3 months before and several months post an invasive procedure, to reduce the risk of seeding in case of cyst rupture during the procedure. Praziquantel may be used in combination with albendazole, especially post cyst rupture or where surgery is not possible, and long-term suppressive chemotherapy is required.[53]

Helminths: Trematodes

LIVER FLUKE INFECTION

Fascioliasis is caused by the liver trematodes *Fasciola hepatica* and *F. gigantica*. Humans become infected after ingesting the metacercariae on water plants, such as watercress, after their lifecycle involving freshwater snails and livestock, particularly sheep. The metacercariae will excyst, and the larvae migrate through the host before maturing in the bile ducts. The disease is present worldwide but is especially common in sheep-rearing areas. Disease is common in the Andes, with prevalence around 90% in some parts of Bolivia.

Clinical Features

The migratory phase, 6 to 12 weeks after infection, is often associated with fever, respiratory symptoms, abdominal pain, urticaria, and eosinophilia. Hepatomegaly, transient jaundice, and right upper quadrant (RUQ) pain may also occur. This is usually followed by an asymptomatic phase, although chronic infection can cause anemia and malaise, or recurrent cholangitis or cholecystitis because of obstruction.

Diagnosis

Acute infection is suggested clinically by the triad of hepatomegaly, fever, and eosinophilia where there is a history of consumption of freshwater plants. Eggs may be recovered from stool or duodenal aspirate in established biliary infections. Serology is less reliable than in other trematode infections, especially with *F. gigantica*, but is useful in the late stage of early infection, where serology has become positive but flukes have yet to start producing eggs.

Treatment

Unlike other cestode infections, praziquantel is not reliably effective, and should not be used first line. Triclabendazole 10 mg/kg given once (repeated in heavy infections) is the usual treatment. If unavailable, bithionol—an older drug—or nitazoxanide are also effective, or praziquantel can be tried but follow-up stool microscopy is recommended.

ORIENTAL LIVER FLUKE INFECTION

Clonorchis (also *Opisthorchis*) *sinensis*, and *Opisthorchis viverini* are liver flukes found in Asia. They are flat, hermaphroditic worms that have a complex lifecycle. Humans are infected by ingestion of metacercariae under the scales of uncooked freshwater fish. Larvae migrate through the ampulla of Vater to the pancreatic duct or biliary tree, releasing eggs into the bile when mature. Most cases are found in China, Japan, Korea, and Vietnam, where fish rearing and consumption practices contribute to transmission.

Clinical Features

Most patients are asymptomatic but heavy infection can present acutely as anorexia, epigastric pain, and diarrhea with an eosinophilia and, occasionally, jaundice. Helminths in the biliary tract can cause recurrent bouts of ascending cholangitis, jaundice, and pancreatitis. Cholangiocarcinoma is associated with chronic infection and is a public health problem in areas with high prevalence, such as NE Thailand.

Diagnosis

Characteristic operculated eggs are visible on stool microscopy.

Treatment

Praziquantel 25 mg/kg tds (repeated for 2–3 days in heavy infections) is effective.

PARAGONIMIASIS

Paragonimus species, most commonly *P. westermani,* are lung flukes, zoonotic trematodes which can cause respiratory symptoms. The lifecycle is complex, but humans are most commonly infected when eating or handling uncooked crabs or crayfish. The disease is most common in Asia, although foci of disease are found in Africa and the Americas. Local consumption patterns, for example, eating live crabs dipped in rice wine, drive transmission.

Clinical Features

Initial exposure can result in an acute phase (particularly with heavy infections) causing fever, sweats, eosinophilia, and urticarial rash. Lung disease causes a chronic cough, productive of red-brown sputum, often with breathlessness and chest pain. Pleural effusions or empyema may complicate the infection. Ectopic disease can cause CNS pathology.

Investigations

Chest x-rays may demonstrate infiltrates, nodules, cavities, and pleural effusions. It may mimic TB. CT appearances are often diagnostic. Eosinophilia is common and the diagnosis can be confirmed by visualization of the characteristic operculated eggs in sputum, pleural fluid, or stool (because of swallowed eggs). Specialist laboratories offer serologic tests that are sensitive and specific.

Treatment

Praziquantel 25 mg/kg po tds for 3 days is the treatment of choice. Patients usually improve within a few days although radiological improvement can take months. Concomitant steroid therapy is used in CNS disease.

SCHISTOSOMIASIS

The trematodes *Schistosoma haematobium, S. mansoni,* and *S. japonicum* cause schistosomiasis, a globally distributed helminth infection. It has a complex lifecycle with eggs expelled in the stool or urine of humans. Eggs hatch into ciliated miracidia in freshwater and penetrate the body of an appropriate snail intermediate host. Weeks later, a cercariae emerges from the snail, and will penetrate the exposed skin of the human definitive host. The parasite, now named a schistosomulum, migrates via the lungs to the liver, before migrating, sexually paired, to terminal venules, the lower mesenteric veins, to lay eggs in the rectum for *mansoni* and *japonicum*, and the vesicular plexus to lay eggs in the bladder for *haematobium.* There are around 200 million people infected with schistosomiasis worldwide, with approximately 200,000 deaths per year. The distribution is patchy depending on appropriate water sources (with dams causing emerging foci) and intermediate hosts. *Mansoni* is present in Africa and South America, *haematobium* throughout Africa, especially along the major river systems and lakes, and *japonicum* in SE Asia, but no longer in Japan, because of control efforts.

Clinical Features

The trematodes can cause disease at each stage in their migration. Swimmer's or fisherman's itch, an intensely itchy, papular rash, is caused by penetration through the skin, most commonly in migrants or travelers rather than those that dwell in endemic areas. Acute schistosomiasis, also known as Katayama fever, occurs 2 to 6 weeks after exposure, with fever, eosinophilia, malaise, and weight loss. Again it is commoner in travelers. Cough and wheeze as the trematodes migrate through the lungs is often also present. Established infections cause disease according to the species. Established *haematobium* infection causes hematuria and anemia in proportion to the worm and egg burden. An inflammatory response can lead to masses, and an obstructive uropathy. Squamous cell carcinoma can result from long-term infection. Established mansoni or japonicum infection initially causes diarrhea, which may be bloody. However, most of the pathology and morbidity is a result of a granulomatous response to the eggs, which leads to intrahepatic portal vein occlusion, and in turn massive hepatosplenomegaly, bleeding from esophageal varices, and eventually cirrhosis. Ectopic schistosomiasis is where a worm pair accidentally migrates outside of its usual habitat. The most important manifestation of this is in the CNS, where focal neurology may result.

Diagnosis

Direct demonstration of the typically shaped eggs on simple microscopy of stool or urine is diagnostic. As shedding of eggs may be intermittent or low in number in light infections, the yield of microscopy can be increased by repeated examination and concentration methods including sedimentation and filtration of urine. Histologic specimens may be diagnostic, commonly of bladder biopsies performed in returning travelers with hematuria, because of the characteristic histology or visualization of eggs surrounded by granulomas. Serology is diagnostic but is not usually positive until 3 months, so is negative during acute infections. Previous exposure may cause false positives in those living in endemic areas.

Treatment

Praziquantel is the drug of choice, usually given at 40 mg/kg as a stat dose, although some regimes recommend 20 mg/kg with a second dose repeated later. In acute schistosomiasis, the treatment should be repeated after 3 months to eradicate any worms that were immature (and not killed with praziquantel) during the initial dose. Steroids may help with both Katayama fever and neuroschistosomiasis.[54]

Viral Infections

A note on virus classification: There are many ways to classify viruses. Purists will use a taxonomic approach, grouping the viruses into related families such as adenoviruses or herpesviruses based on shared characteristics, most importantly their genomic structure. This overlaps with the well-known Baltimore classification. Clinicians may prefer classifying according to clinical effects such as the viral hemorrhagic fevers (VHFs) or viruses that cause gastroenteritis. Classifying into ecological niche is also useful, with "arboviruses," viruses spread by arthropods (e.g., dengue spread by the *Aedes* mosquito), the best known of these. Here we have used a combination of the classification schemes. Although this may not please purists, and does leave some viruses in overlapping groups from different schemes (e.g., Crimean-Congo hemorrhagic fever could appear in either the arboviruses or VHFs, or a putative entry on nairoviridae), it should be convenient and familiar to the users, and feels appropriate for a field manual where the ease of finding information on a disease outweighs the drive for virologic purity. We have included a taxonomic classification scheme with some major viruses for reference (Table 3.6).

TABLE 3.6 ■ Major Virus Families Causing Human Disease

Virus Family	Genetic Structure	Viruses	Clinical Features	Notes
Adenovirus	dsDNA	Various serotypes	Respiratory disease; conjunctivitis; gastroenteritis	
Hepadnaviridae	DNA; partially ds	Hepatitis B	Acute and chronic hepatitis	
Herpesviridae	ssDNA (+)	Herpes simplex; varicella; cytomegalovirus; Epstein-Barr virus	Oral and genital ulcers; chickenpox and shingles; pneumonia and diarrhea in immunosuppressed; glandular fever and oncovirus	Persistent infection typical
Papoviruses	dsDNA	Papilloma viruses	Warts; cancers including cervical	Vaccination for some serotypes available
		Polyoma viruses e.g., JC virus; BK virus	Nephropathy in transplant patients; progressive multifocal leukoencephalopathy	
Poxviridae	dsDNA	Smallpox, cowpox, orf	Smallpox	Smallpox was the first infectious disease to be eradicated
Arenaviridae	ssRNA (−)	Lassa virus, Junin, Machupo, Guanarito	Various hemorrhagic fevers	Various geographical ranges
Astroviridae	ssRNA (+)	Astrovirus	Gastroenteritis	
Bunyaviridae	ssRNA (−)	Crimean-Congo hemorrhagic fever; hantavirus	Hemorrhagic fever; hemorrhagic fever and pulmonary syndrome	
Calciviridae	ssRNA (+)	Norovirus	Gastroenteritis	Often outbreaks
Coronaviridae	ssRNA (+)	SARS and MERS	(Severe) respiratory illness	Emergent viral diseases in 21st century
Filoviridae	ssRNA (−)	Ebola and Marburg	Hemorrhagic fever	
Flaviridae	ssRNA (+)	Yellow fever, dengue, Zika, West Nile	Arbovirus syndromes: fever-arthralgia-rash, encephalitis, and hemorrhagic fever	
		Hepatitis C	Chronic hepatitis, cirrhosis and hepatocellular carcinoma	
Hepeviridae	ssRNA (+)	Hepatitis E	Hepatitis	
Orthomyxoviridae	ssRNA (−)	Influenza A, B and C	Respiratory illness	Pandemics occur

Continued

TABLE 3.6 ■ Major Virus Families Causing Human Disease—cont.

Virus Family	Genetic Structure	Viruses	Clinical Features	Notes
Paromyxo-viridae	ssRNA (–)	Measles; mumps; RSV and parain-fluenza viruses	Rash, coryza, and fever; parotitis and orchitis; respiratory illness esp. children	
Picornaviri-dae	ssRNA (+)	Polio	Acute flaccid paralysis	Global eradica-tion possible
		Rhinovirus	Mild respiratory illness	Cause of the common cold
		Coxsackie and echovirus	Febrile illness, gastro-intestinal illness, and myocarditis	
		Hepatitis A	Diarrhea and hepatitis	
Rhabdoviri-dae	ssRNA (–)	Rabies	Characteristic fatal encephalitis	
Reoviridae	dsDNA	Rotavirus	Gastroenteritis	Especially children
Retroviridae	ssRNA (ret-rovirus)	HIV-1 and HIV-2; HTLV-1 and HTLV-2	Immunodeficiency and opportunistic infection; tropical spastic para-paresis	
Togaviridae	ssDNA (+)	Alphaviruses, e.g., Ross river, equine encephalovi-ruses, sindbis virus	Arboviruses causing fever-arthralgia-rash or encephalitis	
		Rubella	Rash and fever	Infection during pregnancy can cause fetal abnormalities

(–), Negative sense; (+), positive sense; *BK,*; *ds,* double stranded; *HIV,* human immunodeficiency virus; *HTLV,* human T-lymphotropic virus 1; *JC,*; *MERS,* Middle East respiratory syndrome; *RSV,* respiratory syncytial virus; *SARS,* severe acute respiratory syndrome; *ss,* single-stranded.

ARTHROPOD-BORNE VIRAL DISEASES (ARBOVIRUSES)

"Arbovirus" is an ecological classification and covers viruses spread by an arthropod vector. Arthropods include the insects, in this context the most important of which are the mosquitoes, as well as ticks. There are over 500 arboviruses, from four viral groups, some of which have a large endemic range and are medically important, such as dengue fever, and some of which have a small geographic range and are of limited importance (such as Barmah Forest virus, limited to some forested areas of Australia). Clinically, arboviral diseases present as one of three clinical syndromes: (1) fevers of an undifferentiated type with or without a maculopapular rash, usually known as fever-arthralgia-rash (FAR); (2) encephalitis, often with a high case fatality rate; and

(3) hemorrhagic fevers, also frequently severe and fatal. Arboviruses may be associated with more than one syndrome (e.g., dengue), and the presentation can depend on host age, immunity, and comorbidities. Intensity of viral burden and predominant tissue involvement can vary significantly, and individual arboviruses can result in a mild illness in one case, with profound illness in another. Malaise, headache, nausea, vomiting, and myalgia frequently accompany fever, which is an invariable symptom and sometimes the only one. The illness may stop at this stage, recur with or without a rash, or reveal hemorrhagic manifestations secondary to vascular abnormalities; in epidemics, however, one clinical picture usually predominates. We will only consider the most important arboviruses here, although readers are encouraged to understand their own local epidemiology, and suspect an arboviral infection in people presenting from an endemic area with FAR, encephalitis, or a hemorrhagic fever.

DENGUE FEVER

Dengue fever is a flavivirus transmitted by the *Aedes aegypti* mosquito, largely in urban settings, across the globe (Fig. 3.12). The mosquito breeds in standing water, typically in artificial water containers around the home, and bites during the day. It has a wide geographic range, with hyperendemicity in many areas of SE Asia, and is present widely in the Americas, Africa, and Oceania, including the Caribbean and India. Climate change may be responsible for dengue encroaching into southern Europe. There are an estimated 40 million symptomatic cases per year. Dengue has four serotypes, all of which cause disease. Interestingly, infection with one serotype is not only not protective of infection from another serotype, but increases the risk of severe dengue. The widely accepted antibody-dependent enhancement hypothesis posits that neutralizing antibodies produced in response to the first serotype infection bind to the new serotype virions, increasing uptake into blood monocyte and tissue macrophages, enhancing viral replication, and leading to a higher viral load and thus severity. Dengue outbreaks occur when populations previously are nely exposed to a serotype. This may be as vector numbers increase, for example, after flooding.

Clinical Features

Dengue infection presents with a spectrum of illness, from asymptomatic or subclinical illness (especially in younger children) to dengue fever and severe dengue fever. The WHO classification has dispensed with a previous division between dengue fever, dengue shock syndrome, and dengue hemorrhagic fever, and now categorizes clinical dengue into dengue fever (which can be with or without warning signs) and severe dengue fever. Warning signs include abdominal pain, persistent vomiting, fluid accumulation, mucosal bleeding, lethargy, an increase in hematocrit with decrease in platelet count, and an enlarged liver. Severe dengue is characterized by severe plasma leakage leading to shock or fluid accumulation and respiratory compromise; or severe hemorrhage; or severe organ involvement with impaired consciousness, AST greater than 1000, or other organ dysfunction.

Generally, dengue fever follows three phases in its course. Some 4 to 7 days after being bitten by an infected mosquito, the febrile phase begins. Sudden-onset high fever, backache, myalgia, arthralgia, and malaise are typical. There may be a transient macular rash, sore throat, nausea, and vomiting. Most patients will recover as they defervesce after some 3 to 7 days but some, especially those with comorbidities, previous dengue fever, or the elderly, may progress to the critical phase. This is characterized by an increase in capillary permeability resulting in pleural effusions, ascites, and a decrease in circulating plasma volume leading to hypotension and shock. Visceral pain is common. The hematocrit rises with hemoconcentration and the platelets fall, often as low as 20×10^9/L. Hemorrhagic manifestations are common, including petechiae, bruising, and mucosal bleeding, with GI and other significant bleeding more likely to occur in the elderly. Some 24 to 48 hours after onset of the critical phase, patients usually enter the recovery

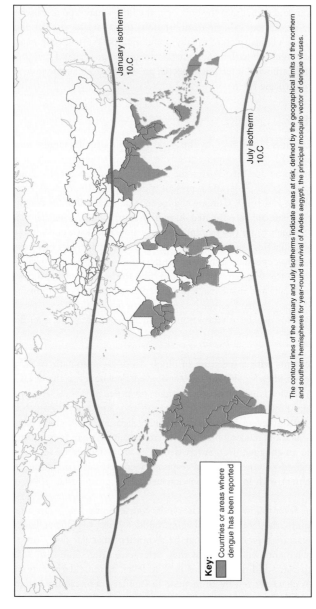

Fig. 3.12 Map of dengue distribution. (From Nabarro L, Morris-Jones S, Moore DAJ. Arthropod-borne diseases. In: Nabarro L, Morris-Jones S, Moore DAJ, eds. *Peters' Atlas of Tropical Medicine and Parasitology*. 7th ed. London, UK: Elsevier Ltd; 2019:1–108.)

January isotherm
10.C

July isotherm
10.C

The contour lines of the January and July isotherms indicate areas at risk, defined by the geographical limits of the northern and southern hemispheres for year-round survival of *Aedes aegypti*, the principal mosquito vector of dengue viruses.

Key:
Countries or areas where dengue has been reported

phase. Capillary permeability returns to normal, fluid is resorbed, and shock and coagulopathy resolve. This is often accompanied by a vivid erythematous blanching rash which may resolve with desquamation.

Diagnosis

Early in the illness (first 5 days) diagnosis is via real-time (RT)-PCR, or antigen detection methods, including detection of nonstructural protein 1 (NS1). However, post day 5, serologic methods, including ELISAs for IgM, and then IgG, are required. There can be cross-reaction with other flaviviruses (such as yellow fever, including vaccination, West Nile virus, and Zika), so a single result in a patient resident in an area endemic with other flaviviruses should be treated with caution. Demonstration of rising titers is more specific, but the illness may have subsided by this point. RDTs for dengue are available that identify NS1, IgM/IgG, or a combination, which are sensitive and specific and can be used at the patient bedside, so are useful in outbreaks and epidemics. However, there are cost and storage issues, and tests based on single detection may not be positive throughout the disease course. Thrombocytopenia and leukopenia are common, as is mildly elevated liver enzymes.

Treatment

Most cases of dengue fever, even those with severe dengue fever, will self-resolve and make a full recovery. There are no specific therapeutic agents for dengue. Treatment should focus on good supportive care, including temperature control, analgesia, and repeated assessment. Fluid management is crucial in severe dengue, as increased capillary permeability leads to loss of circulating plasma volume, but overreplacing this can worsen edema. Crystalloid fluids should be given judiciously to maintain circulating volume and reverse shock, but beware of fluid overload. Blood product replacement may be needed in severe dengue syndrome, and although thrombocytopenia is common, generally platelet replacement should be limited to those who are also actively bleeding.[55]

YELLOW FEVER

Yellow fever is caused by a flavivirus and is transmitted by mosquitoes in two cycles: a jungle cycle involving a monkey reservoir and canopy-dwelling mosquitoes where it is a zoonosis; and an urban cycle involving person-to-person transmission, typically by *Aedes aegypti*. Historically, yellow fever is of huge public health and economic importance, contributing to the failure of the French efforts to build the Panama canal and causing epidemics throughout the globe, such as those recorded amongst colonial settlers in the Caribbean and Americas. Global control efforts following development of a vaccine reduced its importance throughout the 20th century but various changes, including urbanization in many areas of Africa and the Americas, has resulted in an upsurge in cases more recently with perhaps 200,000 cases and 30,000 deaths per year across 47 countries. Large outbreaks in Brazil and the DRC were seen in 2017, and unvaccinated travelers remain at risk (Fig. 3.13).

Clinical Features

Most cases are mild, with only 1 in 20 infections resulting in the classic picture of jaundice that gives this flavivirus its name. After an incubation period of 3 to 5 days, disease manifests with sudden fever, chills, headache, backache, myalgia, nausea, vomiting, and often prostration. A relative bradycardia, Faget's sign, and conjunctivitis may be present. In severe disease, yellow fever is biphasic and a temporary remission may occur before progressive liver failure develops resulting in jaundice, coagulopathy, metabolic acidosis, renal failure, coma, and death. Where jaundice develops the prognosis is poor with a 50% fatality rate.

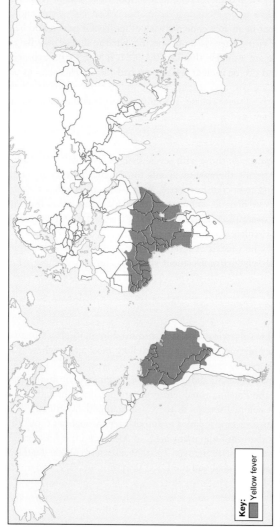

Key:
■ Yellow fever

Fig. 3.13 Map of yellow fever distribution. (From Nabarro L, Morris-Jones S, Moore DAJ. Arthropod-borne diseases. In: Nabarro L, Morris-Jones S, Moore DAJ, eds. *Peters' Atlas of Tropical Medicine and Parasitology.* 7th ed. London, UK: Elsevier Ltd; 2019:1–108.)

Diagnosis

Although PCR is positive in the early stages, it is not widely available. Serology becomes positive late in the disease, but beware of cross-reactions with other flaviviruses. Diagnosing on clinical grounds can be difficult, especially early in the disease, so close attention to epidemiologic exposure is warranted. In the latter stages, leukopenia or thrombocytopenia with renal and hepatic dysfunction may provide clues, although acute viral hepatitis, severe leptospirosis, severe dengue fever, and the VHFs may all present in a similar fashion.

Treatment

Treatment is supportive with no specific therapy available. Close monitoring and intensive care including organ support such as dialysis may be required. The vaccine is effective and should be given to those traveling to endemic areas, or may be used in response to an outbreak. It is a live viral vaccine and has some contraindications including extremes of age, pregnancy, and immunosuppression, although these may be relative in the context of an epidemic.[56,57]

ZIKA VIRUS INFECTION

Zika virus is a flavivirus spread by *Aedes* mosquitoes. It was first described in 1947 in the Zika forest in Uganda and remained an obscure arbovirus until the recent outbreaks in Oceania in 2013–2014, and then in the Americas from 2015 onwards. Currently Zika is widespread in parts of Central America and the Caribbean and Oceania, and foci exist in SE Asia, South Asia, and parts of Africa. Part of the recent increase in distribution may be because of an increase in awareness and testing. Up-to-date epidemiologic information can be found from the Public Health England and Centers for Disease Control websites, and elsewhere.

Clinical Features

After a short incubation period of 3 to 12 days, Zika causes a typical arbovirus syndrome with fever, rash, headache, and myalgia. It is benign and usually self-limiting. However, rarely it may trigger Guillain-Barré syndrome, and when acquired by pregnant women there is a risk of microcephaly. Data on the precise risks of these is accumulating with the current unprecedented outbreaks.

Diagnosis

PCR is diagnostic early in disease, and serology will become positive later. However, interpretation, particularly of unpaired samples, can be hampered by cross-reaction with other flavivirus serology.

Treatment/Advice

There is no specific treatment for Zika infection. Symptomatic care will suffice, and the disease is self-limiting. Potential exposure to Zika for pregnant women, or men or women who are hoping to conceive, is more problematic. Zika has been detected in semen for many weeks after infection, and sexual transmission is well reported. Relevant national guidelines should be consulted.[58-60]

CHIKUNGUNYA VIRUS INFECTION

Chikungunya is an alphavirus spread by the day-biting *Aedes* mosquito. Epidemics occur in urban areas, during the rainy season in particular. The disease has a wide geographic distribution, which may become even wider if climate change increases the distribution of the *Aedes* vector. South America, Africa, southern and SE Asia, including China, the Caribbean, and even southern Europe have all seen transmission. A recent outbreak caused over 1.4 million cases in India, the Indian Ocean islands, and Kenya.

Clinical Features

The incubation period is usually short, typically 2 to 4 days, followed by fever and arthralgia. Rash, often maculopapular, follows in 50% a few days later. The arthralgia is particularly pronounced, and often affects the small joints of the hands and feet. This may last months, and as it is often associated with effusions patients are frequently investigated for an inflammatory arthropathy.

Diagnosis

PCR is diagnostic during the first week, when there is a viremia. Subsequently, antibodies are detectable.

Treatment

No specific treatment is required and the illness is self-limiting. Diagnosis is helpful in those with arthropathy, to prevent extended investigation for other causes. Prevention by bite avoidance or vector control is the key to preventing or terminating outbreaks.

SANDFLY FEVER VIRUS INFECTION

Sandfly fever or Pappataci fever is caused by several bunyaviruses of the *Phlebovirus* genus. It is present in the Mediterranean region but also east into India, Pakistan, Afghanistan, and southern Russia. After a 2- to 6-day incubation period it causes fever and headache, often associated with photophobia. It is self-limiting and no deaths have been reported.

COLORADO TICK FEVER

Colorado tick fever is caused by a *Coltivirus* (Order: *Reoviridae*), which is transmitted from an animal reservoir, including rodents and deer, to humans by a variety of ticks, the most important of which is *Dermacentor andersoni*. It is found in the western and northwestern parts of North America, with cases peaking in May to July.

Clinical Features

The incubation period is 4 to 6 days and disease presents with sudden-onset chills, fever, and myalgia. Headache and backpain are common, but only 1 in 8 will develop a rash. The disease usually lasts 10 to 14 days. Meningism, coagulopathy, and myocarditis all occur occasionally. There may be a biphasic "saddleback" fever pattern.

Diagnosis

Diagnosis is by antigen or PCR detection early in the disease, with antibody detection useful in the second week.

Treatment

No specific therapy is available and treatment is supportive.

JAPANESE ENCEPHALITIS

Japanese encephalitis is a flavivirus with a distribution across rural areas of Asia, including India, the Pacific, and Nepal (Fig. 3.14). The reservoir hosts are water birds, typically found in paddy fields, and the disease in spread to humans by *Culex* mosquitoes. Pigs act as an amplifying host peridomestically. Children are most commonly affected, and in temperate areas the disease is seasonal. There are an estimated 50,000 to 70,000 cases of encephalitis per year.

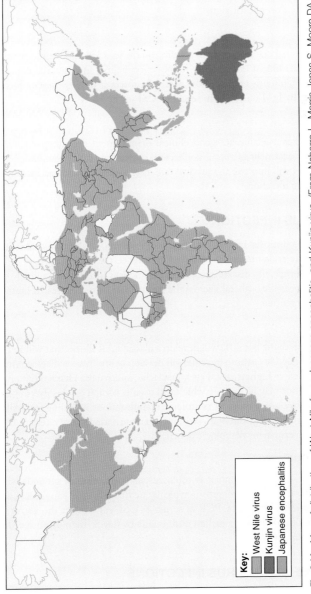

Fig. 3.14 Map of distribution of West Nile fever, Japanese encephalitis, and Kunjin virus. (From Nabarro L, Morris-Jones S, Moore DAJ. Arthropod-borne diseases. In: Nabarro L, Morris-Jones S, Moore DAJ, eds. *Peters' Atlas of Tropical Medicine and Parasitology.* 7th ed. London, UK: Elsevier Ltd; 2019:1–108.)

Key:
West Nile virus
Kunjin virus
Japanese encephalitis

Clinical Features

Most infections are not symptomatic. Following a 6- to 16-day incubation period there is usually a prodromal illness with high fever, headache, cough, and nausea. Patients may then develop neurologic symptoms including seizures, and a reduced consciousness level. Parkinsonian features, cranial nerve palsies, and acute flaccid paralysis may also occur. Prolonged convulsions and respiratory depression are poor prognostic signs.

Diagnosis

There is a wide differential diagnosis that, depending on the location, may include cerebral malaria, other arboviruses presenting as encephalitis, herpes encephalitis, and bacterial meningoencephalitis. A lymphocytic meningitis with a mildly elevated protein is usually present. Definitive diagnosis is usually made by IgM detection in serum or CSF, or by PCR.

Treatment

No specific treatment is available but good clinical management including nutritional support, seizure management, treatment of secondary bacterial infection (e.g., pneumonia), and management of pressure areas will improve the survival rate. Bite avoidance and vaccination are effective methods of preventing infection.[61]

WEST NILE VIRUS INFECTION

West Nile virus is a zoonotic flavivirus with a wild bird reservoir. It is transmitted to man by *Culex* mosquitoes. Previously endemic in the Middle East (hence the name), parts of Africa, eastern Asia, and southern Europe, the disease spread to the Americas in 1999 attributed to a confluence of factors and causes periodic outbreaks across the continental United States, in southern Canada, and as far south as Argentina.

Clinical Features

Most cases are asymptomatic but 20% will develop a classic FAR illness that will self-resolve in 3 to 6 days. Approximately 1% of those infected will develop neuroinvasive disease, with the elderly and immunosuppressed at highest risk. Fever, headache, and nausea characterizes neuroinvasive disease. Meningitis alone may be present, which will usually completely resolve, but in those with encephalitis, which can cause a range of neurologic manifestations including acute flaccid paralysis, parkinsonism, radiculopathy, and brain stem involvement, case fatality rates are 10% and up to half may be left with permanent neurologic deficit.

Diagnosis and Treatment

The differential diagnosis is wide, but it is often suspected on clinical grounds where there is known epidemiologic risk. The meningitis is typically neutrophilic early in disease and lymphocytic later. Confirmation is usually by PCR of serum or CSF early in the disease, or detection of antibodies by ELISA. IgM develops earliest and usually by day 8. There is no specific treatment and management is supportive.[62]

NEUROINVASIVE ALPHAVIRUS INFECTIONS

Neuroinvasive alphavirus infections such as eastern equine encephalitis, western equine encephalitis, and Venezuelan equine encephalitis are zoonotic infections of the Americas transmitted by mosquitoes. Most infections are subclinical. Some patients develop a fever-arthralgia syndrome and a few sufferers (generally a few percent of adults and slightly higher percentage of children) will develop encephalitis. Diagnosis is serologic and treatment supportive.

TICK-BORNE ENCEPHALITIS

Tick-borne encephalitis is a flavivirus that causes hundreds of thousands of cases in a belt of temperate countries across the Eurasian continent from the Baltics and Eastern Europe, over the Urals and across Russia to China and Japan. The disease is transmitted by ticks, with cases peaking from April to November. Most patients have a subclinical infection, although when it does cause disease it is usually biphasic. An influenza-like febrile illness for 2 to 7 days is followed by an afebrile (often asymptomatic) phase, and one-third of patients will go on to develop meningoencephalitis with high fevers. The Far Eastern subtype is more likely to cause permanent paralysis and death than the European subtype. Diagnosis is usually made by rising titers of IgM, although PCR is increasingly used. Note there is often serologic cross-reactivity with other flaviviruses. Treatment is supportive only. An effective vaccine is available.

HUMAN IMMUNODEFICIENCY VIRUS

See Chapter 6.

VIRAL HEMORRHAGIC FEVERS

The VHFs are a diverse group of zoonotic viruses, grouped clinically, which cause fever, and may cause hemorrhage. They come from four different viral groups, arenaviridae, filoviridae, bunyaviridae, and flaviviridae. They are transmitted in a number of ways, including via arthropod vectors, from animal feces and urine, and from exposure to contaminated bush meat, and cause hemorrhage to a greater or lesser extent by a range of pathological mechanisms. Despite their diversity, they are united by the fear they provoke in the population at large, and in healthcare workers particularly, because of the possibility of person-person spread by contaminated body fluids, typically blood, and the high reported case fatality rates. However, the importance of person-person spread, and fatality rate can vary widely according to the context, virus, and host factors.

EBOLA VIRUS DISEASE

Ebola is a filovirus, a large enveloped RNA virus with a bat reservoir, and is present in various forested areas of Central Africa. Bats infect primates causing massive die off of chimpanzees, gorillas, and other species, which often precedes human outbreaks. The index case is usually a hunter, often in a remote, rural area, who is exposed to disease from contaminated blood from a primate. Person-to-person transmission is by contaminated body fluids, especially blood and diarrhea. Transmission while caring for sick relatives, burial practices, and nosocomial infection are important in spreading disease. Outbreaks have varied in size but were generally limited to tens or at worst, hundreds of cases until the West African outbreak, which started in 2014 and caused over 25,000 cases and 10,000 deaths, predominantly in Sierra Leone, Liberia, and Guinea. There were widespread economic consequences and disruption to health care in some of the poorest countries in the world, which resulted in more deaths from HIV, TB, and malaria than from Ebola. A wide-ranging global health response along with local efforts was required to terminate the outbreak.

Clinical Features

After a short incubation period, typically of 4 to 8 days, patients develop a high fever often accompanied by sore throat, myalgia, severe malaise, and conjunctival injection. It can be difficult to distinguish between this and other endemic infections including malaria. Nausea, vomiting, and profuse diarrhea are common, and can lead to dehydration, electrolyte disturbance, and hypotension, as well as putting staff at risk of nosocomial infection. The illness usually lasts some 7 to

14 days. A proportion of patients will go on to develop multiorgan failure, with renal failure, liver impairment, and coagulopathy common. Petechiae, bleeding from the gums, GI bleeding, and other hemorrhagic features occur in around 25%. CNS features such as encephalitis are usually preterminal.

Diagnosis

Diagnosis is usually confirmed by RT-PCR of blood or urine. Early disease has a wide differential diagnosis, including malaria and dengue fever. Care should be taken as occasionally PCR can be negative in the first 48 hours of symptoms, and so PCR testing may need to be repeated after this time. The diagnosis should be considered in febrile patients with a negative malaria test in endemic areas, especially where there are risk factors such as bush meat exposure, an ongoing outbreak, potential nosocomial infection, or specific clinical features including hemorrhage. Many countries provide guidance on when and how to screen returning travelers.

Treatment

Supportive care including good fluid management, monitoring electrolytes, correcting coagulopathy, and nutritional support is likely to reduce mortality. Barrier infection control precautions should be mandated to prevent spread of disease to healthcare workers and other patients. Gloves, aprons, and eye protection are all advocated and detailed guidance is available. Technological solutions including plastic isolators through which patients can be nursed have been used for transport of patients and treatment in developed healthcare settings, but are not practical in an outbreak situation. The 2014 outbreak provided an impetus to developing an evidence base for specific antiviral treatment, although many trials were either unable to fully recruit or used a historical control. ZMapp, a mixture of three monoclonal antibodies against Ebola, remains the most promising treatment, having an observed posterior probability of 90% of being superior to supportive care alone. Brincidofovir, TKM-Ebola, and plasma exchange are all likely not to be effective. An effective Ebola vaccine is available, and ring vaccination of contacts prevents disease and should contribute to the public health response in future. Case fatality rates vary from 60% to 90%, perhaps lower with high-quality supportive care and access to effective antivirals.[63–65]

MARBURG VIRUS INFECTION

Less is known about Marburg virus than its closely related filovirus cousin, Ebola, largely because there have been fewer cases. Similarly, it is a zoonosis with a bat reservoir, which causes cases in humans when exposed to bush meat. It is found in the forested regions of eastern Africa, although cases in Angola in 2005 mean the geographic extent may be throughout sub-Saharan Africa. It produces a clinical disease that is virtually identical to Ebola (see Ebola Clinical Features), and diagnosis is likewise by RT-PCR. It is unknown if specific antiviral measures against Ebola will have cross-effectiveness for Marburg, but the emphasis on meticulous barrier infection control and supportive care with fluid and electrolyte management should remain.

LASSA FEVER

Lassa fever is a zoonotic arenavirus with a small rodent reservoir (*Mastomys natalensis*) and is present in West Africa with cases largely seen in rural Nigeria, Sierra Leone, and Guinea. Lassa is transmitted through direct contact with rodents or aerosolized contaminated urine or feces. There are perhaps 5000 deaths per year but many more clinical cases (perhaps 150,000) and between 300,000 to 500,000 total infections, as most are asymptomatic or subclinical.

Clinical Features

After an incubation period of 7 to 21 days (slightly longer than many other VHFs), Lassa presents with fever, frontal headache, and malaise. A sore throat with pharyngitis is very common, and conjunctival injection and retrosternal chest pain may also help point the alert clinician specifically to Lassa fever. One-third of patients will worsen, become bed-bound, and develop diarrhea and vomiting. Facial and laryngeal edema may also develop. Bleeding manifestations tend to be mild, limited to mucosal surfaces and the GI tract. They and CNS manifestations are poor prognostic signs. Deafness affects nearly one-third of severely affected patients, particularly during convalescence, and may be permanent.

Diagnosis

As with other arenaviruses and VHFs, diagnosis is by PCR early in the disease, or serologic testing later. The differential diagnosis, especially of early disease, is wide, and many cases go undiagnosed.

Treatment

Ribavirin is effective. The earlier it is given the better, and it has been seen to decrease mortality 5 to 10 times when given in the first 6 days of illness. This means it may need to be given empirically. A 2 g IV loading dose is recommended, followed by 1 g qds for 4 days then 500 mg tds for a further 6 days to complete the course. To prevent nosocomial transmission, thorough barrier precautions, including use of aprons, gloves, eye protection, and ideally isolation, are recommended although these can be difficult to enact in some healthcare settings.[66]

OTHER HEMORRHAGIC ARENAVIRUSES

There are a number of other (non-Lassa) arenaviruses including Junin, Machupo, and Guanarito viruses causing Argentine, Bolivian, and Venezuelan hemorrhagic fevers, respectively. These have rodent reservoir hosts, occur over a limited area, typically in epidemics, and person-person transmission is either rare or unreported.

CRIMEAN-CONGO HEMORRHAGIC FEVER

The Crimean-Congo hemorrhagic fever is caused by a bunyavirus of the genus *Nairovirus*. It is found in the Balkans, Middle East, Turkey, western China, and tropical and southern Africa (Fig. 3.15). Many animals can act as a reservoir, including small mammals and livestock. It is transmitted by bite of *Hyalomma* tick most often, but exposure to animal blood during, for example, butchering, crushing ticks, or nosocomial infection all cause disease. Thus farmers, abattoir workers, and healthcare workers are most at risk.

Clinical Features

After an incubation period of 3 to 7 days patients present with abrupt fever, backache, arthralgia, and headache. Vomiting, diarrhea, and abdominal pain may occur. The abdominal pain often mimics an acute abdomen, potentially leading to exposure of the surgical team. Hemorrhagic manifestations are more common than in many other VHFs, with petechiae and ecchymoses common and often extensive. Severe cases develop gum bleeding, epistaxis, and GI and genitourinary tract bleeding. Mortality is 5% to 40%.

Diagnosis

Thrombocytopenia and leucopenia are common. Disease can be confirmed by PCR testing of blood, or by detection of rising Crimean-Congo hemorrhagic fever serologic titers.

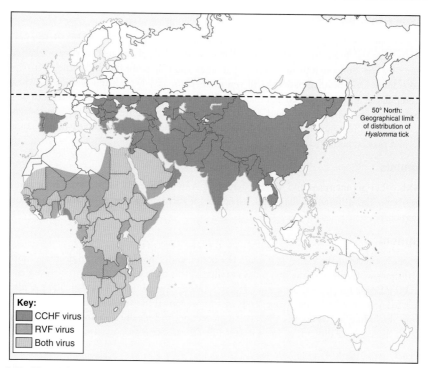

Fig. 3.15 Map of Crimean-Congo hemorrhagic fever (*CCHF*) and Rift Valley hemorrhagic fever (*RVF*). (From Nabarro L, Morris-Jones S, Moore DAJ. Arthropod-borne diseases. In: Nabarro L, Morris-Jones S, Moore DAJ, eds. *Peters' Atlas of Tropical Medicine and Parasitology.* 7th ed. London, UK: Elsevier Ltd; 2019:1–108.)

Treatment

Principles of care include good supportive management, with fluid and electrolyte balance crucial, avoiding nonsteroidal antiinflammatory drugs (NSAIDs) or other drugs that might cause bleeding and preventing nosocomial infection with high-quality barrier nursing. Ribavirin is commonly used to treat Crimean-Congo hemorrhagic fever, although the evidence is not completely clear cut. Oral ribavirin, with a 30 mg/kg loading dose followed by 15 mg/kg qds for 4 days and 7.5 mg/kg tds for 6 days, was the most used dosage in trials.[67]

RIFT VALLEY FEVER

Rift Valley fever is caused by a bunyavirus of the genus *Phlebovirus.* It is predominantly a disease of livestock, with transmission from animal to animal by mosquitoes. Most human infection is from exposure of broken skin to infected animal tissue (e.g., butchering animals and veterinary procedures), although mosquito transmission does occur. There is no reported human-human transmission. As the name suggests it is present in the Rift Valley in Africa, with major outbreaks reported in Kenya, Tanzania, and Egypt. In 2000 it spread to Saudi Arabia and Yemen.

Clinical Features

After a short incubation period of 3 to 6 days, patients develop a febrile illness with headache and arthralgia. Small hemorrhages may be seen on the mucosal membranes and conjunctival injection is common. There may be some features of meningism but for most (>95%) of patients the disease is mild and will self-resolve in a week at most. A few percent of sufferers will develop a more severe form involving hemorrhage, often with DIC and liver and renal impairment, and a high mortality; encephalitis, which may begin after recovery from the initial febrile illness and can result in death; or eye disease which can include macular edema and retinal hemorrhage and may cause permanent loss of vision in up to 50%.

Diagnosis and Treatment

Rift Valley fever is usually diagnosed by PCR or serology. Treatment is supportive with no specific therapy although a vaccine is available (noncommercially) for protection of high-risk individuals. Although person-person transmission has not been reported, barrier precautions are prudent (especially before confirmation of Rift Valley fever as the cause of a hemorrhagic fever).[68]

HANTAVIRUS INFECTIONS

There are four bunyaviruses of the genus *Hantavirus* causing hemorrhagic fever with renal syndrome (HFRS). Hanta virus causes epidemics in the Far East and was first described near the Korean peninsula demilitarized zone. Seoul virus is also present on the Korean peninsula but causes a milder disease more widely including in Europe (and likely wherever *Rattus norvegicus*, the brown rat, is found). Dobrava virus causes a severe HFRS in the Balkans and Puumala virus is present in Scandinavia with a renal predominance. All are zoonoses with a rodent reservoir and humans are infected by aerosolized rodent excreta.

After a 12- to 16-day incubation period, but occasionally longer, disease classically occurs in five phases. A febrile phase, which typically lasts 3 to 7 days and may be accompanied by petechiae and conjunctival hemorrhage, is followed by a hypotensive phase lasting a few hours to days, characterized by shock, and nausea and vomiting, and is responsible for one-third of fatalities. This is followed by an oliguric phase lasting 3 to 7 days associated with anuria and often hemorrhage. Recovery begins with a diuretic phase, followed by a (often prolonged) convalescent phase. PCR and serologic tests are used to confirm the diagnosis. Treatment is supportive, with an emphasis on careful fluid management and renal replacement therapy if required. Severe disease should be treated with ribavirin.

HANTAVIRUS PULMONARY SYNDROME

Hantavirus pulmonary syndrome, although it does not cause hemorrhagic manifestations, is discussed in this section. Caused by hantaviruses in the Americas, of which *Sin nombre* virus was the first and most famously identified, it is a zoonotic disease transmitted by aerosolized excreta from the rodent host. Clinically it causes a prodromal febrile illness of 3 to 6 days followed by cardiogenic shock and ARDS. There is usually thrombocytopenia and hemoconcentration. Treatment is supportive, with two-thirds of patients requiring intubation.[69]

POLIOMYELITIS

Control of polio is one of the success stories of modern medicine and global public health, with a WHO-organized campaign reducing cases from 350,000 cases of paralytic polio in 1988 to just 21 in 2017. The disease is caused by an enterovirus that is usually transmitted fecoorally after contamination of water supplies with feces from infected individuals, most of whom do not have paralysis. Wild type polio is endemic only in Afghanistan and Pakistan, where barriers to immunization remain the greatest hurdle to eliminating the disease. There have been no cases in Nigeria since August 2016, although virus can still be found in the environment there. Circulating vaccine-derived polio virus (cVDPV), where the live oral polio vaccine has been able to circulate in the environment and has mutated and so able to cause disease, remains a potential problem in areas of low vaccine uptake, where the live oral vaccine is used and sanitation poor. This is the case in parts of Nigeria and Syria, where these conditions coexist with civil strife and there have been recent clinical cases of paralysis caused by cVDPV.

Clinical Features

Accidental ingestion of virus leads to multiplication in the gut, then viremia, and later CNS invasion affecting the motor neurons. This leads to flaccid paralysis, particularly of lower extremities. Incubation is 3 to 35 days, with most cases occurring 7 to 14 days after exposure. Most infected individuals are asymptomatic with only 1% of cases developing paralysis, but a minor illness with fever, malaise, headache, nausea, and vomiting may occur in all infected individuals. When flaccid paralysis develops it is usually asymmetrical, with a paralysis of one leg most common in those under 5 years. Polio can involve muscles of swallowing and respiration, which drives the mortality of 2% to 10% in paralytic cases, with mortality and extent of paralysis increasing with age. Recovery of muscle function is often slow and incomplete.

Diagnosis

Diagnosis is usually clinical based on characteristic features, although other neurologic causes must be carefully ruled out. PCR confirms the diagnosis.

Treatment

There is no specific treatment. The acute stage should be carefully managed, observing for paralytic complications including bulbar and respiratory involvement. Physiotherapy will help return to function in survivors. Cases should be reported to WHO officials so control measures can be initiated. Vaccination prevents disease and is the mainstay of global eradication efforts.

A useful website with up-to-date data and analysis of the push for polio eradication is http://polioeradication.org.

HTLV-1 AND HTLV-2 INFECTIONS

HTLV-1 and HTLV-2 are retroviruses with a worldwide distribution. They are not as well known as their retrovirus cousin HIV, which was briefly termed HTLV-3 when first discovered. Humans may be infected by vertical transmission, sexual transmission, and through contaminated blood and blood products. Exposure leads to life-long infection as their RNA is transcribed into DNA and inserted into T-cell chromosomes. Globally, around 20 million people are infected. HTLV-1 is common in southern Japan, with 10% prevalence. There are foci in the Caribbean, Africa (particularly Gabon and Cameroon), and Oceania. HTLV-2 is largely confined to indigenous Americans and Central African pygmy tribes. There are a number of important pathologies associated with HTL-1 and HTLV-2. HTLV-1 is an oncovirus that can cause an aggressive leukemia, adult T-cell leukemia. HTLV-associated myelopathy, known as tropical spastic paraparesis, is a chronic condition causing spastic weakness of the legs, sensory problems, and bowel and bladder dysfunction. HTLV-1 infection should be demonstrated and other causes such as B12 deficiency, spinal cord compression, and demyelination should be ruled out. Infective dermatitis is a chronic dermatitis commoner in children. HTLV-1 is also associated with increased rates of a number of infections including TB, strongyloidiasis, and scabies. HTLV-2 is thought to be less pathogenic but it has been linked to tropical spastic paraparesis, arthritis, and pneumonia. Diagnosis of HTLV infection is serologic. No specific treatments are available for HTLV although various treatments have been used for the complications. The focus is generally on prevention, such as by screening blood supplies.

VIRAL HEPATITIDES

There are five hepatitis viruses lettered A to E. These are unrelated but all are hepatotropic and cause hepatitis. Hepatitis A and E are fecoorally transmitted and can cause a diarrhea, as well as hepatitis. Hepatitis B and C are spread by body fluids, can cause an acute hepatitis (rarely for hepatitis C), but more commonly cause chronic infection leading to cirrhosis and liver cancer years later. Hepatitis D only causes hepatitis in the context of hepatitis B infection. All except hepatitis D are briefly considered here.

HEPATITIS A INFECTION

Hepatitis A is a single-stranded RNA virus that is common in the tropics, and is transmitted fecoorally. In areas where it is highly endemic, children are usually infected, and the major clinical manifestation is diarrheal illness that self-resolves. When adults are infected, commonly travelers from nonendemic areas, there is a risk of hepatitis, which usually develops after a 2- to 6-week incubation period. There is a risk of fulminant hepatitis, and death, which increases with age. Diagnosis is usually serologic with hepatitis A IgM detectable by the onset of symptoms. Care is supportive but there is an effective vaccine available, and improving sanitation will prevent the disease on a population basis. Outbreaks may also occur in areas with good sanitation, usually from an infected food handler or in vulnerable populations, for example, the California outbreak in 2017 that largely affected the homeless.

HEPATITIS B INFECTION

Hepatitis B is an encapsulated DNA virus that is globally widespread. It is transmitted by body fluids, with sexual transmission, injecting drug use, and iatrogenic spread including tattooing and piercing important. In developing-world settings, transmission is in childhood from close contact. The disease is globally widespread with 240 million people currently infected with chronic hepatitis B, and 780,000 deaths annually. Rates are highest in sub-Saharan Africa and East Asia, with other foci in the Artic region and the Amazon.

Clinical Features

The incubation period for hepatitis B is 1 to 6 months. Most people will be asymptomatic during early infection but a few will develop an acute hepatitis. This generally resolves without treatment, although rarely it develops into a life-threatening fulminant hepatitis. The course then depends on what age it was acquired: younger children are likely to develop chronic hepatitis B (80%–90% of infants) with adults much more likely to clear the virus (approximately 5% will develop chronic disease). The disease will be asymptomatic for decades generally, with perhaps the odd flair of hepatitis causing a raised alanine aminotransferase (ALT) ± jaundice, before a proportion will develop cirrhosis, liver failure, and occasionally hepatocellular carcinoma.

Diagnosis

Diagnosis is usually serologic, with the hepatitis B surface antigen (HBsAg) a marker of infection, and chronic infection defined by persistence of HBsAg for more than 6 months.

Treatment

Making decisions about treatment of hepatitis B can be complex. Generally, no treatment is needed for acute hepatitis B and most patients will clear spontaneously. For chronic hepatitis B it depends on the stage of disease, with high ALT or viral DNA levels often a marker of damage and potential progression to liver disease. Interferon provides a life-long cure, but has side effects, long treatment duration, and low efficacy. Antiviral drugs such as tenofovir and entecavir suppress viral replication well, preventing further progression to liver disease, but often need to be taken for years, and are expensive. An effective vaccine is available and is part of the WHO recommended schedule.[70]

HEPATITIS C INFECTION

Hepatitis C is an RNA virus that is bloodborne with infections transmitted by sharing needles, from contaminated blood products, nosocomial spread, and occasionally sexually (especially amongst men who have sex with men). Some 70 million people are affected worldwide with high prevalence usually concentrated within high-risk communities, although there is particular high prevalence in Yemen and Egypt owing to reuse of needles during mass schistosomiasis treatment campaigns.

Clinical Features

Acute hepatitis C is rare, with the early phase usually asymptomatic. Most patients (70%–80%) exposed go on to develop chronic hepatitis C, usually defined as viremia present for more than 6 months. Decades after infection, a subset with chronic hepatitis C will develop significant liver disease, which may lead to cirrhosis and hepatocellular carcinoma. Extrahepatic manifestations, most notably mixed cryoglobulinemia, do occur.

Diagnosis

Hepatitis C antibody detection is the mainstay of diagnosis, and is sensitive and specific. This should be confirmed with hepatitis C PCR and viral load testing because 20% of those infected may have spontaneously cleared the disease but will still have detectable antibodies. In the first 6 months of disease and amongst the immunosuppressed, antibody detection may be negative so for the immunosuppressed (including HIV) and those at recent or ongoing risk of acquisition (e.g., injecting drug users or men who have sex with men) hepatitis C PCR can be a more useful test.

Treatment

Hepatitis C treatment previously required long-term (48-week) treatment with interferon and ribavirin. Side effects were common, treatment completion difficult, and the success rate (usually defined as a sustained viral response, no detectable hepatitis C DNA at 6 months) poor, especially amongst certain hepatitis C genotypes and those with cirrhosis. Direct-acting antivirals have revolutionized the treatment approach, with drugs such as boceprevir, daclatasvir, and now many others, acting directly on the hepatitis C virus and offering rates of SVR of more than 90% across all genotypes, even amongst cirrhotics, and with many interferon-free regimens on offer. However, these are often prohibitively expensive, and access, even in developed healthcare settings, often limited by cost or rationed by need. Consulting up-to-date national guidance and funding bodies when treating patients is important, but even where direct-acting antivirals are unavailable or unaffordable, good management of patients with liver disease, including preventing further hepatic insult with alcohol abstinence and hepatitis B vaccination, screening for hepatocellular carcinoma, and providing health promotion advice to prevent onward spread, for example, by needle exchange schemes or promoting safe sex, is still important.[71]

HEPATITIS E INFECTION

Hepatitis E is spread by the fecooral route in developing countries, often causing epidemics of disease. The Indian subcontinent, Mexico, and parts of Africa are particularly affected. Disease is usually self-resolving but may become persistent in the HIV-positive and immunosuppressed. Pregnant women are also more likely to develop a fulminant hepatitis. Interestingly, hepatitis E cases are on the rise in the developed world, with undercooked pork products responsible. Hepatitis E can be diagnosed by serology or a positive PCR. Treatment is not usually required, although ribavirin has been used in immunosuppressed individuals with persistent infection.[72]

VIRAL GASTROENTERITIS

There are a number of viruses that cause acute vomiting and diarrhea, including the rotaviruses, caliciviruses (which include norovirus), adenoviruses, and astroviruses. Viral gastroenteritis plays an important part in childhood diarrhea, a major killer in the less-developed world. There are 1.7 billion cases of childhood diarrhea a year, with 525,000 deaths in the under 5s, the second-leading cause of death. Viruses (and bacteria) are transmitted via the fecooral route, with rotavirus the most important in this age group. Norovirus is an important cause of outbreaks of diarrheal disease. Cruise ships, hospitals, jails, care homes, and other high-density accommodation are particularly at risk.

Clinical Features

The onset of disease is usually shortly after exposure, and watery diarrhea, with or without vomiting, can last for 4 to 7 days. There may be abdominal cramps, myalgia, and fever. Diarrhea can lead to dehydration and electrolyte disturbance, and even to death, especially in the young or malnourished. Diagnosis is usually clinical in most contexts.

Treatment

Although the diarrhea is self-limiting (except in the immunosuppressed), supportive care is vital. Oral rehydration therapy, a mixture of clean water, sugar, and salt, is cheap, highly effective, and saves lives. IV fluids should be reserved for those unable to tolerate oral fluids or for initial resuscitation of the severely dehydrated. Zinc supplementation reduces duration of diarrhea, and nutritional support after an episode of childhood diarrhea is important in reducing vulnerability to another infection. Prevention methods including provision of adequate sanitation, clean water, and hand washing facilities and are key to reducing the global burden. Breastfeeding can also reduce rates, as it provides excellent nutrition and avoids the need for potentially contaminated water to make formula feeds. Increasing uptake of rotavirus vaccines will prevent diarrheal disease and mortality in many countries.[73]

RESPIRATORY VIRUS INFECTIONS

There are a variety of viruses from several families that cause respiratory tract infections. These include the rhinoviruses, adenoviruses, enteroviruses, coronaviruses, respiratory syncytial virus (RSV), human metapneumovirus, and parainfluenza and influenza viruses. They are transmitted by aerosolized droplets, direct contact, or fomites (surfaces including hands, doorknobs, etc.). Transmission is often seasonal. Generally, there is a short incubation period of a few days before a range of clinical syndromes develop. Coryza, pharyngitis, croup, bronchiolitis, and pneumonia may develop, with clinical syndrome depending on host factors, most importantly age and the virus itself. RSV is an important cause of bronchiolitis and pneumonia in children, hospitalizing 100,000 children annually in the United Stated alone, and influenza and coronaviruses can cause life-threatening pneumonias at all ages, with secondary bacterial infection fairly common.

Diagnosis historically has been with viral culture and/or antigen detection, but these have now been largely replaced by PCR, with near-patient testing of respiratory swabs with multiplex PCR platforms sensitive and specific, but not always affordable.

There are few specific treatment options, with most care supportive, although antibiotics may be needed for secondary bacterial infection. Although many respiratory viruses mostly have nuisance value and are self-resolving, on a global scale they are important causes of morbidity and mortality, with lower respiratory infection (including bacterial infection) the leading cause of death globally from an infectious cause, causing 2.75 million deaths worldwide annually. It is a particularly important cause of infant mortality, causing 12% of deaths in those under 5 years.

INFLUENZA

Influenza is an RNA respiratory virus with marked seasonal transmission. It causes significant morbidity and mortality every year, but also can cause devastating epidemics. The "Spanish flu" epidemic caused around 40 million deaths after World War I and more recently "swine flu" in 2009 caused perhaps 200,000. Antigenic drift and antigenic shift, including reassortments of the viral genome during bird or pig infection, are important as it means any immunological protection after infection is rendered obsolete, as the virus presents a new immunological challenge each influenza season.

Clinical Features

After a short incubation period, onset of fever is abrupt and lasts 1 to 5 days. Myalgia is very common, and most patients will have malaise and be unable to work, or need to take to bed. Coryzal symptoms are usually present. Cough and myalgia may persist for weeks. Complications occur, especially in the extremes of age, with secondary bacterial infection (especially from *Staphylococcus aureus*), myocarditis, and even occasionally encephalitis causing morbidity and mortality.

Diagnosis

Traditionally viral culture was used but now PCR-based approaches, including near-patient multiplex PCR testing, have proved invaluable. In epidemics or when influenza season is at its height, clinical case definitions are used and prevent the laboratory being overwhelmed. Experienced clinicians emphasize the abrupt onset of symptoms, and "feeling too unwell to pick up a $20 note" as useful clinical discriminators.

Treatment

The neuraminidase inhibitors (e.g., oseltamivir) and M2 ion channel blockers (e.g., amantadine) are effective against influenza. Generally, oseltamivir is preferred owing to viral resistance to amantadine in some strains. The earlier administered the better and when given in the first 48 hours they reduce illness duration by 1 to 2 days and may reduce the complication rate. They can also be used for prophylaxis after exposure, for example, on a hematology ward. In the severely ill, intensive care therapy may well be required, and clinicians should have a low threshold for empiric treatment for a secondary bacterial infection, including cover for *S. aureus*.

CORONAVIRUS INFECTIONS

The coronaviruses include severe acute respiratory syndrome (SARS) and Middle East respiratory syndrome (MERS). Both are zoonoses, SARS from bats and MERS from camels, capable of person-person transmission, especially in healthcare settings, and are notable for their high proportion of severe cases and case fatality rate. SARS was responsible for an outbreak of around 8000 cases in 2002 to 2003, largely in China, Hong Kong, and Singapore, and MERS emerged in the Middle East in 2012 with most cases originating in Saudi Arabia. Transmission of MERS is ongoing. A severe respiratory illness with fever and a history of contact with the appropriate area should prompt suspicion and testing. No specific treatments are available, but infection control precautions including the wearing of masks, aprons, and gloves prevent nosocomial infection.

In 2019, a novel coronavirus, SARS-CoV-2, emerged in Wuhan, China, causing a severe respiratory illness, coronavirus disease 2019 (Covid-19). Highly transmissible in community and healthcare settings, the virus rapidly spread around the world causing a pandemic with huge health and economic impacts. Older patients and those with comorbidities such as hypertension, obesity, and cardiovascular disease are particularly severely affected. The disease is characterized by hypoxemic respiratory failure and ARDS, requiring oxygen, or mechanical ventilation in the most severely affected, with characteristic changes on chest x-ray or CT scan. However, most of those infected do not require hospitalization. At the time of writing, extrapulmonary manifestations, including coagulopathy and a cytokine storm, emerged as important in severe disease. Diagnosis is usually from RT-PCR, and a variety of laboratory abnormalities, including transaminitis and a lymphopenia, are well described. Randomized controlled trials to develop the optimal therapeutic strategies, including ventilatory and use of specific antivirals such as remdesivir, are ongoing.[74-76]

MEASLES

Measles is an RNA virus infection spread from human to human by aerosol transmission with no animal reservoir. It is highly contagious with a global spread. Vaccination has reduced the previously estimated 6 million deaths annually substantially. However, measles outbreaks occur in the developed world despite vaccination being offered widely, if not always taken up. In the developing world, low vaccine coverage, especially during complex emergencies, can lead to large epidemics. Overcrowded settings such as refugee camps raise the threshold required for herd immunity meaning outbreaks can occur, even in a previously protected population. Concurrent malnutrition and high rates of secondary respiratory infection, along with immunosuppression from the measles virus itself, leads to significant mortality. The list of priorities of MSF for refugee health puts measles immunization at number two for this reason.

Clinical Features

Some 10 to 14 days after exposure, patients will typically develop a cough, runny nose, and fever, often with conjunctivitis. Koplik's spots, small, bright-red spots on the buccal mucosa develop, early in the disease. A few days after the start of symptoms a morbilliform, erythematous rash spreads over the body, and will later desquamate. Patients typically recover after 7 to 10 days. Measles leaves patients immunosuppressed during the convalescent period, especially those with preexisting malnutrition. Secondary bacterial pneumonia, chronic diarrhea (which may or may not be infective), stomatitis from herpes simplex leading to inability to feed, corneal ulceration in the vitamin A deficient, and pyoderma, which causes deep eroding ulcers known as cancrum oris or noma, may all occur. These contribute to mortality and disability, including blindness. Malnutrition as an exacerbating factor, but also a consequence of measles, is particularly important.

Diagnosis

In most cases measles is diagnosed clinically, based on the typical features in an unimmunized individual in the context of an outbreak. Antigen detection in salivary fluid or measles IgM can confirm the diagnosis where there is doubt.

Treatment

Treatment is based on identifying complications and treating them rapidly. Severe measles or measles in malnourished children requires hospital management. Vitamin A, 100,000 IU for those under 1 year old and 200,000 IU for those older than 1 year, reduces mortality between one-third and one-half and should be given early. Nutritional support and rehydration are vital, and naso-gastric feeding may be required. Systemic antibiotics for pneumonia, topical antibiotics for severe conjunctivitis or eye ulcers, nystatin for oral candidiasis, and acyclovir for oral herpes simplex may all be needed. The live virus measles vaccine is safe and highly effective and should be part of the routine schedule of immunization worldwide. Catch-up campaigns, often in response to an emerging outbreak, or in anticipation of one, for example, during a complex emergency, are effective in limiting the impact of an epidemic.[77-78]

MUMPS

Mumps is a highly infectious virus spread in the saliva of infected individuals. It is largely a disease of childhood, but the older the patient, the more likely complications are. The incubation period is 14 to 18 days and it presents with fever and parotitis, which lasts for 3 to 4 days. Some 4 to 5 days after the parotitis, an orchitis may develop, especially in older patients. Infertility is unusual but well reported. Meningitis and encephalitis both occur rarely, with the encephalitis responsible for much of the mortality from mumps, which is approximately 2 per 1000 cases. Symptoms are distinct enough to make a clinical diagnosis on most occasions but detection of antibody in saliva is positive early in disease, and can prevent surgical exploration of the parotids or testes. Treatment is supportive, with 60 mg prednisolone given for 2 to 3 days in orchitis and occasionally in severe parotitis. Vaccination prevents mumps.

RABIES

Rabies is a zoonotic disease of mammals caused by the lyssaviruses. Bats and other mammals are important reservoirs but most disease in man is caused by bites from rabid canines. The virus is present in the saliva of infected animals. Humans are infected when bitten by infected mammals, or from licks to broken skin or mucosal membranes. After inoculation, the virus is transported in a retrograde fashion along peripheral nerves. When it reaches the CNS, it causes encephalitis which is (almost) universally fatal. Rabies is present in bats worldwide, including the UK, United States, and Australia, although control efforts have rendered many parts of Western Europe, the Caribbean, Oceania, South Korea, and Japan free of terrestrial rabies. There are an estimated 55,000 cases of rabies a year, with most from India (20,000 cases), other parts of Asia (especially Pakistan and Bangladesh), and Africa, where reporting is patchy but the burden of disease high.

Clinical Features

The incubation period in rabies varies considerably according the type and site of exposure, with heavy central exposures, such as a deep bite from a rabid dog on the face, most likely to cause rabies and having the shortest incubation period. A few weeks is typical but it may be as short as 9 days and even as long as years. Hence it is never too late to receive rabies postexposure prophylaxis if indicated. A prodrome of pain, parasthesia, and itching at the site of the wound (even if subsequently healed), sometimes accompanied by fever and myalgia, often preceeds clinical rabies. Clinically, rabies may develop as two forms. Furious rabies is the most common presentation, and the more familiar. There are periods of aggression, agitation, and confusion, with intevening lucid periods. "Hydrophobia," intense painful spasms of the laryngx and respiratory muscles triggered by exposure to water, is pathognomonic. Autonomic disturbances usually develop. Paralytic rabies occurs in around 20%, with an ascending flaccid paralysis often accompanied by sensory impairment, cranial nerve palsies, and sphincter dysfunction. The prognosis is bleak for both forms, with patients dying either during an hydrophobic spasm in the first few days in furious rabies or lapsing into coma and dying after a few weeks.

Diagnosis

Diagnosis usually rests on exposure to the virus along with the characteristic clinical features. Clinicians should note exposure may be months or even years before presentation, and may be relatively trivial or unnoticed (e.g., a lick from a rabid animal). Diagnosis can be confirmed by detection of viral antigen in skin biopsies from the nape of the neck, or PCR in blood, saliva, urine, or CSF. Historically, autopsy of the euthanesed animal responsible for the bite was used. Dogs that are alive 10 days after biting a human will not have caused rabies, as the virus is only found in the saliva of dogs for 3 days before disease presents, and most will die within 7 days. This can be used clinically where postexposure prophylaxis is unaffordable and observation of the dog feasible.

Treatment

Clinical Treatment. Clinical rabies is almost invariably fatal. Even with high-level ITU care and various experimental treatment protocols there have only been eight reported survivors. Treatment should focus on patient's comfort, dignity, and respect. In Western settings, ITU-level supportive care, rabies immunoglobulin, and other elements of the "Milwaukee protocol" may be tried, but are likely to fail. Alhough person-person transmission in healthcare settings has not been documented, treating patients with rabies generates understandable anxiety amongst clinicians. Barrier nursing along with rabies vaccination for staff and visitors should be considered.

Postexposure Prophylaxis. In view of the bleak prognosis of established rabies infection, efforts should be focused on strategies to prevent rabies. This includes postexposure prophylaxis. Appropriate wound management, including debridement, irrigation, and cleaning with alcohol or iodine will limit exposure to rabies virions. The WHO recommends postexposure vaccination for significant exposures (Table 3.7). A four- or five-dose IM regime given over 28 days is typical, but several effective regimes are available including using the intradermal route, which reduces vaccine required and thus cost. WHO recommendations changed in 2018 to endorse the time- and cost-saving two-site intradermal regime at days 0, 3, and 7; but intramuscular regimes are still valid alternatives. Category 3 exposures should also be given rabies immunoglobulin, although this is expensive and can be difficult to source. If patients have previously been vaccinated then an accelerated vaccination regime can be used: either four-site intradermal injection on day 0, or one-site intradermal or intramuscular injection on days 0 and 3. Rabies immunoglobulin is not required in these cases. As rabies may present years after exposure there is no upper limit on the time period during which postexposure prophylaxis should be considered.

TABLE 3.7 ■ **World Health Organization Rabies Postexposure Prophylaxis Recommendations**

Category of Exposure	Description	Postexposure Prophylaxis
I	Touching or feeding animals; licks on intact skin	None required
II	Nibbling of uncovered skin; minor scratches or abrasions (no bleeding)	Vaccine only
III	Bite(s) through the skin; licks on broken skin, contamination of mucus membranes with saliva; exposure to bats	Vaccine + rabies immuno-globulin[a]

[a]Immunoglobulin recommended up to 7 days after exposure.
From World Health Organization. *Rabies Vaccines and Immunoglobulins: WHO Position*. Jan 2018. Available at: http://apps.who.int/iris/bitstream/10665/259855/1/WHO-CDS-NTD-NZD-2018.04-eng.pdf?ua=1. Accessed February 2018; Warrell MJ, Warrell DA. Rabies: the clinical features, management and prevention of the classic zoonosis. *Clin Med*, 2015;15(1):78–81.

Fungal Infections

Fungi cause a range of diseases in humans from the dermatophytoses, which cause disease in keratinized tissue in healthy individuals and are extremely common globally, to those such as *Penicillium marneffei*, which cause disease exclusively in the immunosuppressed in a narrow geographical area (SE Asia). Many fungal diseases are exclusively seen in the immunosuppressed, often in a hospital setting where central venous catheters, urinary catheters, and other instrumentation, along with liberal use of broad-spectrum antibiotics, creates a biological niche for them. Generally, in this section we will cover the major global systemic fungal infections of the immunocompetent in most detail. Superficial fungal diseases such as pityriasis versicolor and the dermatophytoses, and the systemic opportunistic fungal infections such as aspergillosis, invasive candidiasis, and mucormycosis, are covered in detail in other texts, such as the *Oxford Textbook of Medicine: Infection*.

MYCETOMA

Mycetoma, better known as Madura foot, is a chronic infection of skin, subcutaneous tissue, and bone, caused by a range of fungi, including *Madurella mycetomatis*, *M. grisea*, *Scedosporium apiospermum*, and various actinomycetes species. Deep inoculation of soil or soil organisms, typically into the foot, causes a slowly developing infection that can erode deep, even into bone. Mycetoma is common in tropical areas, likely attributed to a lack of footwear and presence of pathogenic organisms in soil, with cases seen in Central and South America, India, and sub-Saharan Africa. Agricultural workers are particularly at risk. The microbiology of mycetoma varies geographically, with some species more important in certain locations.

Clinical Features

Mycetomas usually begin as a hard, subcutaneous nodule enlarging over years. Sinus tracts appear discharging fluid and hard grains. Morbidity is caused by gradual destruction of soft tissue and bone leading to significant disability. Lesions spread slowly, with distant metastasis not usually a problem.

Diagnosis

Diagnosis is a combination of the clinical picture, radiological evidence of mycetoma, and microbiology. Radiologically, cortical erosion is usually the earliest sign. Lytic deposits follow with destruction and deformity later. Plain x-rays may show all this, although MRI, when available, will give more information, especially for early disease. Microscopy of grains mounted in potassium hydroxide can differentiate between fungi and actinomyces, and culture may identify the particular organism, although several samples may be required. Where grains are not present or nondiagnostic, deep biopsy may be required.

Treatment

This depends on the organism responsible. For actinomyces mycetomas, long-term co-trimoxazole or dapsone, often with a second agent such as streptomycin or rifampicin, may produce a response. Treatment often continues for years. Fungal mycetomas generally respond poorly to medical therapy although a trial of itraconazole, ketoconazole, voriconazole, or amphotericin B (ideally tailored to the organism[s] responsible) may have an effect. If there is no response, surgery, often radical or involving an amputation, may be required.[79]

SPOROTRICHOSIS

The fungus *Sporotrix schenkii* (a soil/plant pathogen) causes this infection worldwide in tropical and subtropical regions. It is found in southern and central United States, throughout Latin America, Africa, and Japan, with a few cases in the Far East and Australia. Sporadic outbreaks (often in florists, plant workers, fishermen, and also armadillo hunters) is the rule, but it is hyperendemic in parts of Guatemala, Peru, and South Africa. Inoculation of the soil organism from minor skin trauma is the method of infection.

Clinical Features

The classic form is of an intial nodule which ulcerates, and then spreads along the lymphatic as a series of ulcerating nodules. Solitary nodules are also common. Other patterns such as widespread cutaneous lesions or systemic sporotrichosis do also occur, especially in the immunosuppressed.

Diagnosis

Fungal culture of biopsy or skin scraping is the most usual method of diagnosis although serology is available for systemic sporotrichosis.

Treatment

Saturated solution of potassium iodide orally, start at 1 to 2 mL tds, increased slowly up to a maximum of 4 to 6 mL tds, is effective and cheap. Gradual increase of dosage helps the patient accommodate to the unpleasant taste and other side effects such as nausea, dry mouth, altered taste, and swollen salivary glands. Treatment should be continued until one month after resolution. Alternately, itraconazole may be given. Ambisome may be required for those with systemic sporotrichosis.[80]

CANDIDIASIS

Candida spp. are saprophytic yeast species commonly found as a commensal in the mouth, GI, or genital tract. When host immunological factors change, for example, at extremes of age, in HIV, with chemotherapy, or in diabetes the commensal skin flora is disrupted by, for example, antibiotics, or there is epithelial disturbance, the candida species may increase in number causing superficial candidiasis. Painful, raw mucosa with adherent white plaques are the commonest result. The plaques can be scraped off and will show yeasts under microscopy, or can be cultured. Topical treatments are available, but where there is severe disease or immunosuppression systemic azoles, particularly fluconazole, are favored.

In patients who are hospitalized, particularly the immunosuppressed, with multiple invasive lines (e.g., central lines in situ), and with antibiotic exposure, systemic candidiasis may develop. This is a severe disease, which needs to be treated promptly. Removal of any source material and systemic antifungal therapy is required.[81]

HISTOPLASMOSIS

Histoplasmosis is caused by inhalation of the fungi *Histoplasma capsulatum*, which causes disease in its yeast form. The organism is found in soil, but areas with bird droppings or bat guano, such as chicken coops, caves, barns, etc. are a particular risk. The disease is generally divided into two forms. The classical form caused by *H. capsulatum* var. *capsulatum* is present in the United States, particularly the Ohio and Mississippi areas, the Far East, Central and South America, and Australia. African histoplasmosis, caused by *H. capsulatum* var. *duboisii*, is found in sub-Saharan Africa.

Clinical Features

Histoplasmosis can cause a number of clinical syndromes. Asymptomatic—most patients exposed will be asymptomatic with only a positive serology to show for their caving trip or other exposure. Acute pulmonary histoplasmosis produces a febrile illness with muscle ache, cough, chest pain, hilar lymphadenopathy, and diffuse pulmonary infiltrates on chest x-ray. The disease begins 10 to 14 days after exposure and usually resolves, although some patients will be severely ill and require antifungals. Chronic pulmonary histoplasomosis is more common in those with underlying lung pathology or smokers. Years after infection, nodules, consoliation, and cavitation occur, sometimes with fevers and myalgia. The disease often mimics TB or lung cancer. Relapse despite antifungal treatment is common and surgical treatment may be reuqired. Disseminated histoplasmosis, which can occur early in the disease, especially in those with HIV, or late (where it is often less severe), causes a severe illness with fever, weight loss, and hepatosplenomegaly. The marrow is frequently infiltrated with pancytopenia, and bleeding complications common. Molluscum-like skin lesions may be present and complications such as meningitis or endocarditis may occur. African histoplasmosis usually presents with skin lesions, typically subcutaneous nodules, or skin ulcers, with lymphadenopathy and lytic bone lesions present in the more unwell.

Diagnosis

Culture of typical small yeasts from blood, sputum, bone marrow (most sensitive in disseminated disease), or skin biopsy is ideal, although organisms may also be seen on microscopy. Serologic testing showing a rising antibody titer is helpful.

Treatment

Treatment depends on the clinical syndrome with most cases of acute pulmonary histoplasmosis and 75% of chronic pulmonary histoplasmosis requiring no treatment. For severe disease, or relapse, itraconazole or amphotericin B will be required.[82]

BLASTOMYCOSIS

This systemic fungal infection is caused by *Blastomyces dermatitidis*, a dimorphic fungus. Mainly found in the United States and Canada around the Great Lakes, and Ohio and Mississippi river valleys, cases have been reported in Africa, India, the Middle East, and Europe. When isolated from nature in North America, the organism has come from sites where there is a risk of flooding, such as riverbanks, which fits with the general pattern of epidemiologic exposure.

Clinical Features

Clinically the disease presents similarly to histoplasmosis, although the extent of asymptomatic infection is unclear, and acute infection is less common. The acute pulmonary form presents with cough, pleuritic pain, and fever. Chronic pulmonary disease presents with focal consolidation and cavitation in the lungs accompanied by cough, fever, and weight loss (similar to TB). In disseminated disease the main sites are the skin and bones. The former may develop ulcers, abscesses, granulomas, or crusted plaques which heal, leaving scars behind. The latter involves primarily the axial skeleton (vertebrae), and spinal cord compression may result. Immunocompromised patients are at increased risk for dissemination.

Diagnosis

Direct microscopy of sputum (and other sites) and culture. *B. dermatitidis* is a dimorphic fungus, which is a mold at room temperature, but a yeast at 37°C. Histologic changes of blastomycosis may be diagnostic as the yeasts produce a characteristic broad-based bud.

Treatment

Itraconazole (200–400 mg daily) is usually used for slowly progressive disease with amphotericin B (0.6–1.0 mg/kg daily) for rapidly progressive disease and severely unwell patients.

COCCIDIOIDOMYCOSIS

Coccidioides immitis is a soil organism of the semidesert areas of the United States and parts of Latin America, capable of infecting both healthy and immunocompromised patients. Most cases are from arid regions of California and Arizona. As the fungus is a soil organism, outbreaks may follow dust storms, droughts, or earthquakes with peaks when seasonal rainfall is lowest.

Clinical Features

Around two-thirds of cases are asymptomatic. One to three weeks after exposure patients develop a pulmonary infection with fever, cough, and pulmonary infiltrates clinically similar to other causes of community-acquired pneumonia. An eosinophilia, arthritis, erythema nodusum, or erythema multiforme may give a clue to the true diagnosis. Most will resolve but in a small number cavitation and fibrosis may progressively destroy lung tissue, especially in the immunosuppressed. In a few patients, hematogenous spread occurs months after infection, with joint involvement or meningitis common.

Diagnosis

Direct microscopy of appropriate clinical samples or culture on many media will reveal typically shaped fungi. However, laboratory culture should be undertaken with care as the mycelia readily aerosolize and the infectious dose is low. A wide range of serologic tests are available, with good sensitivity and specificity. In view of the prolonged recovery, and potential for relapse even in immunocompetent patients, in endemic areas consideration should be given to routine testing of all community-acquired pneumonias.

Treatment

A lack of evidence and randomized controlled trials hampers choice of who to treat and what with. Those with primary pulmonary infection with risk factors (immunosuppression, comorbidities, pregnancy, African or Filipino ancestry) are likely to benefit from treatment. The azoles, usually fluconazole starting at 400 mg od for 3 to 6 months, are commonly used first line, with amphotericin reserved for patients who are severely unwell or for second-line therapy. Surgery can be helpful, especially in chronic lung disease.[83]

PARACOCCIDIOIDOMYCOSIS

Paracoccidioidomycosis A is systemic fungal infection confined to Central and South America, caused by the dimorphic fungi *Paracoccidioidomycosis brasiliensis* and *P. lutzii*. It is seen in Colombia, Venezuela, Ecuador, Brazil, and Argentina predominantly, but may also be found to a lesser extent in other Central and South American nations. The disease is most common in agricultural workers and infection is via the respiratory route.

Clinical Features

These can be somewhat variable. In the acute form, progressive lymphadenopathy over months, sometimes with collections, occurs. Lytic bone lesions, small bowel involvement leading to abdominal pain and diarrhea, fever, and weight loss are common. The chronic form has an insidious onset in older people with frequent involvement of the lung. Infiltrates, nodules, and cavities occur with lymphadenopathy often present. Hematogenous spread can cause skin and mucosal lesions with a variety of forms, and ulceration and hemorrhage occur.

Diagnosis

Direct microscopy will demonstrate characteristic yeast forms in sputum smears or biopies. These yeasts form multiple buds, often appearing around the periphery of a parent cell. The organism is a dimorphic fungus that can be isolated in culture of appropriate clinical samples. Serologic tests are sensitive and specific although there are regional variations in antigenicity and local advice should be sought.

Treatment

The azoles such as ketoconazole (200–400 mg daily) or itraconazole (200–400 mg daily) are the treatment of choice for active disease, with a long course of therapy of more than 6 months often required. In severe disease, amphotericin B is usually used in the induction phase followed by oral azoles.

PENICILLIUM MARNEFFEI INFECTION

Penicilium marneffei is a fungal pathogen of bamboo rats in China and SE Asia. The mechanism of human infection is not known but may be from a common environmental source. Few cases were reported before the HIV epidemic and almost all cases seen are in patients profoundly immuno-suppressed because of advanced HIV.

Clinical Features

Fever, lymphadenopathy, and hepatosplenomegaly are frequently seen. Hematogenous dissemination results in molluscum-type cutaneous lesions that ulcerate and bleed. A variety of lung manifestations including cavitary lesions (which may be mistaken for TB) are seen, as is pericarditis, colitis, and abscesses. If not suspected and treated it may be fatal. Given most patients will have advanced HIV, it frequently coexists with other opportunistic infections.

Diagnosis

Direct microscopy of bone marrow, skin lesions, or lymph node biopsy may reveal the character-istic appearance of the fungus with septated yeast cells. Fungal culture, including of blood or skin biopsy specimens, is more sensitive and can be used to confirm microscopy results. Serologic and PCR-based tests have been developed. Where clinical suspicion is high and the patient is critically ill, empiric therapy is often required.

Treatment

A variety of systemic antifungals may be used. Two weeks of amphotericin B followed by 10 weeks of oral itraconazole (400 mg daily) is one recommended regime. HIV-positive patients would require pophylatic itraconazole to continue until highly active antiretroviral therapy (HAART) allows CD4 count to be sustained at more than 100 cells/mm^3.

CRYPTOCOCCOSIS

The encapsulated yeast *Cryptococcus neoformans* causes cryptococcosis. It is found worldwide in soil. Most patients are those who are immunosuppressed, especially HIV-positive patients with a low CD4 count. However, *C. neoformans* var. *gattii*, which is present in Australia, the Philippines, and New Guinea, and has recently been described in the Pacific Northwest of the United States can cause disease in the immunocompetent. The commonest presentation is meningitis, often with high opening pressure, but skin disease, lung disease, and disseminated systemic disease are well described. Even where var. *gatti* is prevalent a diagnosis should lead to investigation for an underlying immune disorder, including HIV. Treatment for meningitis/HIV patients is described elsewhere, but in immunocompetent patients prolonged treatment past 3 to 4 months is gener-ally not required and an isolated pulmonary lesion may be treated with fluconazole alone for 3 to 6 months.[84]

PNEUMOCYSTIS JIVORECI

See Chapter 6 under HIV.

Resources for Further Learning

GENERAL

The following are good general texts which cover tropical medicine and/or infectious diseases. Lecture Notes in Tropical Medicine is particularly recommended as a general, practical guide that is small enough to fit in airplane hand luggage. Also included are a selection of websites that provide reliable, authoritative information on infectious disease, tropical medicine, and travel health:

Beeching N, Gill G. *Lecture Notes in Tropical Medicine.* 7th ed. Oxford, UK: Wiley-Blackwell; 2014.

Warrell D, Cox T, Firth J. *Oxford Textbook of Tropical Medicine: Infection.* Oxford, UK: Oxford University Press; 2010.[85–89]

DISASTER MEDICINE AND COMPLEX EMERGENCIES

The reference/further reading list contains some useful resources covering complex emergencies, disaster medicine, and the importance of infectious disease in this context. There are also some websites that provide accurate, up-to-date information about current ongoing disasters and infectious diseases outbreaks.[90–94]

References and Further Reading

1. Hendricks KA, Wright ME, Shadomy SV, et al. Centers for Disease Control and Prevention Expert Panel Meetings on prevention and treatment of anthrax in adults. *Emerg Infect Dis.* 2014;20(2):e130687.
2. World Health Organization. Tetanus vaccines: WHO position paper—February 2017. *Wkly Epidemiol Record.* 2017;6(92):53–76.
3. Reliefweb. Bangladesh: Diphtheria Outbreak—December 2017. Available at: https://reliefweb.int/disaster/ep-2017-000177-bgd. Accessed February 2017.
4. Allerberger F, Wagner M. Listeriosis: a resurgent foodborne infection. *Clin Microbiol Infect.* 2010; 16(1):16–23.
5. Shallcross LJ, Fragaszy E, Johnson AM, et al. The role of the Panton-Valentine leucocidin toxin in staphylococcal disease: a systematic review and meta-analysis. *Lancet Infect Dis.* 2013;13(1):43–54.
6. Thwaites GE, Edgeworth JD, Gkrania-Klotsas E, et al. Clinical management of *Staphylococcus aureus* bacteraemia. *Lancet Infect Dis.* 2011;11(3):208–222.
7. Mitjà O, Asiedu K, Mabey D. Yaws. *Lancet.* 2013;381:763–773.
8. Mitjà O, Houinei W, Moses P, et al. Mass treatment with single-dose azithromycin for yaws. *New Engl J Med.* 2015;372(8):703–710.
9. Sejvar J, Bancroft E, Winthrop K, et al. Leptospirosis in "Eco-Challenge" athletes, Malaysian Borneo, 2000. *Emerg Infect Dis.* 2003;9(6):702–707.
10. Bharti AR, Nally JE, Ricaldi JN, et al. Leptospirosis: a zoonotic disease of global importance. *Lancet Infect Dis.* 2003;3(12):757–771.
11. Stanek G, Wormser GP, Gray J, Strle F. Lyme borreliosis. *Lancet.* 2012;379(9814):461–473.
12. Anstead GM, Shanks GD. War and infectious disease. *Lancet.* 2016;237(9955):e164–e172.
13. Larsson C, Andersson M, Bergström S. Current issues in relapsing fever. *Curr Opin Infect Dis.* 2009; 22(5):443–449.
14. Wain J, Hendriksen RS, Mikoleit ML, et al. Typhoid fever. *Lancet.* 2015;385(9973):1136–1145.
15. Typhoid fever—Syria (03) (Damascus) Refugee Camp. Available at: http://www.promedmail.org/post/3670433. Accessed January 2018.
16. Parker LA, Rumunu J, Jamet C, et al. Adapting to the global shortage of cholera vaccines: targeted single dose cholera vaccine in response to an outbreak in South Sudan. *Lancet Infect Dis.* 2017;17(4):e123–e127.
17. Orata FD, Keim PS, Boucher Y. The 2010 cholera outbreak in Haiti: how science solved a controversy. *PLoS Pathog.* 2014;10(4).

18. Wiersinga WJ, Currie BJ, Peacock SJ. Melioidosis. *New Engl J Med.* 2012;367(11):1035–1044.
19. Stephens DS, Greenwood B, Brandtzaeg P. Epidemic meningitis, meningococcaemia, and *Neisseria meningitidis. Lancet.* 2007;369(9580):2196–2210.
20. Burdet C, Lepeule R, Duval X, et al. Quinolones versus macrolides in the treatment of legionellosis: a systematic review and meta-analysis. *J Antimicrob Chemother.* 2014;69(9):2354–2360.
21. Feasey NA, Dougan G, Kingsley R, et al. Invasive non-typhoidal salmonella disease: an emerging and neglected tropical disease in Africa. *Lancet.* 2012;379(9835):2489–2499.
22. Tickell KD, Brander RL, Atlas HE, et al. Identification and management of Shigella infection in children with diarrhoea: a systematic review and meta-analysis. *Lancet Glob Health.* 2017;5(12):e1235–e1248.
23. Engels D, Madaras T, Nyandwi S, et al. Epidemic dysentery caused by Shigella dysenteriae type 1: a sentinel site surveillance of antimicrobial resistance patterns in Burundi. *Bull World Health Organ.* 1995;73(6):787–791.
24. Kaper JB, Nataro JP, Mobley HL. Pathogenic *Escherichia coli. Nat Rev Microbiol.* 2004;2(2):123–140.
25. Prentice MB, Rahalison L. Plague. *Lancet.* 2007;369:1196–1207.
26. Reliefweb. Madagascar: Plague outbreak—Sep 2017. Available at: https://reliefweb.int/disaster/ep-2017-000144-mdg. Accessed February 2018.
27. World Health Organization. WHO Guidelines on Tularaemia. 2007. Available at: http://apps.who.int/iris/bitstream/10665/43793/1/9789241547376_eng.pdf. Accessed January 2018.
28. Foucault C, Raoult D, Brouqui P. Randomized open trial of gentamicin and doxycycline for eradication of Bartonella quintana from blood in patients with chronic bacteremia. *Antimicrob Agents Chemother.* 2003;47(7):2204–2207.
29. Corbel MJ. *Brucellosis in Humans and Animals*: World Health Organization; 2006. Available at: http://www.who.int/csr/resources/publications/Brucellosis.pdf?ua=1. Accessed February 2018.
30. Public Health England. *Management of Laboratory Exposure to Brucella Species: Assessing Exposure and Individual Assessment Flowchart*; July 2017. Available at: https://www.gov.uk/government/uploads/system/uploads/attachment_data/file/631714/Brucella_exposure_assessment_and_flowchart.pdf. Accessed February 2018.
31. Hartzell JD, Blaylock JM. Whooping cough in 2014 and beyond: an update and review. *Chest.* 2014;146(1):205–214.
32. Anderson A, Bijlmer H, Fournier PE, et al. Diagnosis and management of Q fever—United States, 2013: recommendations from CDC and the Q Fever Working Group. *MMWR.* 2013;62(3):1–30.
33. World Health Organization. Guidelines for Treatment of Drug-Susceptible Tuberculosis and Patient Care (2017 update). Available at: http://www.who.int/tb/publications/2017/dstb_guidance_2017/en/. Accessed February 2018.
34. Reider HL, Chen-Yuan C, Gie RP, Enarson DA. *Crofton's Clinical Tuberculosis.* 3rd ed. Oxford, UK: International Union Against Tuberculosis and Lung Disease; 2009.
35. Rodrigues LC, Lockwood DNJ. Leprosy now: epidemiology, progress, challenges, and research gaps. *Lancet Infect Dis.* 2011;11(6):464–470.
36. Vogel M, Bayi PF, Ruf MT, et al. Local heat application for the treatment of Buruli ulcer: results of a phase II open label single center non comparative clinical trial. *Clin Infect Dis.* 2016;62(3):342–350.
37. White NJ, Pukrittayakamee S, Hien TT, et al. Malaria. *Lancet.* 2014;383(9918):723–735.
38. Dondorp AM, Fanello CI, Hendriksen ICE, et al. Artesunate versus quinine in the treatment of severe falciparum malaria in African children (AQUAMAT): an open-label, randomised trial. *Lancet.* 2010;376(9753):1647–1657.
39. White NJ. Artesunate versus quinine for treatment of severe falciparum malaria: a randomised trial. *Lancet.* 2005;366(9487):717–725.
    World Health Organization. *Guidelines for the Treatment of Malaria.* 3rd ed. Geneva: WHO; 2015. Available at: http://apps.who.int/iris/bitstream/10665/162441/1/9789241549127_eng.pdf. Accessed February 2018.
40. World Health Organization. *Management of Severe Malaria: A Practical Handbook.* 3rd ed. Geneva: WHO; 2013.
41. Van Griensven J, Diro E. Visceral leishmaniasis. *Infect Dis Clin N Am.* 2012;26(2):309–322.
42. Morillo CA, Marin-Neto JA, Avezum A, et al. Randomized trial of benznidazole for chronic Chagas' cardiomyopathy. *New Engl J Med.* 2015;373(14):1295–1306.
43. Montoya JG, Liesenfeld O. Toxoplasmosis. *Lancet.* 2004;363:1965–1976.
44. Haque R, Huston CD, Hughes M, et al. Amebiasis. *New Engl J Med.* 2003;348(16):1565–1573.

45. Carter ER, Nabarro LE, Hedley L, et al. Nitroimidazole-refractory giardiasis: a growing problem requiring rational solutions. *Clin Microbiol Infect*. 2018;24(1):37–42.
46. Checkley AM, Chiodini PL, Dockrell DH, et al. Eosinophilia in returning travellers and migrants from the tropics: UK recommendations for investigation and initial management. *J Infect*. 2010;60(1):1–20. [A useful reference with details of diagnosis and treatment of a range of helminth infections which cause eosinophilia.]
47. Global Atlas of Helminth Infections. http://www.thiswormyworld.org. [Up-to-date data on worldwide helminth epidemiology.]
48. Bethony J, Brooker S, Albonico M, et al. Soil-transmitted helminth infections: ascariasis, trichuriasis, and hookworm. *Lancet*. 2006;367(9521):1521–1532.
49. Gill GV, Welch E, Bailey JW, et al. Chronic *Strongyloides stercoralis* infection in former British Far East prisoners of war. *QJM*. 2004;97(12):795–798.
50. Gottstein B, Pozio E, Nöckler K. Epidemiology, diagnosis, treatment, and control of trichinellosis. *Clin Microbiol Rev*. 2009. https://doi.org/10.1128/CMR.00026-08.
51. Taylor MJ, Hoerauf A, Bockarie M. Lymphatic filariasis and onchocerciasis. *Lancet*. 2010;376:1175–1185.
52. Garcia HH, Nash TE, Del Brutto OH. Clinical symptoms, diagnosis, and treatment of neurocysticercosis. *Lancet Neurol*. 2014;13(12):1202–1215.
53. McManus DP, Zhang W, Li J, et al. Echinococcosis. *Lancet*. 2003;362(9392):1295–1304.
54. Colley DG, Bustinduy AL, Secor WE, et al. Human schistosomiasis. *Lancet*. 2014;383:2253–2264.
55. Guzman MG, Harris E. Dengue. *Lancet*. 2015;385:453–465.
    World Health Organization. *Dengue: Guidelines for Diagnosis, Treatment, Prevention and Control*. Geneva: WHO; 2009.
56. Monath TP, Vasconcelos PFC. Yellow fever. *J Clin Virol*. 2015;64:160–173.
57. Reliefweb. Nigeria: Yellow Fever Outbreak—Sept 2017. Available at: https://reliefweb.int/disaster/ep-2017-000169-nga. Accessed February 2018.
58. Petersen LR, Jamieson DJ, Powers AM, et al. Zika virus. *New Engl J Med*. 2016;374(16):1552–1563.
59. Public Health England. *Zika Virus: Travel Advice*; August 2017. Available at: https://www.gov.uk/guidance/zika-virus-travel-advice. Accessed February 2018.
60. Centers for Disease Control and Prevention. *Zika Virus*; Feb 2018. Available at: https://www.cdc.gov/zika/index.html. Accessed February 2018.
61. Erlanger TE, Weiss S, Keiser J, et al. Past, present, and future of Japanese encephalitis. *Emerg Infect Dis*. 2009;15(1).
62. Kilpatrick AM. Globalization, land use, and the invasion of West Nile virus. *Science*. 2011;334(6054):323–327.
63. PREVAIL II writing group. A randomized, controlled trial of ZMapp for Ebola virus infection. *New Engl J Med*. 2016;375:1448–1456.
64. Henao-Restrop AM, Camacho A, Longini I, et al. Efficacy and effectiveness of an rVSV-vectored vaccine in preventing Ebola virus disease: final results from the Guinea ring vaccination, open-label, cluster-randomised trial (Ebola Ça Suffit!). *Lancet*. 2017;389(10068):505–518.
65. Advisory Committee on Dangerous Pathogens. *Management of Hazard Group 4 Viral Haemorrhagic Fevers and Similar Infectious Diseases of High Consequence*; November 2015. Available at: https://www.gov.uk/government/uploads/system/uploads/attachment_data/file/534002/Management_of_VHF_A.pdf. Accessed February 2018. [UK guidance on risk assessment, testing, and protective measures for all VHFs.]
66. McCormick JB, King IJ, Webb P, et al. Lassa fever: effective therapy with ribavirin. *New Engl J Med*. 1986;314(1):20–26.
67. Houlihan C, Behrens R. Lassa fever. *BMJ*. 2017;358:j2986.
68. World Health Organization. Rift Valley Fever. *WHO Fact Sheet*. July 2017. Available at: http://www.who.int/mediacentre/factsheets/fs207/en/. Accessed February 2018.
69. Duchin JS, Koster FT, Peters CJ, et al. Hantavirus pulmonary syndrome: a clinical description of 17 patients with a newly recognized disease. The Hantavirus Study Group. *New Engl J Med*. 1994;330:949–955.
70. Trépo C, Chan HLY, Lok A. Hepatitis B virus infection. *Lancet*. 2014;384(9959):2053–2063.
71. Webster DP, Klenerman P, Dusheiko GM. Hepatitis C. *Lancet*. 2015;385:1124–1135.
72. Kamar N, Bendall R, Legrand-Abravanel F, et al. Hepatitis E. *Lancet*. 2012;379(9835):2477–2488.
73. World Health Organization. *The Treatment of Diarrhoea: A Manual for Physicians and Other Senior Health Workers*. Geneva: WHO; 2005. Available at: http://apps.who.int/iris/bitstream/10665/43209/1/9241593180.pdf. Accessed February 2018.

74. Assiri A, Al-Tawfiq JA, Al-Rabeeah AA. et al. Epidemiological, demographic, and clinical characteristics of 47 cases of Middle East respiratory syndrome coronavirus disease from Saudi Arabia: a descriptive study. *Lancet Infect Dis.* 2013;13(9):752–761.
75. Ksiazek TG, Erdman D, Goldsmith CS, et al. SARS Working Group. A novel coronavirus associated with severe acute respiratory syndrome. *New Engl J Med.* 2003;348(20):1953–1966.
76. Guan W, Ni Z, Hu Y, et al. Clinical characteristics of coronavirus disease 2019 in China. *N Engl J Med.* 2020;382:1708–1720.
77. Moss WJ, Griffin DE. Measles. *Lancet.* 2012;379(9811):153–164.
78. Kouadio IK, Kamigaki T, Oshitani H. Measles outbreaks in displaced populations: a review of transmission, morbidity and mortality associated factors. *BMC Int Health Hum Rights.* 2010;10(1).
79. Welsh O, Al-Abdely HM, Salinas-Carmona MC, et al. Mycetoma medical therapy. *PLoS Negl Tropic Dis.* 2014;8(10).
80. Kauffman CA, Bustamante B, Chapman SW, et al. Clinical practice guidelines for the management of sporotrichosis: 2007 update by the Infectious Diseases Society of America. *Clin Infect Dis.* 2007;45:1255–1265.
81. Pappas PG, Kauffman CA, Andes DR, et al. Clinical practice guideline for the management of candidiasis: 2016 update by the Infectious Diseases Society of America. *Clin Infect Dis.* 2015;62(4):e1–e50.
82. Wheat LJ, Freifeld AG, Kleiman MB, et al. Infectious Diseases Society of America. Clinical practice guidelines for the management of patients with histoplasmosis: 2007 update by the Infectious Diseases Society of America. *Clin Infect Dis.* 2007;45(7):807–825.
83. Galgiani JN, Ampel NM, Blair JE, et al. 2016 Infectious Diseases Society of America (IDSA) clinical practice guideline for the treatment of coccidioidomycosis. *Clin Infect Dis.* 2016;63(6):e112–e146.
84. Chen SC, Korman TM, Slavin MA, et al. Antifungal therapy and management of complications of cryptococcosis due to *Cryptococcus gattii. Clin Infect Dis.* 2013;57(4):543–551.
85. Peters W, Pasvol G. *Atlas of Tropical Medicine and Parasitology.* 6th ed. St Louis: Elsevier; 2006.
86. Manson P, Farrar J Hotez P, et al. *Manson's Tropical Diseases.* 23rd ed. Edinburgh: Elsevier; 2013.
87. Centers for Disease Control. Global Health. Available at: https://www.cdc.gov/globalhealth/index.html. Accessed February 2018. [US-based public health resource with wide variety of information and guidelines on global health and infectious diseases. Also see: https://wwwnc.cdc.gov/travel/for travel health advice.]
88. Public Health England. Infectious Diseases. Available at: https://www.gov.uk/topic/health-protection/infectious-diseases. Accessed February 2018. [United Kingdom-based public health resource providing information on clinical management and population control of a wide variety of infectious diseases.]
89. Travel Health Pro. National Travel Health Network and Centre (United Kingdom). Available at: https://travelhealthpro.org.uk. Acccessed February 2018. [UK-based travel health website providing country and disease-specific advice for travellers.]
90. Connolly MA, Gayer M, Ryan MJ, et al. Communicable diseases in complex emergencies: impact and challenges. *Lancet.* 2004;364(9449):1974–1983.
91. Watson JT, Gayer M, Connolly MA. Epidemics after natural disasters. *Emerg Infect Dis.* 2007;13(1).
92. Médecins Sans Frontières. *Refugee Health: An Approach to Emergency Situations.* Geneva: MSF; 1997. [An excellent, practical handbook with a focus on acute management of health in a refugee population with clear priorities, and detailed planning tools.]
93. http://www.promedmail.org. [An independent monitoring service which collates and disseminates information on infectious diseases outbreaks around the globe. Weekly and daily email alerts are available.]
94. https://reliefweb.int. [A website run by the United Nations Office for the Co-Ordination of Humanitarian Affairs (UNOCHA) providing reliable, up-to-date information on global crises and disasters, and the humanitarian response.]

CHAPTER 4

Laboratory Techniques and Procedures

Fidel Angel Núñez Fernández

Introduction

Although most routine microbiology diagnostic laboratories process specimens for the diagnosis of parasitic infections, there are no best practice guidelines either for processing or for referral to specialist centers. Microscopy for parasites is most often requested on fecal samples, but other biological fluids may be tested. Certain parasitic infections may require other techniques for diagnosis such as serology or polymerase chain reaction (PCR).[1] In this chapter will be described some of parasitological techniques used for the diagnosis of the main parasitic infections associated with disasters, emphasizing malaria, *Schistosoma*, Chagas disease, and intestinal parasitic infections. However, in many other parasitology handbooks or textbooks (Box 4.1) and at many websites, more detailed descriptions of parasitological techniques for these and other parasitic infections may be found.

Parasitological Methods[2]

A. Parasitological methods for intestinal parasitic infections[2–4]

  1. Equipment: microscope:

    a. The use of a good quality microscope with an oil immersion lens is fundamental. This should have a previously calibrated ocular micrometer to help accurately measure objects such as eggs, larvae, or protozoan cysts. Before using, place slide with stage micrometer under lens, then calibrate for each objective lens. Do this by lining up "0" lines of stage and ocular micrometers, and then read to the right until you find another set of perfectly superimposed lines. The number of microns corresponding with one ocular unit for each lens is found by: stage units/ocular units × 1000 = 1 ocular unit.

  2. Preserving samples and wet preparations:

    a. Preservatives: formalin (5% or 10%), polyvinyl alcohol (PVA), or sodium-acetate formalin (SAF). The 5% formalin is ideal for protozoan cysts, and 10% is good for eggs and larvae. Maintain 3:1 fixative:specimen ratio. Formalin is cheap, with a long shelf-life, but not good for trophozoites, and cyst/egg details fade with time. PVA is

BOX 4.1 ■ Recommended Books and Webpages on the Diagnosis of Parasitic Infections

Books and Handbooks

Ash LR, Orihel TC, Bosman A. *Bench Aids for the Diagnosis of Malaria Infections*. Geneva: World Health Organization; 2000.

Ash LR, Orihel TC, Salvioli L. *Bench Aids for the Diagnosis of Intestinal Parasites*. Geneva: World Health Organization; 1994.

Ash LR, Orihel TC. *Atlas of Human Parasitology*. 4th ed. Chicago, IL: American Society of Clinical Pathologists; 1997.

Ash LR, Orihel TC. *Parasites: A Guide to Laboratory Procedures and Identification*. Chicago, IL: American Society of Clinical Pathologists; 1991.

Chiodini PL, Engbaek K, Heuek CC, et al. *Basic Laboratory Methods in Medical Parasitology*. Geneva: World Health Organization; 1991.

Garcia LS. *Diagnostic Medical Parasitology*. 4th ed. Washington, DC: American Society for Microbiology; 2001.

Garcia LS. *Practical Guide to Diagnostic Parasitology*. Washington, DC: American Society for Microbiology; 1999.

Melvin DM, Brooke MM. *Laboratory Procedures for the Diagnosis of Intestinal Parasites*. 3rd ed. US Department of Health and Human Services Publication No. (CDC) 82-8282. Atlanta, GA: Centers for Disease Control and Prevention; 1982.

Melvin DM, Brooke MM. *Morphology of Diagnostic Stages of Intestinal Parasites of Humans*. 2nd ed. US Department of Health and Human Services Publication No. (CDC) 89-8116. Atlanta, GA: Centers for Disease Control and Prevention; 1989.

National Committee for Clinical Laboratory Standards. *Laboratory Diagnosis of Blood-Borne Parasitic Diseases. Approved Guideline M15-A*. Wayne, PA: National Committee for Clinical Laboratory Standards; 2000.

National Committee for Clinical Laboratory Standards. *Procedures for the Recovery and Identification of Parasites from the Intestinal Tract. Approved Guideline M28-A*. Wayne, PA: National Committee for Clinical Laboratory Standards; 1997.

Orihel TC, Ash LR, Ramachandran CP, Ottesen E. *Bench Aids for the Diagnosis of Filarial Infections*. Geneva: World Health Organization; 1997.

Peters W, Gilles HM. *Color Atlas of Tropical Medicine and Parasitology*. 4th ed. London: Mosby-Wolfe; 1995.

Wilcox A. *Manual for the Microscopical Diagnosis of Malaria in Man*. Bethesda, MD: US Department of Health, Education, and Welfare; 1960.

Webpages

http://www.cdc.gov/dpdx/
http://www.diplectanum.dsl.pipex.com/purls/
http://www.southampton.ac.uk/~ceb/
http://www.cdfound.to.it/HTML/atlas.htm

effective (if combined with Schaudinn's solution, called "gold standard"). Good on trophozoites, cysts, eggs. Can do permanent stains (trichrome or iron hematoxylin) afterwards. However, large mercury content, not easy to prepare in the laboratory. SAF is an alternative to gold standard, and it is good for intestinal protozoans. Very good if followed by permanent smears, stained with modified acid-fast. No mercury, cheap, easy to prepare, long shelf-life are some advantages. Can use in concentration procedures, followed by iron hematoxylin staining. With SAF, remember it dilutes specimen, and albumin may be needed to add to slides to aid adhesion.

    b. Buffered water: commonly used for variety of laboratory purposes.

        pH 6.8: 48.6 cc Na_2HPO_4 + 50.4 cc NaH_2PO_4 in 900 cc water.

pH 7.0: 61.0 cc Na_2HPO_4 + 39.0 cc NaH_2PO_4 in 900 cc water.
pH 7.2: 72.0 cc Na_2HPO_4 + 28.0 cc NaH_2PO_4 in 900 cc water.

  c. Conditions for a good fecal sample:
       i. Three stool samples collected on alternate days will increase the sensitivity of parasitological methods.
       ii. Drinking of barium, bismuth, or mineral oil should be avoided because of the ingestion of these liquids can modify the parasitological test results.
       iii. Do not contaminate with water, urine, or other biological fluids.
       iv. Mushy/liquid feces usually have protozoan trophozoites. Cysts have predilection for formed stools. Helminth eggs/larvae variable. First examine exterior for adults, then break up with applicator stick. If adult worms are found can be filtered through a screen.

3. Parasitological techniques for fecal samples:
     a. Direct wet mount:
          i. Saline: small drop of 0.85% saline mix (0.85% NaCl) with small sample should be able to read newsprint through, then place coverslip. Good for helminth eggs and larvae as well as motile protozoan trophozoites.
          ii. 1% Eosin: allows the observation of many protozoa, in general the background is stained pink color in contrast to protozoa, which stain with a white color if they are alive.
          iii. Iodine: use Lugol's iodine in same fashion as saline preparation. Good for protozoan cysts because a good stain of nuclear structures allows better identification.
         - Lugol's iodine:
         Iodine: 1.0 g
         Potassium iodide (KI): 2.0 g
         Distilled water: up to 100 cc
         Dissolve KI in water, then add iodine, store in amber glass bottle out of direct sunlight. Interpretation: positive result—protozoan nuclei take up the iodine and stain pale brown while cytoplasm remains colorless.
         - Some workers prefer to make saline and iodine mounts on separate slides. There is less chance of getting fluids on the microscope stage if separate slides are used. The microscope light should be reduced for low power observations as most organisms will be overlooked by bright light. Illumination should be regulated so that some of the cellular elements in the feces show refraction. Most protozoan cysts will refract light under these conditions. For this method to work effectively, the 1% Lugol's iodine solution should be a fresh preparation (10–14 days).
     b. Formol ether concentration for ova and cysts
          i. To prepare 10% formol saline solution:
         - NaCl: 8.5 g
         - Formaldehyde (37%–41% solution: 100 cc distilled)
         - Water: 900 cc
         - Dissolve NaCl in water; add formaldehyde solution.
         - Add 2 g feces to the bottle, place lid, shake bottle well.
         - Pass this solution through plastic tea strainer into a 15-cc glass centrifuge tube to within 2 cm of the top.
         - Centrifuge at 3000 rpm for 5 minutes. If centrifuge not available, leave to stand out of direct sunlight for 30 minutes.
         - Remove fatty plug at top of solution and discard along with supernatant. Resuspend deposit with saline or iodine over glass slide and examine under microscope.

c. Cellophane (Kato) thick fecal smear technique: fecal egg counts may be useful techniques for research, epidemiology. The previous modified Stoll method described many years ago is more troublesome and time-consuming than Kato-Katz. In fact, the Stoll technique is not effective when the number of eggs is less than 200 ova per gram. This technique is useful for the diagnosis of the main soil transmitted helminthic and *Schistosoma* infections.

   i. With a wood or plastic applicator stick, place 41.7 mg of feces on slide using the template. If sample has excessive amounts of fiber, pass through 105-mesh metal/nylon sieve. Cover sample with previously soaked cellophane coverslip, press against absorbent paper until smear covers area under coverslip, ensuring that the fecal sample does not extend past the edges of the cellophane.

   ii. Leave smear until it clears, usually about 1 hour at room temperature.

   iii. Examine first under 4× objective lens and 40× later.

   iv. Some considerations:

      ■ Hookworm ova visible for up to 30 minutes after preparation. *Schistosoma* ova are best seen about 24 hours later. *Trichuris* and *Ascaris* eggs are visible at any time.

      ■ As the cellophane coverslips are soaked in a malachite green solution, the background will be green, but schistosome and hookworm eggs will remain colorless.

      ■ Cellophane: water wettable cellophane available as 22-mm wide rolls can be cut into rectangles of 22 × 30 mm.

   v. Glycerin-malachite green solution: mix 100 cc glycerol, 100 cc water, and 1.0 cc of 3% aqueous malachite green solution. Place in screw-topped jar, add coverslips, and soak for at least 24 hours before use (Fig. 4.1).

d. Modified cold Ziehl-Neelsen's stain (for *Cryptosporidium* and other coccidian species): This technique is used for the demonstration of oocysts of *Cryptosporidium* species in feces. Alternatively, the modified auramine-phenol stain may be used.

   i. Prepare a medium to thick smear and air dry.

   ii. Fix in methanol for 3 minutes and air dry.

   iii. Flood the slide with modified Kinyoun's acid-fast stain (3% carbol fuchsin) and leave for approximately 15 minutes.

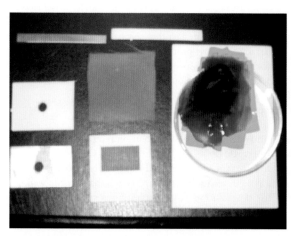

Fig. 4.1 Materials used for Kato-Katz technique: two plastic templates with a hole of 6 mm (for approximately 41.7 mg of feces); two plastic screens, one of them with a cardboard border; two spatulas, one plastic and the other one of aluminum; and strips of hydrophilic cellophane 40- to 50-μm thick, soaked in glycerol-malachite green solution for at least 24 hours before use.

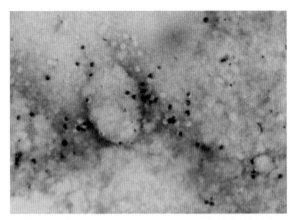

Fig. 4.2 Oocysts of *Cryptosporidium* spp. colored with acid-fast stain in a fecal sample.

    iv. Rinse with tap water.
    v. Flood the slide with 1% acid methanol to decolorize and leave for 15–20 seconds.
    vi. Rinse with tap water.
    vii. Counterstain with 0.4% malachite green or alternative and leave for 30 seconds.
    viii. Rinse with tap water and air dry.
    ix. Examine using 40× or 50× objective and 1× eyepiece lenses. Morphology may be examined closely with a high-power objective.
    x. Positive result: *Cryptosporidium* species are 4–6 µm with a spherical shape; the affinity to fuchsine stain is high, despite some oocysts appearing less stained. *Cyclospora cayetanensis* oocysts stain pinkish red, are spherical, 8–10 µm, and contain a central morula; staining is variable and some oocysts may appear unstained.
    xi. *Cystoisospora belli* species stain red, measure around 31 × 15 µm, and are elongated oval bodies tapered at both ends, containing a granular zygote or two sporoblasts. The oocysts observed in feces are usually unsporulated. Yeasts, other biota, and fecal debris may also take up the stain (Fig. 4.2).

B. Parasitological methods for diagnosis of malaria[2,5–8]

  1. Introduction: The observation of malaria parasites in blood films is the still the gold standard for the diagnosis of malaria. In thick blood, the red blood cells (RBCs) are lysed; consequently, diagnosis is based on the appearance of the parasite. In thick films, organisms tend to be more compact and denser than in thin films. The use of thin films is always required because RBCs are fixed so the morphology of the parasitized cells can be seen, allowing the identification of species and stages. However, malaria parasites may be missed on a thin blood film when there is a low parasitemia. With a thick blood film, the red cells are approximately 6 to 20 layers thick, which results in a larger volume of blood to be observed. Although some technicians stain thick and thin films on separate slides, it is recommended to use both stains in only one slide.

  2. Field's staining method for thick blood films: The method is based in the use of two main components. Field's A is a buffered solution of azure dye and Field's B is a buffered solution of eosin. Both Field's A and B are supplied ready for use by the manufacturers.

    a. Place a drop of blood on a microscope slide and spread to make an area of approximately 1 cm². It should just be possible to read small print through a thick film.
    b. The film is air dried and NEVER fixed in methanol.
    c. The slide is dipped into Field's stain A for 3 seconds.

    d. The slide is then dipped into tap water for 3 seconds and gently agitated.

    e. The slide is dipped into Field's stain B for 3 seconds and washed gently in tap water for a few seconds until the excess stain is removed.

    f. The slide is drained vertically and left to dry.

    g. Dry films upright.

    h. Examine the film at 40× before going to oil immersion (1000× magnification).

    i. Microscopic features of the Field's stained thick blood film:

        i. The end of the film at the top of the slide when it was draining should be looked at. The edges of the film will also be better than the center, where the film may be too thick or cracked.

        ii. In a well-stained film, the malaria parasites show deep-red chromatin and pale-blue cytoplasm.

        iii. White cells, platelets, and malaria pigment can also be seen on a thick film. The leukocyte nuclei stain purple and the background is pale blue. The red cells are lysed and only background stroma remain. The occasional red cell may fail to lyse.

        iv. Schizonts and gametocytes, if present, are also easily recognizable.

        v. A thick film should be examined for at least 10 minutes, which corresponds to approximately 200 oil immersion fields, before declaring the slide negative.

        vi. As a result of hemolysis of the RBC due to staining of an unfixed film, the only elements seen are leukocytes and parasites, the appearance of the latter being altered.

        vii. Consequently:

- The young trophozoites appear as incomplete rings or spots of blue cytoplasm with detached chromatin dots.
- The stippling of *Plasmodium vivax* and *Plasmodium ovale* may be less obvious although occasionally ghost stippling may be seen.
- The cytoplasm of late trophozoites of *P. vivax* and *P. ovale* may be fragmented.

        viii. Caution should be exercised when examining thick blood films, as artifacts and blood platelets may be confused with malaria parasites.

3. Thin blood films: When examining thin blood films for malaria you must look at the infected RBC and the parasites inside the cells.

    a. Rapid Field's stain for thin films: This is a modification of the original Field's stain to enable rapid staining of fixed thin films. This method is suitable for malaria parasites, *Babesia* spp., *Borrelia* spp., and *Leishmania* spp.

        i. Air dry the film.

        ii. Fix in methanol for 1 minute.

        iii. Flood the slide with 1 mL of Field's stain B, diluted 1 in 4 with distilled water.

        iv. Immediately add an equal volume of undiluted Field's stain A, mix well, and allow to stain for 1 minute.

        v. Rinse well in tap water and drain dry.

        vi. Dry films upright.

        vii. Examine the film at 40× before going to oil immersion (1000× magnification).

        viii. Uses: This is a useful method for fast presumptive species identification of malarial parasites. It shows adequate staining of all stages including stippling (mainly Maurer's dots). However, staining with Giemsa is always the method of choice for definitive species differentiation.

4. Giemsa stain for thin films:

    a. Air dry thin films.

    b. Fix in methanol for 1 minute.

    c. Wash in tap water and flood the slide with Giemsa diluted 1 in 10 with buffered distilled water pH 7.2. The diluted stain must be freshly prepared each time.

    d. Stain for 25 to 30 minutes.

    e. Run tap water on to the slide to float off the stain and to prevent deposition of precipitate onto the film.

    f. Dry films upright.

    g. Examine the film at 40× before going to oil immersion (1000× magnification).

    h. Microscopic features of the thin blood film:

        i. Examine the tail end of the slide where the red cells are separated into a one-cell-layer thickness.

        ii. An alkaline buffer pH 7.2 is vital for clear differentiation of nuclear and cytoplasmic material and to visualize inclusions such as Schüffner's/James's dots in the red cells. Acidic buffer is unsuitable.

        iii. The red cells are fixed in the thin film so the morphology of the parasitized cells and the parasites can be seen.

        iv. On a well-stained film the chromatin stains red/purple and the cytoplasm blue. Leukocytes have purple nuclei. The red stippling, if present, should be clearly visible.

    i. Infected RBCs:

        i. Look at the size of the infected RBC.

        ii. Are there any Schüffner's dots present or not?

5. Estimation of percentage parasitemia of *Plasmodium falciparum*: Counting of RBCs infected with parasites of *P. falciparum* is essential and the percentage parasitemia should always be reported as this has implications for prognosis and the pattern of treatment employed.

    a. The recommended procedure for estimating the percentage parasitemia in a thin blood film is by expressing the number of infected cells as a percentage of the RBC, for example, 3 parasitized red cells/100 RBC, or 3% parasitemia.

    b. An RBC infected with multiple parasites counts as one parasitized red cell. The percentage parasitemia should be calculated by counting the number of parasitized RBCs in 1000 cells in a thin blood film.

    c. Alternatively, the World Health Organization recommends a method that compares the number of parasites in a thick blood film with the white blood cell count.

    d. The parasitemia is estimated by first counting the number of parasites per 200 white blood cells in a thick blood film and then calculating the parasite count/μL from the total white blood cell count/μL.

    e. Knowledge of either % parasitemia or total parasite count is essential for the correct clinical management of *P. falciparum* malaria.

6. Effects of anticoagulant on the microscopic diagnosis of malarial parasites

    a. Thin blood films for malaria diagnosis are best prepared from venous or capillary blood taken directly from the patient, without the addition of anticoagulant. However, this is not usually possible in a clinical laboratory, as many samples are received from general practices and other hospitals. All anticoagulants have some effect on the morphology of malaria parasites and the RBC they inhabit. This effect depends on the stage of the parasite, the time taken for the blood to arrive to the laboratory, and the type of anticoagulant used. If it is necessary to use an anticoagulant, the films should be prepared as soon as possible after the blood has been taken.

    b. If the films cannot be made immediately, potassium ethylenediaminetetraacetic acid (EDTA) is the anticoagulant of choice. However, if the blood is left for several hours in EDTA, the following effects may be seen.

        i. Sexual stages may continue to develop and male gametocytes can exflagellate, liberating gametes into the plasma. These can be mistaken for organisms such as *Borrelia*. Gametocytes of *P. falciparum*, which have a characteristic crescent shape, may round up and then resemble those of *Plasmodium malariae*.

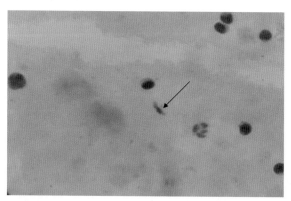

Fig. 4.3 The *arrow* indicates a gametocyte of *Plasmodium falciparum* with a crescent or sausage shape (1000× magnification).

    ii. Accolé forms, which are characteristic of *P. falciparum,* may be seen in *P. vivax* because of attempted reinvasion of the RBC by merozoites.

    iii. Mature trophozoites of *P. vivax* may condense when exposure becomes prolonged and in cases of extreme exposure, RBCs containing gametocytes and mature schizonts may be totally destroyed along with the contained parasites. The malaria pigment, hemozoin, always remains and can provide a clue to the presence and, to an expert eye, identity of the parasite.

    iv. The morphology of the RBCs may be altered by shrinkage or crenation.

  7. Appearance of *Plasmodium* spp. in thin blood films (Figs. 4.3–4.6, Tables 4.1–4.5)

C. Parasitological methods for Chagas disease:

  1. During acute phase:

    a. In the acute phase, motile trypomastigotes can be detected by microscopic examination of fresh anticoagulated blood or buffy coat. Parasites may also be visualized on blood smears stained with Giemsa or other stains and can be grown with the use of hemoculture in a specialized medium.

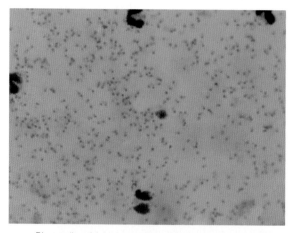

Fig. 4.4 Numerous *Plasmodium falciparum* trophozoites found in blood (1000× magnification).

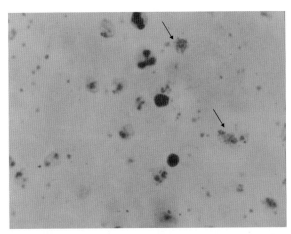

Fig. 4.5 The two *arrows* indicate gametocytes of *Plasmodium vivax*, stages found in blood (1000× magnification).

b. Microhematocrit is the method of choice to identify congenital infection because of its heightened sensitivity and the small amount of blood needed. Microscopic examination of cord blood or peripheral blood of the neonate using this technique is strongly recommended during the first month of life. If the results are repeatedly negative or if the test is not done early in life, the infant should be tested for anti-*Trypanosoma cruzi* immunoglobulin (Ig)G antibodies on several occasions between 6 and 9 months of age (preferentially at 9 months), when transferred maternal antibodies are no longer present in the infant.

c. In specialized centers, assays based on amplification of *T. cruzi* DNA by PCR could also be used for early diagnosis of congenital infection, since in this context the sensitivity of PCR seems to be greater than that of microscopic examination.[9]

2. During chronic phase:

a. During the chronic phase, because parasitemia is scarce, the presence of IgG antibodies against *T. cruzi* antigens needs to be detected by at least two different

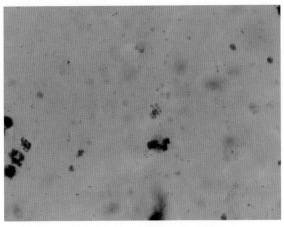

Fig. 4.6 Schizont stages of *Plasmodium malariae* found in blood (1000× magnification).

TABLE 4.1 ■ *Plasmodium falciparum*: Stages Found in Blood, and Appearance of Erythrocyte (Red Blood Cell) and Parasite

Stage Found in Blood	Appearance of Erythrocyte (RBC)	Appearance of Parasite
Ring	Normal; multiple infection of RBC more common than in other species; Maurer's clefts (under certain staining conditions)	Delicate cytoplasm; 1–2 small chromatin dots; occasional appliqué (accolé) forms
Trophozoite	Normal; rarely, Maurer's clefts (under certain staining conditions)	Seldom seen in peripheral blood; compact cytoplasm; dark pigment
Schizont	Normal; rarely, Maurer's clefts (under certain staining conditions)	Seldom seen in peripheral blood; mature = 8–24 small merozoites; dark pigment, clumped in one mass
Gametocyte	Distorted by parasite	Crescent or sausage shape; chromatin in a single mass (macrogametocyte) or diffuse (microgametocyte); dark pigment mass

RBC, Red blood cell.

serologic methods (usually enzyme-linked immunosorbent assay, indirect immuno-fluorescence, or indirect hemagglutination) to confirm diagnosis. No single assay for chronic *T. cruzi* infection has high enough sensitivity and specificity to be used alone; positive results of two tests, preferably based on different antigens (e.g., whole parasite lysate and recombinant antigens), are required for confirmation. Certainly, a proportion of persons tested will have discordant results of the two assays and will need further testing to determine their infection status.

b. PCR is not helpful in routine diagnosis because of the need for specific laboratory facilities, poor standardization, potential DNA cross-contamination, and variable

TABLE 4.2 ■ *Plasmodium vivax*: Stages Found in Blood, and Appearance of Erythrocyte and Parasite

Stage Found in Blood	Appearance of Erythrocyte (RBC)	Appearance of Parasite
Ring	Normal to 1.25×, round; occasionally fine Schüffner's dots; multiple infection of RBC not uncommon	Large cytoplasm with occasional pseudopods; large chromatin dot
Trophozoite	Enlarged 1.5–2×; may be distorted; fine Schüffner's dots	Large amoeboid cytoplasm; large chromatin; fine, yellowish-brown pigment
Schizont	Enlarged 1.5–2×; may be distorted; fine Schüffner's dots	Large, may almost fill RBC; mature = 12–24 merozoites; yellowish-brown, coalesced pigment
Gametocyte	Enlarged 1.5–2×; may be distorted; fine Schüffner's dots	Round to oval; compact; may almost fill RBC; chromatin compact, eccentric (macrogametocyte) or diffuse (microgametocyte); scattered brown pigment

RBC, Red blood cell.

TABLE 4.3 ■ *Plasmodium malariae*: Stages Found in Blood, and Appearance of Erythrocyte and Parasite

Stage Found in Blood	Appearance of Erythrocyte (RBC)	Appearance of Parasite
Ring	Normal to 0.75×	Sturdy cytoplasm; large chromatin
Trophozoite	Normal to 0.75×; rarely, Ziemann's stippling (under certain staining conditions)	Compact cytoplasm; large chromatin; occasional band forms; coarse, dark-brown pigment
Schizont	Normal to 0.75×; rarely, Ziemann's stippling (under certain staining conditions)	Mature = 6–12 merozoites with large nuclei, clustered around mass of coarse, dark-brown pigment; occasional rosettes
Gametocyte	Normal to 0.75×; rarely, Ziemann's stippling (under certain staining conditions)	Round to oval; compact; may almost fill RBC; chromatin compact, eccentric (macrogametocyte) or more diffuse (microgametocyte); scattered brown pigment

RBC, Red blood cell.

results across laboratories and countries. However, because of its heightened sensitivity compared with other parasitological methods, PCR could be useful to confirm diagnosis in cases of inconclusive serology, and as an auxiliary method to monitor treatment. PCR is useful to identify treatment failure from positive detection of *T. cruzi* DNA, but not treatment success because even repeated negative PCR results do not necessarily indicate parasitological cure. At best, such results are indicative of the absence of parasite DNA at the time of the test.

TABLE 4.4 ■ *Plasmodium ovale*: Stages Found in Blood, and Appearance of Erythrocyte and Parasite

Stage Found in Blood	Appearance of Erythrocyte (RBC)	Appearance of Parasite
Ring	Normal to 1.25×, round to oval; occasionally Schüffner's dots; occasionally fimbriated; multiple infection of RBC not uncommon	Sturdy cytoplasm; large chromatin
Trophozoite	Normal to 1.25×; round to oval; some fimbriated; Schüffner's dots	Compact with large chromatin; dark-brown pigment
Schizont	Normal to 1.25×, round to oval, some fimbriated, Schüffner's dots	Mature = 6–14 merozoites with large nuclei, clustered around mass of dark-brown pigment
Gametocyte	Normal to 1.25×; round to oval, some fimbriated; Schüffner's dots	Round to oval; compact; may almost fill RBC; chromatin compact, eccentric (macrogametocyte) or more diffuse (microgametocyte); scattered brown pigment

RBC, Red blood cell.

TABLE 4.5 ■ *Plasmodium knowlesi*: Stages Found in Blood, and Appearance of Erythrocyte and Parasite

Stage Found in Blood	Appearance of Erythrocyte (RBC)	Appearance of Parasite
Ring	Normal to 0.75×; multiple infection not uncommon	Delicate cytoplasm; 1–2 prominent chromatin dots; occasional appliqué (accolé) forms
Trophozoite	Normal to 0.75×; rarely, Sinton and Mulligan's stippling (under certain staining conditions)	Compact cytoplasm; large chromatin; occasional band forms; coarse, dark-brown pigment
Schizont	Normal to 0.75×; rarely, Sinton and Mulligan's stippling (under certain staining conditions)	Mature = up to 16 merozoites with large nuclei, clustered around mass of coarse, dark-brown pigment; occasional rosettes; mature merozoites appear segmented
Gametocyte	Normal to 0.75×; rarely, Sinton and Mulligan's stippling (under certain staining conditions)	Round to oval; compact; may almost fill RBC; chromatin compact, eccentric (macrogametocyte) or more diffuse (microgametocyte); scattered brown pigment

RBC, Red blood cell.

    c. Quantitative PCR assays are useful in monitoring for reactivation (e.g., after heart transplantation); a positive PCR result does not prove that reactivation has occurred, but a rising parasite load over time is the earliest and most sensitive indicator.[9]

Methods for Rapid Diagnosis of Parasitic Diseases

Although some common parasitic infections can be managed syndromically without the need for diagnostic tests, this approach cannot be appropriate for many other parasitic diseases, in which a positive diagnostic test is needed before treatment can be given. In that sense, many molecular and point-of-care (POC) tests have been created, all of them allowing a rapid diagnosis for many parasitic infections, a valuable characteristic for disasters.

Molecular tests: PCR has become an important diagnostic tool in the detection of parasitic pathogens. Many PCR tests have been validated, harmonized, and commercialized to make PCR a standard tool used by microbiology laboratories to detect parasitic pathogens. Current PCR technology allows for rapid detection of pathogens in real time.[10] In addition, real-time PCR can provide qualitative, as well as quantitative, information. In fact, during the last times have increased the number of laboratories where the multiplex PCR panel is being used as a first-line screening diagnostic method.[10]

Table 4.6 shows real-time PCR and other molecular methods useful for the diagnosis of some parasitic diseases.

Rapid tests: Although the field of molecular diagnostics in the clinical laboratory has escalated in the past two decades, simple, rapid immunoassays that are highly sensitive and specific, cost effective, and easy to use still remain as the methods of choice for quick and accurate results.

Rapid, reliable, and affordable POC tests, requiring no equipment and minimal training, are now available for some parasitic diseases such as malaria and filarial infections.[11] Table 4.7 reveals various rapid tests used for the diagnosis of some parasitic diseases and their main references.

TABLE 4.6 ■ Various Molecular Tests Used for the Fast Diagnosis of Parasitic Diseases, With References

Parasite Species/Parasitic Disease	Type of Molecular Test	Publication (Authors, Year)
Entamoeba histolytica, Entamoeba dispar, Entamoeba moshkovskii, Giardia lamblia, Cryptosporidium spp.	Multiplex PCR and real-time quantitative polymerase chain reaction with melting-curve analysis (qPCR-MCA) for simultaneous detection and differentiation in human fecal samples	Tajebe et al., 2016[21]
Giardia lamblia	Real-time PCR assays targeting the (SSU) rRNA and gdh genes	Boadi et al., 2014[22]
Cryptosporidium spp., Cyclospora cayetanensis, Entamoeba histolytica, Giardia lamblia	Multiplex FilmArray GI panel	Binnicker, 2015[23]
Cryptosporidium spp.	Genus-specific DNA dot blot hybridization assay; PCR; real-time PCR assay	Khalil et al., 2016[24]
Cryptosporidium spp., Cyclospora cayetanensis, Cystoisospora belli, Entamoeba histolytica	qPCR, TaqMan Array Card (Thermo Fisher, Carlsblad, CA, USA)	Liu et al., 2014[25]
Entamoeba histolytica, Cryptosporidium parvum/hominis, Giardia lamblia, Dientamoeba fragilis	Multiplex real-time PCR	Bruijnesteijn van Coppenraet et al., 2015[26]
Cryptosporidium spp., Cyclospora cayetanensis, Entamoeba histolytica, Giardia lamblia	Multiplex FilmArray GI panel; multiplex Luminex xTag GPP	Khare et al., 2014[27]
Human African trypanosomiasis	SL-RNA molecule for its diagnostic potential using reverse transcription followed by real-time PCR	González-Andrade, 2014[28]
Schistosoma mansoni	SYBR green real-time qPCR	Eraky et al., 2016[29]
	TaqMan qPCR technique	Espírito-Santo et al., 2014[30]
Echinococcus granulosus	Real-time loop-mediated isothermal amplification (LAMP) assay	Ahmed et al., 2016[31]
Chagas disease	Real-time qPCR	Ramírez et al., 2015[32]
	Multiplex real-time PCR assay	Cura et al., 2015[33]
Leishmania	Leishmania infantum kinetoplast DNA detection by real-time qPCR	Pessoa-E-Silva et al., 2016[34]
	Leishmania-specific real-time PCR	Opota et al., 2016[35]
	High-resolution melting-curve real-time PCR	Zampieri et al., 2016[36]
Malaria	Real-time PCR targeting the 18S rRNA gene	Diallo et al., 2016[37]
	Real-time fluorescence LAMP assay	Patel et al., 2014[38]
	SYBR Green I-based real-time PCR	Eroglu et al., 2014[39]
Schistosoma mansoni, Schistosoma haematobium	7500 Fast real-time PCR system (Applied Biosystems, Inc.; Foster City, CA, USA) with high-resolution melting-curve (HRM Master Mix) assay (Applied Biosystems, Inc.)	Sady et al., 2015[40]

TABLE 4.7 ■ **Various Rapid Tests Used for the Diagnosis of Parasitic Diseases, With References**

Species of Parasite	Type of Rapid Test (Company, Country)	Publication (Authors, Year)
Giardia lamblia	CORIS Giardia-Strip test (CORIS Bioconcepts, Gembloux, Belgium)	Oster et al., 2006[41]
Entamoeba histolytica, *Entamoeba dispar*	ImmunoCardSTAT CGE (Meridian Bioscence, Milan, Italy)	Formenti et al., 2015[42]
Cryptosporidium spp.	CoproStrip Cryptosporidium kit (Savyon Diagnostics Ltd., Israel)	Shimelis et al., 2014[43]
	ImmunoCard STAT (Meridian Bioscience Inc., Cincinnati, OH, USA)	El-Moamly et al., 2012[44]
Giardia lamblia, *Cryptosporidium* spp.	ImmunoCard STAT! *Cryptosporidium/Giardia* rapid assay (Meridian Bioscience, Inc., USA)	Minak et al., 2012[45]; Sadaka et al., 2015[46]
	Crypto-Giardia antigen rapid test (CA-RT) (DIA. PRO, Diagnostic Bioprobes, Milano, Italy)	Zaglool et al., 2013[47]
	Giardia/Cryptosporidium Quik Chek immunoassay (TechLab, Inc., USA). Quik Chek immunoassay (TechLab, Inc., USA).	Minak et al., 2012;[48] Alexander et al. 2013;[45] Van den Bossche et al., 2015[49]
	sdc Xpect *Giardia/Cryptosporidium* (Remel, Inc., USA)	Minak et al., 2012[45]
	Crypto/Giardia Duo-Strip (CORIS Bioconcepts, Gembloux, Belgium)	Van den Bossche et al., 2015[49]
Giardia lamblia, Entamoeba histolytica/Entamoeba dispar, and *Cryptosporidium* spp.	RIDA®QUICK *Cryptosporidium/Giardia/Entamoeba* Combi (R-BioPharm, Darmstadt, Germany)	Van den Bossche et al., 2015[49]
	ImmunoCardSTAT!®CGE (Meridian Bioscience Inc., Cincinnati, OH, USA)	Van den Bossche et al., 2015[49]
	Triage Micro Parasite Panel (Biosite Diagnostics, Inc., San Diego, CA, USA)	Sharp et al., 2001[50]
Human African trypanosomiasis	Card Agglutination Test for Trypanosomiasis (CATT)	Magnus et al., 1978[51]
	Immunochromatographic test (ICT) SD BIOLINE HAT	Bisser et al., 2016[52]
Echinococcus granulosus	ICT kit for CE (ADAMU-CE test; Saitama, Japan)	Santivañez et al., 2015[53]
	VI Rapid HYDATIDOSIS (Vircell, Salamanca, Spain); *Echinococcus* DIGFA (Unibiotest, Wuhan, China); ADAMU-CE (ICST, Japan)	Tamarozzi et al., 2016[54]

TABLE 4.7 ■ **Various Rapid Tests Used for the Diagnosis of Parasitic Diseases, With References—cont.**

Species of Parasite	Type of Rapid Test (Company, Country)	Publication (Authors, Year)
Chagas disease	Electrochemical magnetic microbeads-based biosensor (EMBIA) platform	Cortina et al., 2016[14]
	ICT Chagas Detect Plus (CDP) (InBios, Seattle, WA, USA).	Shah et al., 2014[55]
	ICT Operon (Operon S.A., Spain)	Flores-Chavez et al., 2012[56]
	Chagas STAT-PAK (Chembio Diagnostic Systems, Medford, NY, USA)	Chappuis et al., 2010[57]
	ICT-SD (Bioline Chagas Ab Rapid, Korea)	Ji et al., 2009[58]
Leishmania	ICT Signal-KA (Span Diagnostics, Ltd., Surat, India); ICT Crystal-KA (Span Diagnostics, Ltd., Surat, India); ICT Onsite Leishmania Ab (CTK Biotech, Inc., San Diego, CA, USA); ICT Rev A & Rev B rapid test (CTK Biotech, Inc., San Diego, CA, USA); ICT Kala-azar Detect (InBios International, Inc. (Seattle, WA, USA); ICT Bio-Rad Laboratories (Marnes-la-Coquette, France).	Kumar et al., 2013[59]; Ghosh, 2015[60]
Malaria	ICT-BinaxNOW Malaria (Binax, Inc., Inverness Medical Professional Diagnostics, Scarborough, ME, USA); ICT-SD Bioline (Standard Diagnostics Inc., Korea); ICT-Carestart (Access Bio Inc., Monmouth, USA); ICT-First Response (Premier Medical Co. Ltd., India)	Wanja et al., 2016;[61] Tadesse et al., 2016;[62] Abba et al., 2014;[63] Murray et al., 2008[64]
Lymphatic filariasis	ICT cards (AMRAD ICT, NSW, Australia)	Rebollo et al., 2015[65]
Schistosoma mansoni	Circulating Cathodic Antigen (POC-CCA) assay (Rapid Medical Diagnostics, Pretoria, South Africa)	Casacuberta et al., 2016[66]

It is important to highlight that the lack of regulation of diagnostic tests in many countries has resulted in the widespread use of substandard POC tests, especially for malaria, making it difficult for manufacturers of reliable POC tests to compete.

Other Diagnostic Methods and Conclusions

Some modern technologies depend on stable energy supplies, which can be problematic in disaster conditions; nevertheless, the current use of qualified portable energy supplies and powerful backups might fulfill this condition. Matrix-assisted laser desorption ionization-time of flight mass spectrometry (MALDI-TOF MS) is currently being used for rapid and reproducible identification of bacteria, viruses, and fungi in clinical microbiological laboratories; however, studies have also reported the use of this technique for identification of parasites such as *Giardia*, *Cryptosporidium*, *Entamoeba*, and *Leishmania*. In fact, MALDI-TOF MS is considered a promising technology that may replace/augment molecular methods in many clinical parasitology laboratories.[12]

Power cuts may occur during disasters because of difficulties in energy generation or temporary elimination of regional networks. Therefore, there is an unmet need to develop portable, simple, rapid, and accurate methods for detection of infections. Loop-mediated isothermal amplification assays do not require a source of electricity, and these technologies have proved useful where resources are limited.[13]

A portable, robust, and inexpensive electrochemical magnetic microbeads-based biosensor (EMBIA) platform for serodiagnosis of infectious diseases such as Chagas disease has been developed and validated; this technology platform could potentially be applicable to diagnosing other parasitic diseases.[14]

Taking into account the unmet need to develop portable, simple, rapid, and accurate methods for detection of infections, full laboratory-quality immunoassays have been developed and validated to run on smartphone accessories, and this advance can make certain laboratory-based diagnostics accessible to almost any population with access to smartphones.[15]

Other studies have highlighted the potential of smartphones as relatively sophisticated, inexpensive, and portable medical diagnostic devices. A field-portable and cost-effective platform for detection and quantification of *Giardia lamblia* cysts in environmental samples of drinkable and recreational water has been created; the platform consists of a smartphone coupled with an optomechanical attachment that uses a hand-held fluorescence microscope design aligned with the camera unit of the smartphone to image custom-designed disposable water sample cassettes. Each sample cassette is prepared to capture the individual *Giardia* cysts, which are fluorescently labeled.[16] Other studies have shown that a cellular smartphone can be used as an inexpensive device for imaging fluorescent eggs, and which, by harnessing the computational power of the phone, can perform image analysis to count the eggs.[17,18]

Disasters may place major strain on energy infrastructure in affected communities. Advances in renewable energy and microgrid technology offer the potential to improve mobile disaster medical response capabilities.[19] In the process of disaster preparedness, all personnel who work in infectious disease diagnostic laboratories should be adequately qualified.[20] Parasitology laboratories will be prepared to provide a capable response to disasters according to availability of technologies and other laboratory resources; but the most important factor for every catastrophe will be always accessibility to qualified and skilled human resources.

Suggested Reading

Ash LR, Orihel TC. *Atlas of Human Parasitology*. 4th ed. Chicago, IL: American Society of Clinical Pathologists; 1997.

Bailey MS, Thomas R, Green AD, Bailey JW, Beeching NJ. Helminth infections in British troops following an operation in Sierra Leone. *Trans R Soc Trop Med Hyg*. 2006;100(9):842–846.

Bern C. Chagas' disease. *N Engl J Med*. 2015;373(5):456–466.

Garcia LS. *Practical Guide to Diagnostic Parasitology*. Washington, DC: American Society for Microbiology; 1999.

Guzman-Tapia Y, Ramírez-Sierra MJ, Escobedo-Ortegon J, Dumonteil E. Effect of Hurricane Isidore on *Triatoma dimidiata* distribution and Chagas disease transmission risk in the Yucatán Peninsula of Mexico. *Am J Trop Med Hyg*. 2005;73(6):1019–1025.

Ketai L, Currie BJ, Alva Lopez LF. Thoracic radiology of infections emerging after natural disasters. *J Thorac Imaging*. 2006;21(4):265–275.

Krishnamoorthy K, Jambulingam P, Natarajan R, Shriram AN, Das PK, Sehgal SC. Altered environment and risk of malaria outbreak in South Andaman, Andaman & Nicobar Islands, India affected by tsunami disaster. *Malar J.* 2005;4:32.

Li XH, Hou SK, Zheng JC, Fan HJ, Song JQ. Post-disaster medical rescue strategy in tropical regions. *World J Emerg Med.* 2012;3(1):23–28.

Lora-Suarez F, Marin-Vasquez C, Loango N, et al. Giardiasis in children living in post-earthquake camps from Armenia (Colombia). *BMC Public Health.* 2002;2:5.

Melvin DM, Brooke MM. *Morphology of Diagnostic Stages of Intestinal Parasites of Humans.* 2nd ed. US Department of Health and Human Services Publication No. (CDC) 89-8116. Atlanta, GA: Centers for Disease Control and Prevention; 1989.

National Committee for Clinical Laboratory Standards. *Laboratory Diagnosis of Blood-Borne Parasitic Diseases. Approved Guideline M15-A.* Wayne, PA: National Committee for Clinical Laboratory Standards; 2000.

National Committee for Clinical Laboratory Standards. *Procedures for the Recovery and Identification of Parasites From the Intestinal Tract. Approved Guideline M28-A.* Wayne, PA: National Committee for Clinical Laboratory Standards; 1997.

Orihel TC, Ash LR, Ramachandran CP, Ottesen E. *Bench Aids for the Diagnosis of Filarial Infections.* Geneva: World Health Organization; 1997.

Oztürk CE, Sahin I, Yavuz T, Oztürk A, Akgünoğlu M, Kaya D. Intestinal parasitic infection in children in post-disaster situations years after earthquake. *Pediatr Int.* 2004;46(6):656–662.

Peters W, Gilles HM. *Color Atlas of Tropical Medicine and Parasitology.* 4th ed. London: Mosby-Wolfe; 1995.

Setzer C, Domino ME. Medicaid outpatient utilization for waterborne pathogenic illness following Hurricane Floyd. *Public Health Rep.* 2004;119(5):472–478.

Suner S. History of disaster medicine. *Turk J Emerg Med.* 2016;15(suppl 1):1–4.

Tajebe A, Magoma G, Aemero M, Kimani F. Detection of mixed infection level of *Plasmodium falciparum* and *Plasmodium vivax* by SYBR Green I-based real-time PCR in North Gondar, north-west Ethiopia. *Malar J.* 2014;13:411.

Townes D, Existe A, Boncy J, et al. Malaria survey in post-earthquake Haiti—2010. *Am J Trop Med Hyg.* 2012;86(1):29–31.

Wannasan A, Uparanukraw P, Songsangchun A, Morakote N. Potentially pathogenic free-living amoebae in some flood-affected areas during 2011 Chiang Mai flood. *Rev Inst Med Trop Sao Paulo.* 2013;55(6):411–416.

Wu XH, Zhang SQ, Xu XJ, et al. Effect of floods on the transmission of schistosomiasis in the Yangtze River valley, People's Republic of China. *Parasitol Int.* 2008;57(3):271–276.

References

1. Francis J, Barrett SP, Chiodini PL. Best Practice No. 174. Best practice guidelines for the examination of specimens for the diagnosis of parasitic infections in routine diagnostic laboratories. *J Clin Pathol.* 2003;56(12):888–891.

2. Garcia LS. *Diagnostic Medical Parasitology.* 4th ed. Washington, DC: American Society for Microbiology; 2001.

3. Ash LR, Orihel TC, Salvioli L. *Bench Aids for the Diagnosis of Intestinal Parasites.* Geneva: World Health Organization; 1994.

4. Melvin DM, Brooke MM. *Laboratory Procedures for the Diagnosis of Intestinal Parasites.* 3rd ed. US Department of Health and Human Services Publication No. (CDC) 82-8282. Atlanta, GA: Centers for Disease Control and Prevention; 1982.

5. Ash LR, Orihel TC, Bosman A. *Bench Aids for the Diagnosis of Malaria Infections.* Geneva: World Health Organization; 2000.

6. Ash LR, Orihel TC. *Parasites: A Guide to Laboratory Procedures and Identification.* Chicago, IL: American Society of Clinical Pathologists; 1991.

7. Chiodini PL, Engbaek K, Heuek CC, et al. *Basic Laboratory Methods in Medical Parasitology.* Geneva: World Health Organization; 1991.

8. Wilcox A. *Manual for the Microscopical Diagnosis of Malaria in Man.* Bethesda, MD: US Department of Health, Education, and Welfare; 1960.

9. Rassi A Jr, A Rassi A, Marin-Neto JA. Chagas disease. *Lancet.* 2010;375(9723):1388–1402.

10. Verweij JJ. Application of PCR-based methods for diagnosis of intestinal parasitic infections in the clinical laboratory. *Parasitology.* 2014;141(14):1863–1872.
11. Peeling RW, Mabey D. Point-of-care tests for diagnosing infections in the developing world. *Clin Microbiol Infect.* 2010;16(8):1062–1069.
12. Singhal N, Kumar M, Virdi JS. MALDI-TOF MS in clinical parasitology: applications, constraints and prospects. *Parasitology.* 2016;143(12):1491–1500.
13. Hattori T, Chagan-Yasutan H, Shiratori B, et al. Development of point-of-care testing for disaster-related infectious diseases. *Tohoku J Exp Med.* 2016;238(4):287–293.
14. Cortina ME, Melli LJ, Roberti M, et al. Electrochemical magnetic microbeads-based biosensor for point-of-care serodiagnosis of infectious diseases. *Biosens Bioelectron.* 2016;80:24–33.
15. Laksanasopin T, Guo TW, Nayak S, et al. A smartphone dongle for diagnosis of infectious diseases at the point of care. *Sci Transl Med.* 2015;7(273):273.
16. Koydemir HC, Gorocs Z, Tseng D, et al. Rapid imaging, detection and quantification of *Giardia lamblia* cysts using mobile-phone based fluorescent microscopy and machine learning. *Lab Chip.* 2015;15(5):1284–1293.
17. Slusarewicz P, Pagano S, Mills C, et al. Automated parasite faecal egg counting using fluorescence labelling, smartphone image capture and computational image analysis. *Int J Parasitol.* 2016;46(8): 485–493.
18. Sowerby SJ, Crump JA, Johnstone MC, Krause KL, Hill PC. Smartphone microscopy of parasite eggs accumulated into a single field of view. *Am J Trop Med Hyg.* 2016;94(1):227–230.
19. Callaway DW, Noste E, McCahill PW, et al. Time for a revolution: smart energy and microgrid use in disaster response. *Disaster Med Public Health Prep.* 2014;8(3):252–259.
20. Nekoie-Moghadam M, Kurland L, Moosazadeh M, Ingrassia PL, Della Corte F, Djalali A. Tools and checklists used for the evaluation of hospital disaster preparedness: a systematic review. *Disaster Med Public Health Prep.* 2016;10(5):781–788.
21. Tajebe A, Magoma G, Aemero M, et al. Simultaneous detection and differentiation of *Entamoeba histolytica, E. dispar, E. moshkovskii, Giardia lamblia* and *Cryptosporidium* spp. in human fecal samples using multiplex PCR and qPCR-MCA. *Acta Trop.* 2016;162:233–238.
22. Boadi S, Polley SD, Kilburn S, Mills GA, Chiodini PL. A critical assessment of two real-time PCR assays targeting the (SSU) rRNA and gdh genes for the molecular identification of *Giardia intestinalis* in a clinical laboratory. *J Clin Pathol.* 2014;67(9):811–816.
23. Binnicker MJ. Multiplex molecular panels for diagnosis of gastrointestinal infection: performance, result interpretation, and cost-effectiveness. *J Clin Microbiol.* 2015;53(12):3723–3728.
24. Khalil S, Mirdha BR, Paul J, et al. Development and evaluation of molecular methods for detection of *Cryptosporidium* spp. in human clinical samples. *Exp Parasitol.* 2016;170:207–213.
25. Liu J, Kabir F, Manneh J, et al. Development and assessment of molecular diagnostic tests for 15 enteropathogens causing childhood diarrhoea: a multicentre study. *Lancet Infect Dis.* 2014;14:716–724.
26. Bruijnesteijn van Coppenraet LE, Dullaert-de Boer M, Ruijs GJ, et al. Case-control comparison of bacterial and protozoan microorganisms associated with gastroenteritis: application of molecular detection. *Clin Microbiol Infect.* 2015;21(6):592e9–592e19.
27. Khare R, Espy MJ, Cebelinski E, et al. Comparative evaluation of two commercial multiplex panels for detection of gastrointestinal pathogens by use of clinical stool specimens. *J Clin Microbiol.* 2014;52(10):3667–3673.
28. González-Andrade P, Camara M, Ilboudo H, Bucheton B, Jamonneau V, Deborggraeve S. Diagnosis of trypanosomatid infections: targeting the spliced leader RNA. *J Mol Diagn.* 2014;16(4):400–404.
29. Eraky MA, Aly NS. Diagnostic and prognostic value of cell free circulating *Schistosoma mansoni* DNA: an experimental study. *J Parasit Dis.* 2016;40(3):1014–1020.
30. Espírito-Santo MC, Alvarado-Mora MV, Dias-Neto E, et al. Evaluation of real-time PCR assay to detect *Schistosoma mansoni* infections in a low endemic setting. *BMC Infect Dis.* 2014;14:558.
31. Ahmed ME, Eldigail MH, Elamin FM, Ali IA, Grobusch MP, Aradaib IE. Development and evaluation of real-time loop-mediated isothermal amplification assay for rapid detection of cystic echinococcosis. *BMC Vet Res.* 2016;12:202.
32. Ramírez JC, Cura CI, da Cruz Moreira O, et al. Analytical validation of quantitative real-time PCR methods for quantification of *Trypanosoma cruzi* DNA in blood samples from Chagas disease patients. *J Mol Diagn.* 2015;17(5):605–615.

33. Cura CI, Duffy T, Lucero RH, et al. Multiplex real-time PCR assay using TaqMan probes for the identification of *Trypanosoma cruzi* DTUs in biological and clinical samples. *PLoS Negl Trop Dis*. 2015;9(5):e0003765.

34. Pessoa-e-Silva R, Mendonça Trajano-Silva LA, Lopes da Silva MA, et al. Evaluation of urine for *Leishmania infantum* DNA detection by real-time quantitative PCR. *J Microbiol Methods*. 2016;131:34–41.

35. Opota O, Balmpouzis Z, Berutto C, et al. Visceral leishmaniasis in a lung transplant recipient: usefulness of highly sensitive real-time polymerase chain reaction for preemptive diagnosis. *Transpl Infect Dis*. 2016;18(5):801–804.

36. Zampieri RA, Laranjeira-Silva MF, Muxel SM, Stocco de Lima AC, Shaw JJ, Floeter-Winter LM. High resolution melting analysis targeting hsp70 as a fast and efficient method for the discrimination of *Leishmania* species. *PLoS Negl Trop Dis*. 2016;10(2):e0004485.

37. Diallo MA, Badiane AS, Diongue K, et al. Non-falciparum malaria in Dakar: a confirmed case of *Plasmodium ovale wallikeri* infection. *Malar J*. 2016;15(1):429.

38. Patel JC, Lucchi NW, Srivastava P, et al. Field evaluation of a real-time fluorescence loop-mediated isothermal amplification assay, RealAmp, for the diagnosis of malaria in Thailand and India. *J Infect Dis*. 2014;210(8):1180–1187.

39. Eroglu F, Uzun S, Koltas IS. Comparison of clinical samples and methods in chronic cutaneous leishmaniasis. *Am J Trop Med Hyg*. 2014;91(5):895–900.

40. Sady H, Al-Mekhlafi HM, Ngui R, et al. Detection of *Schistosoma mansoni* and *Schistosoma haematobium* by real-time PCR with high resolution melting analysis. *Int J Mol Sci*. 2015;16(7):16085–16103.

41. Oster N, Gehrig-Feistel H, Jung H, Kammer J, McLean JE, Lanzer M. Evaluation of the immunochromatographic CORIS Giardia-Strip test for rapid diagnosis of *Giardia lamblia*. *Eur J Clin Microbiol Infect Dis*. 2006;25(2):112–115.

42. Formenti F, Perandin F, Bonafini S, Degani M, Bisoffi Z. Evaluation of the new ImmunoCard STAT!® CGE test for the diagnosis of amebiasis [Article in French]. *Bull Soc Pathol Exot*. 2015;108(3):171–174.

43. El-Moamly AA, El-Sweify MA. ImmunoCard STAT cartridge antigen detection assay compared to microplate enzyme immunoassay and modified Kinyoun's acid-fast staining technique for detection of *Cryptosporidium* in fecal specimens. *Parasitol Res*. 2012;110(2):1037–1041.

44. Shimelis T, Tadesse E. Performance evaluation of point-of-care test for detection of *Cryptosporidium* stool antigen in children and HIV infected adults. *Parasit Vectors*. 2014;7:227.

45. Minak J, Kabir M, Mahmud I, et al. Evaluation of rapid antigen point-of-care tests for detection of *Giardia* and *Cryptosporidium* species in human fecal specimens. *J Clin Microbiol*. 2012;50(1):154–156.

46. Sadaka HA, Gaafar MR, Mady RF, Hezema NN. Evaluation of ImmunoCard STAT test and ELISA versus light microscopy in diagnosis of giardiasis and cryptosporidiosis. *Parasitol Res*. 2015;114(8):2853–2863.

47. Zaglool DA, Mohamed A, Khodari YA, Farooq MU. Crypto-Giardia antigen rapid test versus conventional modified Ziehl-Neelsen acid fast staining method for diagnosis of cryptosporidiosis. *Asian Pac J Trop Med*. 2013;6(3):212–215.

48. Alexander CL, Niebel M, Jones B. The rapid detection of *Cryptosporidium* and *Giardia* species in clinical stools using the Quik Chek immunoassay. *Parasitol Int*. 2013;62(6):552–553.

49. Van den Bossche D, Cnops L, Verschueren J, Van Esbroeck M. Comparison of four rapid diagnostic tests, ELISA, microscopy and PCR for the detection of *Giardia lamblia*, *Cryptosporidium* spp. and *Entamoeba histolytica* in feces. *J Microbiol Methods*. 2015;110:78–84.

50. Sharp SE, Suarez CA, Duran Y, Poppiti RJ. Evaluation of the Triage Micro Parasite Panel for detection of *Giardia lamblia*, *Entamoeba histolytica/Entamoeba dispar*, and *Cryptosporidium parvum* in patient stool specimens. *J Clin Microbiol*. 2001;39(1):332–334.

51. Magnus E, Vervoort T, Van Meirvenne N. A card agglutination test with stained trypanosomes (CATT) for the serological diagnosis of *T. b. gambiense* trypanosomiasis. *Ann Soc Belg Med Trop*. 1978;58(3):169–176.

52. Bisser S, Lumbala C, Nguertoum E, et al. Sensitivity and specificity of a prototype rapid diagnostic test for the detection of *Trypanosoma brucei gambiense* infection: a multi-centric prospective study. *PLoS Negl Trop Dis*. 2016;10(4):e0004608.

53. Santivañez SJ, Rodriguez ML, Rodriguez S, et al. Evaluation of a new immunochromatographic test using recombinant antigen b8/1 for diagnosis of cystic echinococcosis. *J Clin Microbiol*. 2015;53(12):3859–3863.

54. Tamarozzi F, Covini I, Mariconti M, et al. Comparison of the diagnostic accuracy of three rapid tests for the serodiagnosis of hepatic cystic echinococcosis in humans. *PLoS Negl Trop Dis.* 2016;10(2):e0004444.
55. Shah V, Ferrufino L, Gilman RH, et al. Field evaluation of the InBios Chagas detect plus rapid test in serum and whole-blood specimens in Bolivia. *Clin Vaccine Immunol.* 2014;21(12):1645–1649.
56. Flores-Chavez M, Cruz I, Nieto J, et al. Sensitivity and specificity of an operon immunochromatographic test in serum and whole-blood samples for the diagnosis of *Trypanosoma cruzi* infection in Spain, an area of nonendemicity. *Clin Vaccine Immunol.* 2012;19(9):1353–1359.
57. Chappuis F, Mauris A, Holst M, et al. Validation of a rapid immunochromatographic assay for diagnosis of *Trypanosoma cruzi* infection among Latin-American migrants in Geneva, Switzerland. *J Clin Microbiol.* 2010;48(8):2948–2952.
58. Ji MJ, Noh JS, Cho BK, Cho YS, Kim SJ, Yoon BS. Evaluation of SD BIOLINE Chagas Ab Rapid kit [Article in Korean]. *Korean J Lab Med.* 2009;29(1):48–52.
59. Ghosh P, Hasnain MG, Ghosh D, et al. A comparative evaluation of the performance of commercially available rapid immunochromatographic tests for the diagnosis of visceral leishmaniasis in Bangladesh. *Parasit Vectors.* 2015;8:331.
60. Kumar D, Khanal B, Tiwary P, et al. Comparative evaluation of blood and serum samples in rapid immunochromatographic tests for visceral leishmaniasis. *J Clin Microbiol.* 2013;51(12):3955–3959.
61. Abba K, Kirkham AJ, Olliaro PL, et al. Rapid diagnostic tests for diagnosing uncomplicated non-falciparum or *Plasmodium vivax* malaria in endemic countries. *Cochrane Database Syst Rev.* 2014;12:CD011431.
62. Murray CK, Gasser RA Jr, Magill AJ, Miller RS. Update on rapid diagnostic testing for malaria. *Clin Microbiol Rev.* 2008;21(1):97–110.
63. Tadesse E, Workalemahu B, Shimelis T. Diagnostic performance evaluation of the SD Bioline Malaria Ag Pf/Pan Test (05FK60) in a malaria endemic area of southern Ethiopia. *Rev Inst Med Trop Sao Paulo.* 2016;58:59.
64. Wanja EW, Kuya N, Moranga C, et al. Field evaluation of diagnostic performance of malaria rapid diagnostic tests in western Kenya. *Malar J.* 2016;15:456.
65. Rebollo MP, Sambou SM, Thomas B, et al. Elimination of lymphatic filariasis in the Gambia. *PLoS Negl Trop Dis.* 2015;9(3):e0003642.
66. Casacuberta M, Kinunghi S, Vennervald BJ, Olsen A. Evaluation and optimization of the Circulating Cathodic Antigen (POC-CCA) cassette test for detecting *Schistosoma mansoni* infection by using image analysis in school children in Mwanza Region, Tanzania. *Parasite Epidemiol Control.* 2016;1(2):105–115.

CHAPTER 5

Nutritional Diseases of Low- and Middle-Income Countries

Bradley Boetig ▉ Lorna Renner

Introduction

Nutrition is a fundamental domain of global health; it is fundamental to the health of individuals, the stability of populations, and the academic discipline that is global health.

Nutrition is also a domain of global health where military forces are likely to be called upon to assist. Undernourishment is chronic in many less-developed regions across the globe, and many more people are acutely vulnerable to undernourishment with even the slightest perturbation in their local economy or community. War and conflict often serve as major disruptors that push vulnerable populations into acute states of undernourishment, and already-undernourished individuals into the most desperate of circumstances. This chapter will begin with an overview of the fundamentals of nutrition as should be understood from the perspective of a global health practitioner, and then transition to a discussion of the relationship between nutrition and security.

The Global Burden of Malnutrition

It is important to comprehend the scope and depth of the problem of malnutrition if one aspires to assist in combating the problem. There are currently 795 million people in the world who are undernourished.[1] Although hunger and food insecurity can be found even in the wealthiest countries, the overwhelming majority of clinically undernourished people reside in developing countries. Of all people who live in developing countries, 12.9% are undernourished.[1] The following figure (Fig. 5.1a) from the World Food Program illustrates the prevalence of undernourishment in various parts of the world.

Undernourishment represents such an enormous burden to global health and development that it is the subject of the second Sustainable Development Goal: "End hunger, achieve food security and improved nutrition and promote sustainable agriculture." In the era of the Millennium Development Goals (MDGs), undernourishment was represented by goal number 1c: "Halve, between 1990 and 2015, the proportion of people who suffer from hunger."

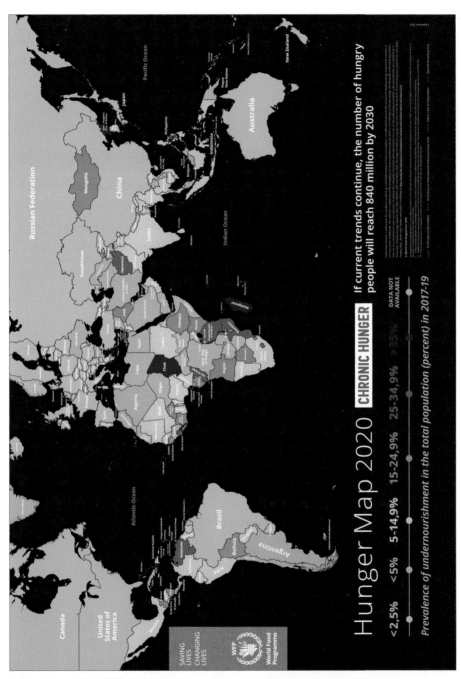

Fig. 5.1a   Hunger Map 2020. From https://www.wfp.org/publications/hunger-map-2020.

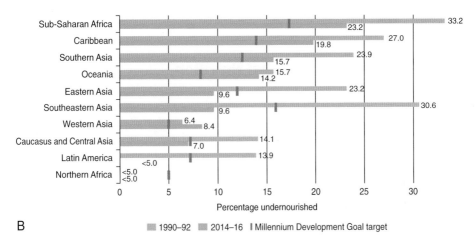

B

▨ 1990–92 ▨ 2014–16 ❙ Millennium Development Goal target

Fig. 5.1b Undernourishment trends: progress made in almost all regions but at very different rates.

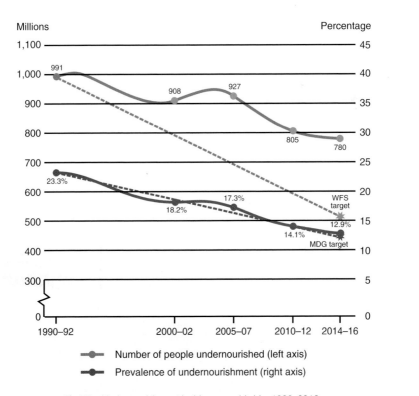

Fig. 5.2 Undernourishment incidence worldwide, 1990–2016.

Despite the profound challenges and diverse obstacles to addressing undernourishment, significant progress was made in most regions of the world during the period of the MDGs. Fig. 5.1b shows that all regions have made positive progress toward addressing undernourishment, with Western Asia being an unfortunate but lone exception. Fig. 5.2 shows the general decline in overall undernourishment worldwide from 1990 through 2016. It is important to consider, however, that despite progress in the right direction, 795 million people suffering chronic undernourishment is a tragic burden on an enormous scale.

Basic Terminology in Global Nutrition

It is important to have a precise understanding of the basic terms used in this subfield. Nutrition challenges are large, complex, and require multidisciplinary teams working together toward common goals. A common lexicon understood by all is therefore of significant import. This section will precisely define the most common terms used within this subfield and highlight the relationships between these terms that give them meaning to global health planners and practitioners.

Proper nourishment for all is the goal, and improperly nourished individuals are said to be "malnourished." Malnourished is a term that includes both "undernourished" and "overnourished" (Fig. 5.3). The phenomenon of overnourishment is creating a rapidly increasing health burden, particularly in middle-income countries, as it leads to costly secondary conditions such as obesity, heart disease, diabetes, and stroke, among others. Those conditions of overnourishment (sometimes referred to as "noncommunicable diseases") are not the focus of this chapter. This chapter will focus on the challenge of undernourishment because it is believed that although the two subfields have some overlap, they generally require different approaches and strategies to work toward solutions. The problems of undernourishment are also thought to be more closely linked to security and instability.

"Undernourishment" is further divided into two major categories: macronutrient deficiency (sometimes called "PEM" for "protein-energy malnutrition") and micronutrient deficiency (sometimes referred to as vitamin-mineral deficiency). The "macronutrients" are carbohydrates, proteins, and fats—the large molecules that provide energy, measured in kilocalories. An acute shortage of macronutrients leads to wasting (extreme thinness), whereas chronic deficiency leads to stunting (poor growth) among many other problems discussed later in this chapter. "Micronutrients" are vitamins, minerals, and other small molecules that serve as catalysts in various chemical processes in the human body; they are an essential component of healthy growth and development and result in a wide manifestation of unique symptoms as will be discussed later in this chapter. The most common micronutrient deficiencies in stable populations are iron, vitamin A, zinc, and iodine deficiency. In unstable populations, attention needs to additionally be paid to thiamine, niacin, vitamin C, and riboflavin deficiencies.

The category macronutrient deficiency (PEM) subdivides into two categories based on time/duration of deficiency: acute ("wasting") and chronic ("stunting"). Acute or "short-term" deficiency in macronutrients results, predictably, in "thinness" which, when excessive, is referred to as

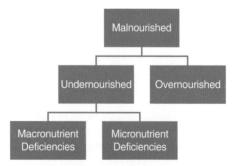

Fig. 5.3   Malnourished individuals may be undernourished or overnourished.

> **BOX 5.1 ■ Kilocalories**
>
> Energy in food is most often measured in "kilocalories." In the United States, a kilocalorie is often referred to simply as a "calorie," but that is not technically correct. Sometimes kilocalorie is written as "Calorie" (with a capital C) to signify that it represents 1000 calories, or 1 kilocalorie. In general, a calorie is such a small unit of energy that it has no practical value in nutrition, thus energy in food is measured in kilocalories.

wasting. Someone who is "wasted" will be thin and will have low "weight-for-height" and probably also low "weight-for-age" measurements, but will typically have a normal "height-for-age." In other words, the short duration of the macronutrient deficiency precludes any measurable effect on the child's linear growth measurement. A patient is said to be wasted when their weight-for-height measurement is greater than two standard deviations (SDs) below the mean. High numbers of cases of wasting are typically seen in populations experiencing conflict, natural disaster, or displacement for any reason.

"Chronic" macronutrient deficiency is a long-term phenomenon that is most common in least developed countries but also prominent in poorer, usually rural areas of middle-income countries. Children who suffer chronic macronutrient deficiency will become "stunted" as measured by a low height-for-age. Stunting is defined as greater than two SDs below the mean for height for that patient's age. Patients certainly can be stunted and wasted (suffering from both chronic and acute macronutrient deficiency), in which case they would be both short-for-age and very thin. Children can also be stunted without being wasted, which is the case when they have previously suffered long periods of chronic macronutrient deficiency (and are now stunted) but are not acutely experiencing undernourishment (so they are no longer wasted).

Macronutrient deficiency also has three recognized subtypes: marasmus, kwashiorkor, and marasmic-kwashiorkor. Marasmus refers to a deficiency of energy, usually measured in kilocalories (Box 5.1). Marasmus implies that a person is suffering from deficiency of all the macronutrients—proteins, fats, and carbohydrates. Patients with marasmus are thin, with skinny arms and legs. They often have soft, sparse hair; extra skin around the buttocks (referred to as the "baggy pants" effect); and a look that is described as "old man facies." These patients can be either apathetic or alert and are often hungry.

Kwashiorkor refers to a deficiency of protein specifically. Patients with kwashiorkor have often been eating a diet that is exclusively carbohydrate in composition, such as rice or potatoes, without meat or other protein source. In contrast to the patient with marasmus, patients with kwashiorkor often have a poor appetite. Most significantly, they often have edema (in the abdomen, as well as the hands, feet, and elsewhere) that disguises their otherwise thin stature.

The combination of lack of appetite and edematous appearance can cause these patients to be overlooked when one is screening for malnutrition. In addition to disguising their thinness, the edema also increases these patients' weight measurements, and therefore they are easy to overlook. Physical examination to include assessment for edema (particularly of the abdomen, hands, and feet) is therefore an essential component of screening for malnutrition. Patients with kwashiorkor are also often irritable; sometimes have what is described as "moon facies"; and often present with pale, sparse, sometimes reddish hair and sometimes an enlarged liver.

Perhaps the most distinctive features of kwashiorkor (other than edema) are the "flag sign" and the "flaky-paint" rash. The flag sign refers to a distinct band of pale or blonde hair in an otherwise dark-haired individual. This stripe of blond hair represents a period of time when the patient suffered from severe protein deficiency (kwashiorkor). All-blonde hair in a patient of a genetic makeup that would not be expected to have blonde hair is a sign that is concerning for kwashiorkor. Patients with kwashiorkor often have a rash that looks like the skin has peeled or flaked off as would old paint from a wall. The rash, when present, is therefore referred to as the flaky-paint rash.

Marasmus and kwashiorkor have traditionally been thought of as separate entities, the former being a global deficiency in all macronutrients (fats, protein, and carbohydrates) and latter a severe deficiency specific to protein. There was clinical value in recognizing these as separate conditions because they call for different treatment plans, and because it is important to not overlook patients with kwashiorkor who, because of the edema, might not appear malnourished to the untrained eye. As the subfield advanced its understanding of undernourishment, however, it was recognized that a significant number of severely malnourished children actually suffer from both marasmus and kwashiorkor and therefore require specific attention and treatment for both clinical syndromes. These patients are said to have "marasmic-kwashiorkor." Patients suffering from marasmic-kwashiorkor are in a particularly dangerous physical state and need urgent skilled, comprehensive care (see section Treatment of Severe Acute Malnutrition).

Assessing Malnutrition

Four basic measurements used to rapidly assess for malnutrition are height, length, weight, and middle-upper arm circumference (MUAC). The related terms height and length actually have an important clinical distinction when assessing for malnutrition: height is measured with the patient standing, and length is measured with the patient lying down. Although the distinction might sound trivial, the difference in measurement technique is clinically significant when assessing toddlers and young children. In general, children under the age of 2 years should have their length measured (lying down); children over 3 years of age should have their height measured; and between 2 and 3 years of age children can be measured by either method, but the clinician must ensure that their chosen method is the same as that used to generate the reference table or growth chart of normal values. Plotting a 2.5-year-old child's length, for example, on a chart where the standard values are height measurements will decrease the sensitivity of the assessment.

In contrast to height and length, weight measurements are intuitive and can be assessed with a variety of scale types. Once height (or length) and weight are known, standard World Health Organization (WHO) growth charts can be used to plot weight-for-age, height-for-age, and even weight-for-height. A particularly low weight-for-length implies acute macronutrient deficiency. A very low height-for-age suggests likely chronic macronutrient deficiency. A patient with low weight-for-age can be suffering from either (or both) acute or chronic macronutrient deficiency.

Measuring and plotting weight-for-height, height-for-age, and weight-for-age is not particularly difficult, but it does require an amount of time and effort, which can be particularly burdensome when there is a need to assess a large population in a short period of time with very limited staff. MUAC is therefore an alternative measurement that was developed for these more time-limited situations. MUAC is a simple measurement that involves the use of a flexible tape to measure the circumference of the midportion of the upper arm. MUAC measurements are so simple that one does not even need to consider a young child's age when taking the measurement because it is theorized that the mid-upper arm circumference is stable enough from 6 months through 5 years of age—particularly when one is assessing for severe acute malnutrition in a distressed population. MUAC measurements are therefore argued to have reasonable sensitivity and specificity for use in time-pressed situations. International organizations have established cutoff values for severe, moderate, and mild malnutrition, and children are sometimes simply classified according to this one metric.

Worth noting, however, is that international organizations have not always agreed on what MUAC measurement constitutes severe, acute, or mild malnutrition. For example, Médecins

Sans Frontières (MSF) defines severe acute malnutrition as any child with a MUAC of less than 125 mm, but the United Nations Children's Fund (United Nations International Children's Emergency Fund [UNICEF]) uses 115 mm as its cutoff. UNICEF actually increased its cutoff from 110 to 115 after it determined that 115 mm correlates approximately with SDs below the mean on weight-for-height measurements. Despite these disagreements over cutoff values, however, the use of MUAC to assess malnutrition has advantages that include ease of use, speed of assessment, and minimal training requirements, and only a minimal amount of equipment (just the tape) is needed.

There are several disadvantages to using MUAC measurements, however. It has been shown, for example, that the norms for MUAC actually do differ somewhat between 6 months and 5 years of age, despite prior claims to the contrary. MUAC has been shown to have more measurement error than height and weight measurements—and this error applies to both individual and interuser variability in measurements. In addition, in general, MUAC has been shown to be less specific than height-for-weight measurements when assessing for wasting.

Perhaps as a result of these recognized limitations, a practical compromise has been reached when it comes to MUAC measurements: their use should be limited to situations when rapid screening is needed to quickly determine admission to treatment facilities, but they should not be used for prevalence studies, and they are not to be interpreted as a predictor of mortality. Even better, MSF has adopted a two-step protocol: they use a fairly high cutoff value (125 mm instead of 115 mm) to assess for severe malnutrition (thus ensuring adequate sensitivity of their screening process), and then all patients with less than 125 mm MUAC measurement receive follow-up testing via the more conventional methods of weight-for-height and weight-for-age (ensuring adequate specificity).

Height, length, weight, and MUAC are all categorized as anthropometric measurements—measurement of the human individual. "Assessment" and screening for malnutrition, however, requires assessment beyond pure measurements. There are physical findings related to kwashiorkor, for example, that must be recognized when present. Edema, particularly of the hands, feet, and abdomen; flaky-paint rash; and flag sign in the hair are all signs of kwashiorkor for which anthropometric screening tests do not have adequate sensitivity and must be recognized on an individual basis by clinical assessment. Beyond kwashiorkor, there are several important micronutrient deficiencies (vitamin A, thiamine, iodine, and iron) that each cause a spectrum of signs and symptoms that must be assessed. These signs and symptoms of micronutrient deficiency are discussed in the section on micronutrient deficiencies later.

The treatment of severe acute malnutrition differs from that of moderate acute malnutrition; it is important, therefore, to first properly assess and triage the patient into the appropriate category. The three criteria of symmetrical edema, weight-for-height measurement, and height-for-age measurement will allow one to do this (Table 5.1).

Any patient with symmetrical edema is considered severely malnourished; this underscores the grave danger of kwashiorkor and the importance of prompt recognition and treatment. In addition, any patient with a weight-for-height or height-for-age less than three SDs below the mean is considered severely malnourished. Children between two and three SDs below the mean are classified as moderately malnourished. Additional important medical history and clinical examination findings relevant to assessment of malnutrition are provided in Box 5.2.

Treatment of Severe Acute Malnutrition

Treatment of severe acute malnutrition requires attention to several principles that are critically important to maximizing favorable outcomes. These principles include immediate treatment for dehydration; immediate assessment and treatment as needed for any hypoglycemia or hypothermia; immediate correction of any electrolyte imbalances; empiric treatment of infection; attention

TABLE 5.1 ■ Classification of Malnutrition[a] (Moderate Versus Severe)

	Classification	
	Moderate Malnutrition	Severe Malnutrition (Type)[b]
Symmetrical edema	No	Yes (edematous malnutrition)[c]
Weight-for-height	−3 ≤ SD score < −2[d] (70%–79%)[e]	SD score < −3 (<70%) (severe wasting)[f]
Height-for-age	−3 ≤ SD score < −2 (85%–89%)	SD score < −3 (<85%) (severe stunting)

[a]For further information about anthropometric indicators, see reference 1.
[b]The diagnoses are not mutually exclusive.
[c]This includes kwashiorkor and marasmic-kwashiorkor in older classifications. However, to avoid confusion with the clinical syndrome of kwashiorkor, which includes other features, the term "edematous malnutrition" is preferred.
[d]Below the median National Center for Health Statistics (NCHS)/World Health Organization (WHO) reference; the SD-score is defined as the deviation of the value for an individual from the median value of the reference population, divided by the standard deviation of the reference population. S-score observed value median reference value standard deviation of reference population, D = ( )–( ).
[e]Percentage of the median NCHS/WHO reference (see footnote in Appendix 1).
[f]This corresponds to marasmus (without edema) in the Wellcome clinical classification (2, 3) and to grade III malnutrition in the Gomez system (4). However, to avoid confusion, the term "severe wasting" is preferred.
Modified from World Health Organization. *Management of Severe Malnutrition: A Manual for Physicians and Other Senior Health Workers*. Geneva, Switzerland: World Health Organization; 1999.

to micronutrient deficiencies; and a progressive, stepwise advancement of feedings. Table 5.2 lists these interventions along with suggested timelines for implementation.

Intravenous (IV) rehydration and feedings should be avoided whenever possible. Even when available, IV treatments are very taxing on limited healthcare staff; the patient is often in an environment where laboratory monitoring of electrolyte disturbances (a common complication of IV treatments) is limited; there is increased risk of infection; and it is important to begin activating the gastrointestinal (GI) tract as early as possible. IV feedings (and even fluids) should be avoided whenever possible, therefore, and methods such as oral rehydration solutions fed via syringe should be heavily favored. Signs or symptoms of shock, however, would be an exception to this rule and a time when IV fluids (and antibiotics) should be administered when available.

Most patients with severe acute malnutrition can be rehydrated via oral means. If available, there are commercially available packages such as ReSoMal which, when mixed with water, provide appropriate concentrations of salts, minerals, and sugars. Otherwise, standard WHO oral rehydration salts (ORS) packets mixed with 2 L of water (instead of the usual 1 L) along with 50 g of sucrose and 40 mL of a mineral mix solution can be used.

Rehydration solutions should be fed to a child at a rate of approximately 70 to 100 mL/kg of body weight over 12 hours; this approximates to about 1 liter of fluid for a toddler and 1 to 2 L for a typical 4- to 5-year-old child. Caregivers will often need to begin these feedings very slowly, sometimes at a rate of only 1 teaspoon per kilogram of body weight every 30 minutes. These fluids may need to be given via nasogastric (NG) tube in children who repeatedly vomit, are breathing too fast, or are just too exhausted to feed orally. Patients also need to be monitored at least every hour for signs of fluid intolerance, to include edema (newly puffy eyelids, hands, or feet), distention of the jugular veins, or an increase in pulse or respiratory rates.

After correction of dehydration, hypoglycemia, hypothermia, electrolyte imbalance, and initiation of antibiotics, patients should begin liquid feedings with formulas that are lighter in protein,

---

BOX 5.2 ■ Checklist of Points for Medical History and Physical Examination Related to Assessment of Malnutrition

Checklist of points for taking the child's medical history and conducting the physical examination

Medical History

- Usual diet before current episode of illness
- Breastfeeding history
- Food and fluids taken in past few days
- Recent sinking of eyes
- Duration and frequency of vomiting or diarrhea, appearance of vomit or diarrheal stools
- Time when urine was last passed
- Contact with people with measles or tuberculosis
- Any death of siblings
- Birth weight
- Milestones reached (sitting up, standing, etc.)
- Immunizations

Physical Examination

- Weight and length or height
- Edema
- Enlargement or tenderness of liver, jaundice
- Abdominal distension, bowel sounds, "abdominal splash" (a splashing sound in the abdomen)
- Severe pallor
- Signs of circulatory collapse: cold hands and feet, weak radial pulse, diminished consciousness
- Temperature: hypothermia or fever
- Thirst
- Eyes: corneal lesions indicative of vitamin A deficiency
- Ears, mouth, throat: evidence of infection
- Skin: evidence of infection or purpura
- Respiratory rate and type of respiration: signs of pneumonia or heart failure
- Appearance of feces

Modified from World Health Organization. *Management of Severe Malnutrition: A Manual for Physicians and Other Senior Health Workers.* Geneva, Switzerland: World Health Organization; 1999.

---

fat, and sodium than typical formulas. Younger children who are able should breastfeed when possible, but otherwise formulas such as "F-75" and "F-100" are commercially available, and equivalent formulas can also be constituted locally using basic ingredients of dried skim milk, sugar, cereal flower, and oil. When constituting formula locally, it is also important to provide vitamin and mineral mixes, specifically for added potassium and magnesium.

Loose stools or even diarrhea for several weeks is not uncommon when refeeding severely malnourished children. This is definitely not a reason to use IV fluids, and it is also important not to overdiagnose lactose intolerance. The loose stools are a result of atrophy of the intestinal microvilli resulting in loss of surface area for absorption, as is also seen commonly after viral gastroenteritis. This condition typically resolves slowly as the microvilli gradually regenerate and the intestine regains its full absorptive function.

Treatment of Moderate Acute Malnutrition

Attending to the health of vulnerable populations requires attention to the nutritional needs of all the people, many of whom will either be experiencing, or will be at risk for, moderate acute malnutrition. One must ensure that everyone is getting at least a general ration, which is defined

TABLE 5.2 ■ Timeframe for the Management of a Child With Severe Malnutrition

Activity	Initial Treatment		Rehabilitation	Follow-Up
	Days 1–2	Days 3–7	Weeks 2–6	Weeks 7–26
Treat or prevent:				
Hypoglycemia	⟶			
Hypothermia	⟶			
Dehydration	⟶			
Correct electrolyte imbalance	⟶			
Treat infection	⟶			
Correct micronutrient deficiencies	←without iron→ | ←without iron→			
Begin feeding	⟶			
Increase feeding to recover lost weight (catch-up growth)			⟶	
Stimulate emotional and sensorial development	⟶			
Prepare for discharge			⟶	

Modified from World Health Organization. *Management of Severe Malnutrition: A Manual for Physicians and Other Senior Health Workers.* Geneva, Switzerland: World Health Organization; 1999.

as a minimum of 2100 kilocalories per person per day (kcal/d), 10% to 12% of which should come from protein, and about 17% of which should come from fat. Adjustments should be made upward by 100 kcal/d for every 5°C that the temperature is less than 20°C. Additionally, anywhere that people are required to have higher activity levels (perhaps to fetch water, or perform manual work), the ration needs to be increased by an additional 140 to 350 kcal/d.

It is essential to ensure that everyone in a vulnerable population is receiving a general ration. Beyond that, there are two strategies for providing supplementary feedings to specific individuals or groups. Targeted supplementary feeding programs are programs that provide a supplement (in addition to the general ration) to the moderately malnourished individuals within particular groups—usually children and pregnant or lactating women. Blanket supplementary feeding programs are programs that provide a supplement to all members of a particular group—again, usually children under 5 years of age, as well as pregnant or lactating women.

Both the World Food Program (WFP) and the UN High Commissioner for Refugees (UNHCR) emphasize the importance of not using either of these supplementary feeding programs in place of a general ration program for the entire population. Whether one uses the targeted supplementary feeding or blanket supplementary feeding approach, they must always be supplementary to a program that provides at least a general ration to all.

The means by which rations can be provided to individuals suffering or at risk of moderate malnutrition has undergone a renaissance in the past 20 years. Specifically, the development of ready-to-use therapeutic foods (RUTFs) has enabled the provision of a palatable food to adults and children at a reasonable cost, with minimal-to-no onsite preparation required, and with good shelf-life without refrigeration. First developed by Nutriset and marketed as "Plumpynut," RUTFs are now often manufactured locally using local ingredients. Typically, a cereal is mixed with a protein supplement (beans, nuts, milk, meat, or eggs), a vitamin and mineral supplement, and an energy supplement (fat, oil, and/or sugar). Among many other benefits, the use of RUTFs has been shown to reduce the amount of time moderately malnourished children must remain in feeding facilities, and instead, children can be monitored once daily on an outpatient basis.

Micronutrient Deficiencies

Micronutrients are the vitamins and minerals that the human body requires, often only in trace amounts, to perform its normal functions. Deficiency of any of the essential micronutrients represents a serious threat to health. The micronutrient deficiencies responsible for the greatest health burden worldwide are iron, vitamin A, and iodine, followed closely by thiamine and zinc. Micronutrients do not provide energy, but rather serve as catalysts that facilitate the essential chemical processes required to maintain health. Awareness of the signs and symptoms of each of these micronutrient deficiencies and attention to supplementation of these micronutrients into the diet are critical elements of the practice of global nutrition.

Iron is required in the human diet as an essential component of hemoglobin, the metalloprotein found in red blood cells (RBCs) responsible for the transport of oxygen. People suffering from iron deficiency develop a type of anemia characterized by low levels of hemoglobin and an inability of RBCs to transport appropriate amounts of oxygen to the tissues that need it. Over 1 billion people worldwide suffer some level of iron deficiency anemia. Iron deficiency is caused by a lack of intake and/or absorption of iron and is exacerbated by conditions such as malaria, human immunodeficiency virus (HIV)/acquired immunodeficiency syndrome (AIDS), hookworm infestation, schistosomiasis, tuberculosis, and others.

Consequences of iron deficiency include acute and chronic fatigue, poor growth, increased maternal mortality, and irreversible impaired cognitive development in children. Foods rich in iron include red meat, pork, poultry, some seafood, beans, dark green leafy vegetables, and any cereals, breads, or pastas that may have been fortified with iron. Unfortunately, rice, corn, and potatoes (the most common staples in low-income regions) are not good sources of dietary iron. Supplementation with iron can sometimes be challenging, as it is not as easily absorbed by the GI system relative to some of the other micronutrients. Small doses of iron supplemented daily over relatively long periods of time (weeks to months) are required to treat a single patient with iron deficiency. On a population level, therefore, a multipronged approach that includes improvement to the overall quality of the diet, fortification of foods with iron, direct iron supplementation, and control of any comorbid infections is the preferred strategy.

Vitamin A deficiency is one of two leading causes of preventable blindness worldwide. Mild cases of vitamin A deficiency will cause night blindness, as vitamin A is a critical component of rhodopsin, a chemical in the retina necessary for low-light vision. More severe vitamin A deficiency will lead to complete blindness, often caused by xeropthalmia, a condition where the eyes fail to produce tears, eventually leading to various degrees of disease on the surface of the eye.

In addition to its role in ensuring proper vision, vitamin A is also a micronutrient that is essential to the proper functioning of the immune system. Vitamin A is necessary for the proper formation and function of the epithelial cell layers of the mucous membranes of the respiratory tract and the intestines. In global health practice, people who are deficient in vitamin A suffer significantly worse morbidity and mortality from infectious outbreaks such as measles virus. It is for this reason that clinical guidelines call for blanket supplementation of entire populations with vitamin A when there is any risk of measles infection. Likewise, clinical guidelines for the treatment of measles also call for empiric administration of vitamin A.

In contrast to the challenges with direct supplementation of iron, Vitamin A supplementation is remarkably easy and inexpensive. A single gel cap containing vitamin A, given orally and costing approximately three US cents per capsule, provides enough vitamin A to prevent deficiency for 6 months.

Iodine deficiency is the number one cause of brain damage worldwide. Iodine is a micronutrient required for multiple functions within the body, proper nervous system development being just one. Cretinism, the most severe form of iodine deficiency, is a profound, irreversible form of mental retardation with characteristic features that include very short stature and decreased muscle tone. Other consequences of iodine deficiency include spontaneous abortion, stillbirth, and congenital anomalies. Most of the symptoms of iodine deficiency actually manifest as a result of thyroid deficiency because iodine is an essential micronutrient in the production of thyroid hormones.

Iodine deficiency is easily prevented on the population level by a strategy of iodinization of salt. Much progress has been made in the past three decades to provide iodine in salt, but this progress is still incomplete because 54 countries worldwide still have large populations suffering from iodine deficiency.

Secondary Consequences of Malnutrition

The natural inclination to address nutritional needs is usually so spontaneous and compelling that discussion of the long-term implications of why attention should be paid to nutritional issues is often overlooked. But the impact that malnutrition has on immune function, maternal mortality, cognitive abilities, economic growth, and even security is worth some discussion.

Undernutrition (both micro- and macronutrient deficiencies) impairs immune function in a variety of ways through an assortment of different mechanisms. The overall impact of malnutrition on immune function has been characterized now by its own syndrome: nutritionally acquired immune dysfunction (NAID). It is estimated that NAID plays a role in up to 54% of all child deaths under 4 years of age; children who are malnourished suffer greater mortality from threats as varied as diarrhea to malaria and pneumonia.

Pregnant women suffer increased mortality throughout their pregnancy as a consequence of NAID, whereas specific micronutrients such as iron deficiency specifically put women at greater risk of death during delivery and the immediate peripartum period. Malnutrition also leads to low birth weight and slow growth and development of newborns, infants, and toddlers. Stunted growth during the first 2 years of life also puts children on a path toward short stature that is irreversible, regardless of any future nutritional opportunities. This significant decrease in stature in turn results in increased morbidity and mortality when that woman becomes pregnant, as the incidence of obstetric fistula and need for emergency cesarean delivery are inversely proportional to maternal height. Safe cesarean delivery is, of course, often not available in rural and low-income regions.

The pernicious effects of malnutrition on cognition are also widespread and grossly underappreciated. The causal link between malnutrition and impaired cognitive development is self-evident to clinicians, and the body of research literature confirming this association is also substantial. In one study of children in the Philippines, for example, an 11-point IQ differential was measured between stunted and nonstunted children. In addition to having less cognitive mental capacity, however, malnourished children also have a much harder time paying attention and learning while in school, if they are afforded the opportunity to attend school at all. Very commonly, the point of malnourishment is often the point when families make the choice not to send their children to school. Blanket school-lunch feeding programs, therefore, such as the world's largest program in India, are looked upon favorably as an important step in the right direction.

The economic argument for prioritizing nutritional interventions is also strong. Malnutrition negatively impacts economic growth in several ways. Decreased per-worker productivity secondary to fatigue, secondary to either macronutrient deficiency or iron deficiency, is just one example.

Even more pernicious, however, is the loss of productivity and innovation because of lowered cognitive abilities secondary to poor nutrition. In many poor regions, iodine and iron deficiencies combine to cause a decrease in cognitive ability across large portions of the population, decreasing economic growth on a macroeconomic scale. Pakistan, for example, is estimated to suffer a 3.3% lower gross domestic product (GDP) secondary to iodine deficiency alone. Vietnam is estimated to suffer a decrease of 1.1% from iron deficiency, 1% secondary to iodine deficiency, and another 0.3% owing to macronutrient deficiency (PEM). Bangladesh is estimated to lose 1.9% of GDP, as a result of decreased cognitive ability and loss of manual work, from iron deficiency alone.

Security is yet another consideration in global nutrition and one that is particularly relevant to state interests. If one defines security broadly, for example, by using the broader notion of "human security," then the important role that nutrition plays in security is explicit and contained within the domain of "freedom from want." In addition, the United Nations Development Program (UNDP) specifically identifies "food security" as a category unto itself in its landmark 1994 definition of human security.

Even if one defines security more narrowly, with a focus more limited to stability and protection from violent conflict, nutrition plays an often overlooked but very prominent role. Food insecurity has for millennia been a reason for groups outside a state's territory to violently invade its borders. Food insecurity certainly plays a role in the many violent conflicts erupting in the Sahel region of Africa today. And food (and economic) security is a driving force for migration in the Western hemisphere, too, from Central America into Mexico and the United States. With regard to internal threats, providing for the basic health needs of a population is well recognized as one of the major obligations of a state, and failure to provide such provisions is widely recognized as a threat to state security. Counterinsurgency theorists recognize this distinctly and therefore explain the need for adequate nutrition as not just a humanitarian but also a security necessity.

Appendix: Specific Malnutrition Conditions

A. Protein-Energy Malnutrition (PEM)
  1. Classically divided into three forms: marasmus, kwashiorkor, and marasmic-kwashiorkor.
  2. A spectrum of disease, multifactorial in origin, onset usually around weaning age, often precipitated by a health event (flu, diarrhea, etc.).
  3. Marasmus:
     a. Defined as "nutritional deficiency state associated with a weight-for-age of less than 5th percentile by National Center for Health Statistics (NCHS) standards or less than 50% of the median NCHS standard." Classically, patients are weak and emaciated, and may look anxious, with little interest in their environment. Usually little to no muscle mass or subcutaneous (SQ) fat, appearing with "skin draped over bones" look. Usually no skin lesions as with kwashiorkor, and hair, although sparse, is usually qualitatively normal. Diet typically good qualitatively, but low in kcals. Diarrhea on account of (a/o) GI infections are common. Hypoglycemia, hypothermia not uncommon.
  4. Kwashiorkor: "deprived child" (for each type give clinical presentation—do diagnosis [dx] and treatment [tx] together):
     a. Diet low in protein, but often adequate kcals from carbohydrates. Clinically, the salient features are failure to grow, edema, skin/hair changes, diarrhea, and mental status changes. Classically, onset is during second year of life, precipitated by a bout of diarrhea or measles or displacement from mother. Infants may also be affected if fed excessive sugar a/o starches in proportion to breast milk.
     b. Failure to gain appropriate weight may herald onset.
     c. Edema is pitting and may progress to anasarca; may appear deceptively "plump," only to reveal emaciation when recovery begins and fluids are taken back into circulation.

    d. Some degree of skin atrophy is almost invariably present. Lesions may begin as erythema that dries, darkens, and becomes hyperkeratotic or start off dark and hyperkeratotic and expand to confluence. Result is decreased immunocompetence, low weight (wt), osteoporotic bone, and poor muscle tone.

    e. Liver function is well preserved until late. Pancreas is atrophic and may calcify; may contribute to tropical pancreatitis. Gut atrophy may lead to lactose/glucose intolerance.

    f. Cardiac output is reduced, with risk of circulatory overload with aggressive hydration.

    g. Skin may be hyperpigmented, exfoliating, atrophic, hypopigmented, with ulcers, fissures, a/o hyperkeratosis; nails are usually thin and soft.

    h. Damage of glomeruli and convoluted tubules can produce albuminuria, worsening protein deficiency.

    i. Normocytic, normochromic anemia is the rule, which generally responds to refeeding and tx of infections.

    j. Edema is quintessential, which is multifactorial, but largely dependent upon albumin levels.

    k. The patient (pt) may have abnormal glucose metabolism; hypoglycemia is frequently seen. Poor fat metabolism may also exist and lead to steatorrhea.

    l. Markedly abnormal protein metabolism is reflected in inverted albumin:globulin ratio, and high bromsulphthalein retention by the liver. Blood urea nitrogen and urinary excretion of urea are both low. Both T-cell and B-cell immunity are depressed.

    Note that fluid overload and edema are most striking, often with falsely healthy-appearing weights. Edema is pitting and may be limited to feet or be frank anasarca. Patients are often anorexic, often with diarrhea, compounded by malabsorption from villous atrophy a/o pancreatic insufficiency.

    Note that skin changes are common, manifesting as hyper/hypopigmented areas, sometimes with hyperkeratosis, and most common in areas of irritation. Skin may peel, leaving raw areas vulnerable to secondary infection. After several months of disease, hair changes are common, such as straightening of kinky hair, dark hair lightening (to orange or brown).

5. Marasmic-kwashiorkor:

    a. Children appear marasmic, yet with some edema, and are less than 5th percentile wt-for-age.

    b. Diagnosis: history (hx) and physical exam (PEx) most important, few lab tests helpful. Kwashiorkor has hypoalbuminemia and a (often factitious) hyponatremia.

    c. Treatment of life-threatening PEM:

        i. Fluid and electrolytes: per os (PO)/naso-gastric (NG) tube fluids with WHO rehydration solution, giving maintenance fluids of 100 cc/kg per day divided q 1 to 2 hours to start, increasing *pari passu* with diarrheal or emesis losses. If pt is strictly marasmic with no diarrhea and a good appetite, milk-based formula may be started immediately instead.

        ii. Bacterial infections: maintain high index of suspicion, may manifest as hypothermia, hypoglycemia, lethargy, tachypnea, or tachycardia. Fever and leukocytosis may be suppressed by poor reserves. Kwashiorkor is especially predisposing to gram-negative sepsis and overwhelming pneumococcal sepsis.

        iii. Vitamin A deficiency: may become evident as nutrition is augmented/restarted, resulting in keratomalacia (can be blinding). Most often, 200,000 units of vitamin A is given (po) initially, to be repeated in 48 hours or when taking milk/formula po.

        iv. Look for and treat congestive heart failure (CHF), anemia, hypothermia, hypoglycemia

    d. Nutritional restoration:
- i. Many pts anorexic, especially those with kwashiorkor, use NG tube if otherwise inad. feeds.
- ii. Feeds should have 3 to 4 g protein and 135 to 145 kcal per 100 cc.
- iii. Acceptable feeds are various milks (cow, goat, camel, buffalo, ewe, etc.) with varying amounts of sucrose, oil, and water, or:
  - K-Mix 2 = 17% calcium caseinate, 28% skimmed milk powder, 55% sucrose, with vitamin A (distributed by UNICEF)
  - ICSM = 63% cornmeal, 24% defatted soy flour, 5% skimmed milk powder, 5% soy oil, 3% vitamin/mineral mix (distributed by US Agency for International Development [US AID], Care International [CARE])
  - Incaparina = 58% lime-treated corn flour, 38% cottonseed flour, 4% lysine vitamin/mineral/lysine mix (developed by INCAP)

B. Thiamine/B1 (Beri-Beri)
1. Epidemiology (epid.): thiamine deficiency most common in areas of rice-based diet. Vitamin B1 found in cereals, fish, meat, eggs, specific legumes, and pork. It functions as a cofactor for carbohydrate metabolism.
2. Symptoms (sx): in infants of thiamine-deficient mothers, may manifest at 2 to 4 m, with anorexia, vomiting, restlessness, progressing to CHF (tachycardia, tachypnea, edema).

    May produce bouts of muscular rigidity and head retraction, may be perceived as meningeal sx.

    Laryngeal m. paralysis may produce aphonia. Noninfantile disease (dz) "dry," "wet," or "dry and wet." Dry = peripheral neuropathy with extremity weakness, lower extremity (LE) paresthesias a/o hypo-/hyperreflexia. Wet = CHF, edema, tachycardia, tachypnea, hepatomegaly, etc.

    Dry and wet = peripheral (esp. LE) neuropathy with CHF. "Cerebral beri-beri" (Wernicke's encephalopathy) is associated most strongly with alcoholism; confusion, recent amnesia/memory loss, nystagmus, ophthalmoplegia, ataxia, peripheral neuropathy are suggestive.
3. Diagnosis: usually clinical. Erythrocyte transketolase and thiamine pyrophosphate (TPP) levels useful. If suspected, can try therapeutic trial of thiamine of 25 to 50 mg for infants and 50 to 100 mg for others.
4. Treatment: thiamine, 40 mg IM injection daily until resolved (typically <1 week). Maintenance 2.5 to 5.0 mg po daily.

C. Niacin (Pellagra)
1. Epid: available to humans as niacin or derived from tryptophan. Maize contains no niacin, is low in tryptophan, and is high in leucine, which may antagonize nicotinamide function.
2. Sx: deficiency may lead to the "three D's": diarrhea, dermatitis, and dementia. Inflammation of oral mucous membranes and GI tract result in glossitis and diarrhea with dysphagia and nausea and vomiting (N/V). Dermatitis initially presents as erythema, progressing to hyperpigmentation and cracking in sun-exposed areas. Dementia, a late finding, presents as apathy, depression, irritability, insomnia, possibly with psychotic features.
3. Diagnosis: clinical. No useful lab tests. If suspected, therapeutic trial of nicotinamide, 10 to 25 mg in children, 100 to 200 mg in adults, tid. Within 48 hours diarrhea should stop, and within 7 days dermatitis and dementia should improve.
4. Treatment: niacin, nicotinic acid, tryptophan.

D. Iodine (Endemic Goiter, Endemic Cretinism)
1. Epid: most individuals need at least 20 μg/d to avoid goiters, as 60 to 70 μg/d is marginal steady state (no growth period). Ingestion of goitrogens (cassava, cabbage, mustard, etc.) may accelerate goiter development.

    2. Sx: endemic goiter is mostly seen in central Africa, Indonesia, and New Guinea. Diffuse hypertrophy can progress to independently functioning nodules, fibrosis, cystic changes, and degenerative changes.

        a. Irreversible enlargement eventually. Mass effect can lead to tracheal compression or laryngeal nerve paralysis.

        b. Endemic cretinism is generally clustered in areas of endemic goiter (usually [us.] < 20 µg/d). It is most often from iodine deficiency during intrauterine or early postnatal life. In "nervous cretinism," eye squint and proximal spasticity are generally seen, often with growth and mental retardation. With "myxedematous cretinism," (us. in Africa, China), mental retardation is prominent, accompanied by growth delay (short stature, delayed bony maturation), with goiters or deafness rarely seen; all have signs/symptoms of hypothyroidism.

    3. Diagnosis: a clinically enlarged thyroid is de facto a goiter. Iodine deficiency may be suggested by urine daily iodine excretion assays. Thyroid function tests (TFTs) are warranted if dz is suspected.

    4. Treatment: iodine may be given as tablets, drops (Lugol's solution, saturated solution of potassium iodide [SSKI]), or iodinized oil injections. Caveat: excess iodine can also cause goiters as well. Dosage of 1 to 2 µg of iodine/kg per day is appropriate. If reversible, change will come within weeks. No tx for cretinism; ensure fecund or lactating females have adequate dietary iodine.

  E. Vitamin A

    1. Epid: retinol can be procured in animal products such as liver, fish liver oils, butter, and egg yolk; vegetable sources include green vegetables, yellow fruit, and red palm oil. It is necessary for epithelial cell maintenance as well as retinal photopigments. Generally, children need 400 µg, adult females need 500 µg, and adult males need 600 µg/d. In the developed world, deficiency only seen with malabsorption or alcoholism or other liver dz. In the developing world, fairly common, resulting in night blindness a/o xerophthalmia; mucous membranes of respiratory and GI tract also affected.

    2. Sx: night blindness, conjunctival dryness (xerosis), Bitot's spots, corneal xerosis, corneal ulceration, a/o corneal scars may be the ocular effects.

    3. Diagnosis: clinical:

        a. Treatment: in areas of risk, prophylactic vitamin A at 50,000 to 200,000 IU q 6 m for children over 1 year of age (halve this dosage for children <1 year). Children with measles, malabsorption syndromes, a/o PEM are at particular risk. In emergent situations (i.e., malnourished child with keratomalacia or xerophthalmia), consider IM vitamin A, ensuring the water-soluble form (vitamin A palmitate) is used, not the oil-based form, which is poorly absorbed. If not available, children with xerophthalmia should get 200,000 IU (or 10,000 IU/kg) po or via NG tube once, repeated during the first day, then once/day × 5 days. Give with some source of fat, such as milk-based nutrition with vegetable oil, if possible.

  F. Vitamin D (Rickets—Children, Osteomalacia—Adult Females)

    1. Epid: fat-soluble, absorbed in duodenum and jejunum. Important hormone for calcium and phosphorus metabolism. Fatty fish is rich (salmon, mackerel, etc.), whereas human milk is poor. Significant amounts are provided by cutaneous photosynthesis. Deficiency a problem in India, the Middle East, and Northern Africa, and to a lesser degree in the Caribbean, southern Europe, and South Africa; housing, diet, and clothing customs are most often implicated.

    2. Sx: in congenital cases, craniotabes (softening of skull bones) is common. In children, rickets affects growth plates and spongiosa. Late rickets may manifest during pubertal growth spurts, causing back or leg pain, a/o weakness. Adult deficiency commonly leads to bone pain, followed by leg bowing, gibbous, pectus carinatum, kyphoscoliosis, a/o

diminished trunk height. Proximal muscle weakness, if present, may accompany these sx or stand alone.

3. Diagnosis: serum 25-(OH) vitamin D concentration sensitive. On x-ray, one may observe widened metaphyses or undercalcified subperiosteal bone resulting in a fuzzy outer shaft margin. In long bones, rarefied zones along the shafts ("Looser's zones") may be seen.

4. Treatment: clinical dz tx with vitamin D, 500 IU/d for several weeks, followed by lower maintenance dosage. Those with (w/) malabsorption may need up to 20,000 IU/d.

Daily supplements of 400 IU/d are frequently used prophylactically.

G. Vitamin C (Scurvy)

1. Epid: ascorbic acid found in several sources, especially citrus fruits. Serves as cofactor for hydroxylation—important for tooth, bone, collagen development.

2. Sx: infantile scurvy presents as failure to thrive, irritability (secondary to subperiosteal hemorrhages), petechiae/ecchymoses, hematuria, a/o bloody diarrhea. Gum bleeding not uncommon; anemia not rare from blood loss. Rarer in adults, scurvy may present as bleeding gums, ecchymoses, a/o hyperkeratosis of hair follicles.

3. Diagnosis: serum ascorbic acid levels are diagnostic, but a therapeutic trial is more common. Ascorbic acid, 100 to 200 mg for infants, and 1 g/d for adults, is recommended.

4. Treatment: same dosage as therapeutic trial of ascorbic acid.

H. Iron

Deficiency:

1. Epid: The most common nutritional deficiency in the world. Heme iron (meat, fish, liver) more readily absorbed than nonheme iron, although vitamin C and amino acids promote absorption of the latter (tea, vegetable fiber inhibit its absorption). Iron absorbed in duodenum and proximal jejunum, and acidification in stomach promotes nonheme iron to be absorbed in ferrous form. Infants, adolescents, fecund women at highest risk of deficiency. Hookworm infestation, GI bleeds (ulcers, tumors, tics, polyps, arteriovenous malformation [AVMs]) can lose significant iron. Poor absorption secondary tropical sprue, achlorhydria, gastric resection can also be causative.

2. Sx: maternal iron deficiency can result in prematurity and low birth wt. Prolonged deficiency in nonanemic children can lead to impaired mental and motor development. Anemic dz leads to fatigue, weakness, dizziness, a/o dyspnea.

3. Diagnosis: low serum ferritin (<12 µg/L), low serum iron, increased total iron binding capacity (TIBC), low transferrin saturation (<10%), peripheral smear hypochromia.

4. Treatment: treat adults with 200 mg of elemental iron per day (i.e., 300 mg $FeSO_4$ po tid). Children should get 5 mg/kg elemental iron per day in tablet or elixir. Iron absorbed better if not given with food. PO tx should correct anemia within 6 weeks but should continue an additional 3 to 6 weeks to replenish stores. Iron-dextran can be given IM or SQ to individuals with malabsorption or noncompliance.

Overload:

1. Epid: different forms geography-dependent, best known is in Africa, related to high iron content in local beer. Hereditary hemochromatosis, thalassemias can also result in iron overload.

2. Sx: liver, heart, pancreas, joints primarily affected. Cirrhosis, cardiomyopathy, diabetes mellitus, arthritis, amenorrhea, impotence may result. Pts with hereditary hemochromatosis at increased risk for hepatoma.

3. Diagnosis: elevated serum iron, transferrin saturation, ferritin, with decreased TIBC. Liver biopsy (bx) procures definitive dx.

4. Treatment: phlebotomy. If dx established, 1 to 2 u/wk removed until stores depleted. In thalassemia, deferoxamine B is used to chelate iron on chronic basis.

I. Folate and Vitamin B12
    1. Folate in leafy vegetables, fruits, liver, human/cow milk: sx of deficiency occur after months of lack. Absorbed in duodenum in brush border. Deficiency usually from poor diet, especially in times of increased need (pregnancy, lactation, hemolytic conditions such as sickle cell disease (SCDz) or poor erythropoiesis such as thalassemia). Less frequently, tropical sprue, Mediterranean lymphoma, or alcoholism may contribute (the first two by malabsorption).
    2. B12 in liver, kidney, bivalves, as well as meats, milk: stores sufficient for 3 to 4 years. Absorbed in terminal ileum, requiring stomach-produced (parietal cells) intrinsic factor. Deficiency usually from malabsorption, specifically "pernicious anemia" from diminished secretion of intrinsic factor (possibly autoimmune, often from gastric resection). Bacterial overgrowth (diverticular, blind loop, fistulas) or infestation with fish tapeworm *Diphyllobothrium latum* can rob body of cobalamin. Malabsorption from regional enteritis, tuberculosis, amebiasis, etc. can likewise cause sx.
    3. Sx: both function in DNA replication, deficiency results in megaloblastic anemia; polymorphonuclear white blood cells (PMNs) are typically hypersegmented also. Cobalamin, but not folate, deficiency also leads to a myelopathy—ataxia, dementia, diminished proprioception/vibration—a/o various motor deficits may result.
    4. Diagnosis: serum folate (or, better, RBC folate), B12 levels most diagnostic. Schilling test used to distinguish low B12 from deficient intrinsic factor versus small bowel problems. Serum antibodies to intrinsic factor identifies pernicious anemia also.
    5. Treatment: folate given 0.5 to 1.0 mg po. Cyanocobalamin, 100 μg/d, IM/SQ × 7 days, then periodic injections to achieve 2000 μg over first 6 weeks. Afterwards, maintain by 100 μg IM q m. If unavailable parentally, B12 can be given as 1000 μg/d po to overcome pernicious anemia.
J. Vitamin E
    1. Epid: a fat-soluble antioxidant, found most in unsaturated vegetable oils. Body stores in adipose and liver good usually good for months, but infants more susceptible.
    2. Sx: deficiency may contribute to infantile hemolytic anemia (esp. if stressed with overly large iron loads) and retrolental fibroplasia (esp. if in overly high oxygen concentrations). Older pts may develop myopathies or neuropathies (esp. along sensory pathways).
    3. Diagnosis: dx by therapeutic trial.
    4. Treatment: 300 mg (400 IU) po qd or bid.
K. Vitamin K
    1. Epid: a fat-soluble vitamin required for synthesis of clotting factors II (prothrombin), VII, IX, X, and the coagulation inhibitors protein C and protein S. Although some vitamin K is produced in the gut by bacteria, green leafy vegetables are the best sources. Infants are born with low stores; adults may become depleted from fat malabsorption, antibiotics that alter gut flora, dietary lack, total parenteral nutrition (TPN), biliary obstruction or diversion, or megadoses of vitamins A or E. Coumadin-type drugs act as vitamin K antagonists.
    2. Sx: abnormally prolonged bleeding, oozing of blood from puncture sites.
    3. Diagnosis: prothrombin time (PT) is prolonged, as is activated partial thromboplastin time (PTT) usually. Correction within 24 hours by therapeutic trial confirms dx.
    4. Treatment: phylloquinone (K1) is the preferred form; may give 1 mg parenterally for newborns and up to 10+ mg for reversal of anticoagulants in adults.
L. Zinc
    1. Epid: found in meats, milk products, crustaceans, mollusks, whole grains, leafy and root vegetables, and nuts; important for RBC membranes and immunity. Unrefined cereal grains and legumes contain fiber and phytic acid, inhibitors of zinc absorption. Can be

absorbed anywhere along GI tract but preferentially in jejunum. Increased needs during pregnancy, lactation, certain tumors; excess losses may occur through feces, sweat, or urine.

2. Sx: growth retardation, delayed sexual maturation, hypospermia/hypogonadism, alopecia, skin lesions, diarrhea, glucose intolerance, depression, impaired wound healing, night blindness, hypogeusesthesia may result. Acute deficiency in infants may present with circumoral rash, diarrhea, aberrant behavior, a/o immunodeficiency.

3. Diagnosis: zinc levels in serum, white blood cells (WBCs), nails, and hair useful.

4. Treatment: zinc salts, 150 mg po qd, for acute tx. Ongoing supplementation should not exceed 45 mg po qd (can produce copper deficiency).

M. Copper

Deficiency:

1. Epid: found in oysters and other shellfish, tuna and other fish, legumes, whole-grain products; part of redox enzymes in humans. Most often seen in children of India and Andean highlands.

2. Sx: microcytic, hypochromic anemia, neutropenia, skin/hair depigmentation, arterial aneurysms secondary defective elastin, central nervous system aberrancies, hypotonia, hypothermia, skeletal demineralization, subperiosteal hemorrhages, a/o epiphyseal separation may develop.

3. Diagnosis: serum copper levels below 50 µg/dL, decreased WBC and RBC copper, and decreased RBC superoxide dismutase activity.

4. Treatment: elemental copper, 2 mg po, repeated several times daily; ionic copper is an emetic, thus do not "lump" doses together.

Overload:

1. Epid: may occur with Wilson's dz (sublenticular degeneration), resulting in deposition in brain, liver, cornea, kidney. Also seen with Indian childhood cirrhosis, a familial dz seen most in Pakistan, Burma, India, and Sri Lanka, with onset between birth and 10 years.

2. Sx: hepatic dz leads to cirrhosis, cholestasis, and death from portal hypertension.

3. Diagnosis: clinical, serum tests, bx.

4. Treatment: penicillamine is given to acutely reverse symptoms.

N. Selenium

1. Epid: an important antioxidant and player in cytochrome P-450 detox system. Most concentrated in certain fish (tuna, haddock), marine mollusks, organ meats, skeletal muscle, grains from certain regions. Low selenium in soil of regions in Australia, China (home of Keshan's dz and Kashin-Beck dz), Finland, New Zealand, United States, Thailand, Guatemala, and Zaire. PEM, and TPN may all lead to selenium deficiency.

2. Sx: deficiency leads to myalgias and myositis, cardiomyopathy, hemolytic anemia, decreased WBC bactericidal efficacy, decreased cellular immunity. Keshan's dz is a progressive myocardiopathy of childhood and adolescence; Kashin-Beck dz is a deforming osteoarthropathy with diffuse siderosis.

3. Diagnosis: selenium levels in plasma, whole blood, RBCs, and activity of serum creatine kinase and creatine phosphokinase helpful.

4. Treatment: sodium selenite or torula yeast tablets po, to give 100 to 400 µg of selenium daily.

O. Chromium

1. Epid: important in insulin function and nucleic acid metabolism. Found in brewer's yeast, mushrooms, prunes, nuts, asparagus, beer, wine. Pediatric cases are only seen with PEM.

2. Sx: hyperglycemia, glucose intolerance, hyperinsulinemia, hyperlipidemia, peripheral neuropathy, and encephalopathy have all been described.
3. Diagnosis: plasma, RBC, whole blood, and hair chromium concentrations, as well as 24-hour urinary chromium concentration, may be used.
4. Treatment: brewer's yeast (1.1 µg chromium/g yeast), given to accomplish 100 to 200 µg chromium daily.

References

1. Goal 2: End hunger, achieve food security and improved nutrition and promote sustainable agriculture. Sustainable Development Goals. UN Web Services Section. Accessed July 15, 2016. https://unstats.un.org/sdgs/report/2016/goal-02/.
2. World Health Organization. *Management of Severe Malnutrition: A Manual for Physicians and Other Senior Health Workers*. Switzerland: Geneva World Health Organization; 1999.

Sexually Transmitted Diseases

Kaku Tamura

Diseases Characterized by Genital, Anal, or Perianal Ulcers

1. General Management
   a. Genital herpes, syphilis, and chancroid have been associated with an increased risk for human immunodeficiency virus (HIV) acquisition and transmission. Because early treatment decreases the possibility of transmission, public health standards require healthcare providers to presumptively treat any patient with a suspected case of infectious syphilis at the initial visit, even before test results are available.
2. Chancroid
   a. Caused by *Haemophilus ducreyi*. Infection might still occur in some regions of Africa and the Caribbean.
   b. The combination of a painful genital ulcer and tender suppurative inguinal adenopathy suggests the diagnosis of chancroid.
   c. A definitive diagnosis of chancroid requires the identification of *H. ducreyi* on special culture media that are not widely available from commercial sources; even when these media are used, sensitivity is <80%. A probable diagnosis of chancroid can be made if all of the following criteria are met: (1) the patient has one or more painful genital ulcers; (2) the clinical presentation, appearance of genital ulcers and, if present, regional lymphadenopathy are typical for chancroid; (3) the patient has no evidence of *Treponema pallidum* infection by darkfield examination of ulcer exudate or by a serologic test for syphilis performed at least 7 days after onset of ulcers; and (4) a herpes simplex virus (HSV) polymerase chain reaction (PCR) test or HSV culture performed on the ulcer exudate is negative.
   d. Azithromycin 1 g orally in a single dose or ceftriaxone 250 mg intramuscular (IM) in a single dose or ciprofloxacin 500 mg orally twice a day for 3 days or erythromycin base 500 mg orally three times a day for 7 days. Azithromycin and ceftriaxone offer the advantage of single-dose therapy. Worldwide, several isolates with intermediate resistance to either ciprofloxacin or erythromycin have been reported. Patients should be reexamined 3 to 7 days after initiation of therapy. If treatment is successful, ulcers usually improve symptomatically within 3 days and objectively within 7 days after

therapy. If no clinical improvement is evident, the clinician must consider whether (1) the diagnosis is correct; (2) the patient is coinfected with another sexually transmitted disease (STD); (3) the patient is infected with HIV; (4) the treatment was not used as instructed; or (5) the *H. ducreyi* strain causing the infection is resistant to the prescribed antimicrobial.

3. Genital HSV Infections
   a. HSV-1 and HSV-2: most cases of recurrent genital herpes are caused by HSV-2.
   b. The painful multiple vesicular or ulcerative lesions typically associated with HSV are absent in many infected persons. Recurrences and subclinical shedding are much more frequent for genital HSV-2 infection than for genital HSV-1 infection.
   c. The clinical diagnosis of genital herpes should be confirmed by type-specific laboratory testing. Both type-specific virologic and type-specific serologic tests for HSV should be available in clinical settings that provide care to persons with or at risk for STDs.
   d. First clinical episode of genital herpes: acyclovir 400 mg orally three times a day for 7 to 10 days or acyclovir 200 mg orally five times a day for 7 to 10 days or valacyclovir 1 g orally twice a day for 7 to 10 days or famciclovir 250 mg orally three times a day for 7 to 10 days.

      Note that treatment can be extended if healing is incomplete after 10 days of therapy. Suppressive therapy for recurrent genital herpes: acyclovir 400 mg orally twice a day or valacyclovir 500 mg orally once a day (valacyclovir 500 mg once a day might be less effective than other valacyclovir or acyclovir dosing regimens in persons who have very frequent recurrences [i.e., ≥10 episodes per year]) or valacyclovir 1 g orally once a day or famciclovir 250 mg orally twice a day.

      Episodic therapy for recurrent genital herpes: acyclovir 400 mg orally three times a day for 5 days or acyclovir 800 mg orally twice a day for 5 days or acyclovir 800 mg orally three times a day for 2 days or valacyclovir 500 mg orally twice a day for 3 days or valacyclovir 1 g orally once a day for 5 days or famciclovir 125 mg orally twice daily for 5 days or famciclovir 1 g orally twice daily for 1 day or famciclovir 500 mg once, followed by 250 mg twice daily for 2 days.

      Daily suppressive therapy in persons with HIV: acyclovir 400 to 800 mg orally twice to three times a day or valacyclovir 500 mg orally twice a day or famciclovir 500 mg orally twice a day.

      Episodic infection in persons with HIV: acyclovir 400 mg orally three times a day for 5 to 10 days or valacyclovir 1 g orally twice a day for 5 to 10 days or famciclovir 500 mg orally twice a day for 5 to 10 days.

      Suppressive therapy of pregnant women with recurrent genital herpes: acyclovir 400 mg orally three times a day or valacyclovir 500 mg orally twice a day.

      Note that treatment is recommended to start at 36 weeks of gestation.

4. Lymphogranuloma Venereum
   a. Caused by *Chlamydia trachomatis* serovars L1, L2, L3.
   b. The most common clinical manifestation of lymphogranuloma venereum (LGV) among heterosexuals is tender inguinal and/or femoral lymphadenopathy that is typically unilateral. A self-limited genital ulcer or papule sometimes occurs at the site of inoculation. However, by the time patients seek care, the lesions have often disappeared. Rectal exposure in women or men who have sex with men can result in proctocolitis mimicking inflammatory bowel disease, and clinical findings may include mucoid and/or hemorrhagic rectal discharge, anal pain, constipation, fever, and/or tenesmus.
   c. Genital lesions, rectal specimens, and lymph node specimens (i.e., lesion swab or bubo aspirate) can be tested for *C. trachomatis* by culture, direct immunofluorescence, or nucleic acid detection. Nucleic acid amplification tests (NAATs) for *C. trachomatis* perform well on rectal specimens.

    d. Recommended regimen: doxycycline 100 mg orally twice a day for 21 days.
Alternative regimen: erythromycin base 500 mg orally four times a day for 21 days.

5. Syphilis

    a. The spirochete *T. pallidum* is causative.

    b. The disease has been divided into stages based on clinical findings, helping to guide treatment and follow-up. Persons who have syphilis might seek treatment for signs or symptoms of primary syphilis infection (i.e., ulcers or chancre at the infection site), secondary syphilis (i.e., manifestations that include, but are not limited to, skin rash, mucocutaneous lesions, and lymphadenopathy), or tertiary syphilis (i.e., cardiac, gummatous lesions, tabes dorsalis, and general paresis). Latent infections (i.e., those lacking clinical manifestations) are detected by serologic testing. *T. pallidum* can infect the central nervous system and result in neurosyphilis, which can occur at any stage of syphilis. Early neurologic clinical manifestations (i.e., cranial nerve dysfunction, meningitis, stroke, acute altered mental status, and auditory or ophthalmic abnormalities) are usually present within the first few months or years of infection.

       Late neurologic manifestations (i.e., tabes dorsalis and general paresis) occur 10 to 30 years after infection.

    c. Darkfield examinations and tests to detect *T. pallidum* directly from lesion exudate or tissue are the definitive methods for diagnosing early syphilis. Although no *T. pallidum* detection tests are commercially available, some laboratories provide locally developed and validated PCR tests for the detection of *T. pallidum* DNA. A presumptive diagnosis of syphilis requires use of two tests: a nontreponemal test (i.e., venereal disease research laboratory [VDRL] or rapid plasma reagin [RPR]) and a treponemal test (i.e., fluorescent treponemal antibody-absorbed [FTA-ABS] tests, the *T. pallidum* passive particle agglutination [TP-PA] assay, various enzyme immunoassays [EIAs], chemiluminescence immunoassays, immunoblots, or rapid treponemal assays). Use of only one type of serologic test is insufficient for diagnosis and can result in false-negative results in persons tested during primary syphilis and false-positive results in persons without syphilis. False-positive nontreponemal test results can be associated with various medical conditions and factors unrelated to syphilis, including other infections (e.g., HIV), autoimmune conditions, immunizations, pregnancy, injection-drug use, and older age. In a person with neurologic signs or symptoms, a reactive cerebrospinal fluid (CSF)-VDRL (in the absence of blood contamination) is considered diagnostic of neurosyphilis. When CSF-VDRL is negative despite the presence of clinical signs of neurosyphilis, reactive serologic test results, and abnormal CSF cell count and/or protein, neurosyphilis should be considered. In this instance, additional evaluation using FTA-ABS testing on CSF may be warranted. The CSF FTA-ABS test is less specific for neurosyphilis than the CSF-VDRL but is highly sensitive.

       Neurosyphilis is highly unlikely with a negative CSF FTA-ABS test, especially among persons with nonspecific neurologic signs and symptoms.

    d. Primary and secondary syphilis in adults: benzathine penicillin G 2.4 million units IM in a single dose.

       Primary and secondary syphilis in children: benzathine penicillin G 50,000 units/kg IM, up to the adult dose of 2.4 million units in a single dose.

       Early latent syphilis in adults: benzathine penicillin G 2.4 million units IM in a single dose.

       Late latent syphilis or latent syphilis of unknown duration in adults: benzathine penicillin G 7.2 million units total, administered as three doses of 2.4 million units IM each at 1-week intervals.

Early latent syphilis in children: benzathine penicillin G 50,000 units/kg IM, up to the adult dose of 2.4 million units in a single dose.

Late latent syphilis in children: benzathine penicillin G 50,000 units/kg IM, up to the adult dose of 2.4 million units, administered as three doses at 1-week intervals (total 150,000 units/kg up to the adult total dose of 7.2 million units).

Tertiary syphilis with normal CSF examination: benzathine penicillin G 7.2 million units total, administered as three doses of 2.4 million units IM each at 1-week intervals.

Recommended regimen for neurosyphilis and ocular syphilis: aqueous crystalline penicillin G 18 to 24 million units per day, administered as 3 to 4 million units IV every 4 hours or continuous infusion, for 10 to 14 days.

Alternative regimen for neurosyphilis and ocular syphilis: procaine penicillin G 2.4 million units IM once daily plus probenecid 500 mg orally four times a day, both for 10 to 14 days.

Note that persons with HIV infection and neurosyphilis should be treated according to the recommendations for HIV-negative persons with neurosyphilis.

Primary and secondary syphilis in persons with HIV infection: benzathine penicillin G, 2.4 million units IM in a single dose.

Recommended regimen for early latent syphilis in persons with HIV infection: benzathine penicillin G, 2.4 million units IM in a single dose.

Recommended regimen for late latent syphilis in persons with HIV infection: benzathine penicillin G, at weekly doses of 2.4 million units for 3 weeks.

6. Granuloma Inguinale (Donovanosis)
   a. The intracellular gram-negative bacterium *Klebsiella granulomatis* (formerly known as *Calymmatobacterium granulomatis*).
   b. Painless, slowly progressive ulcerative lesions on the genitals or perineum without regional lymphadenopathy; subcutaneous granulomas (pseudobuboes) also might occur.
   c. Visualization of dark-staining Donovan bodies on tissue crush preparation or biopsy.
   d. Recommended regimen: zithromycin 1 g orally once per week or 500 mg daily for at least 3 weeks and until all lesions have completely healed.

   Alternative regimens: doxycycline 100 mg orally twice a day for at least 3 weeks and until all lesions have completely healed or ciprofloxacin 750 mg orally twice a day for at least 3 weeks and until all lesions have completely healed or erythromycin base 500 mg orally four times a day for at least 3 weeks and until all lesions have completely healed or trimethoprim-sulfamethoxazole one double-strength (160 mg/800 mg) tablet orally twice a day for at least 3 weeks and until all lesions have completely healed.

Diseases Characterized by Urethritis and Cervicitis

1. General Management
   a. If point-of-care diagnostic tools are not available, drug regimens effective against both gonorrhea and chlamydia should be administered. Further testing to determine the specific etiology is recommended to prevent complications, reinfection, and transmission, because a specific diagnosis might improve treatment compliance, delivery of risk reduction interventions, and partner notification.
2. Nongonococcal Urethritis
   a. Nongonococcal urethritis (NGU) is a nonspecific diagnosis that can have many infectious etiologies. NGU is caused by *C. trachomatis* in 15% to 40% of cases. *Mycoplasma genitalium*, which can be sexually transmitted, is associated with symptoms of urethritis as well as urethral inflammation and accounts for 15% to 25% of NGU cases in the United States. *Trichomonas vaginalis* can cause NGU in heterosexual men, but the

prevalence varies substantially by region of the United States and within specific sub-populations. In some instances, NGU can be acquired by fellatio, sometimes because of specific pathogens such as HSV, Epstein-Barr virus, and adenovirus; data supporting other *Mycoplasma* species and *Ureaplasma* as etiologic agents are inconsistent.

b. Symptoms, if present, include dysuria; urethral pruritis; and mucoid, mucopurulent, or purulent discharge. Signs of urethral discharge on examination can also be present in persons without symptoms.

c. NGU is confirmed in symptomatic men when staining of urethral secretions indicates inflammation without gram-negative or purple diplococci. All men who have confirmed NGU should be tested for chlamydia and gonorrhea even if point-of-care tests are negative for evidence of gonorrhea. NAATs for chlamydia and gonorrhea are recommended because of their high sensitivity and specificity; a specific diagnosis can potentially reduce complications, reinfection, and transmission.

Testing for *T. vaginalis* should be considered in areas or populations of high prevalence.

d. Recommended regimens: azithromycin 1 g orally in a single dose or doxycycline 100 mg orally twice a day for 7 days.

Alternative regimens: erythromycin base 500 mg orally four times a day for 7 days or erythromycin ethylsuccinate 800 mg orally four times a day for 7 days or levofloxacin 500 mg orally once daily for 7 days or ofloxacin 300 mg orally twice a day for 7 days.

3. Cervicitis

a. When an etiologic organism is isolated in the presence of cervicitis, it is typically *C. trachomatis* or *Neisseria gonorrhoeae*. Cervicitis also can accompany trichomoniasis and genital herpes (especially primary HSV-2 infection). However, in most cases of cervicitis, no organism is isolated, especially in women at relatively low risk for recent acquisition of these STDs. Limited data indicate that infection with *M. genitalium* or bacterial vaginosis (BV) and frequent douching might cause cervicitis.

b. A purulent or mucopurulent endocervical exudate visible in the endocervical canal or on an endocervical swab specimen (commonly referred to as mucopurulent cervicitis) or sustained endocervical bleeding easily induced by gentle passage of a cotton swab through the cervical os. Either or both signs might be present. Cervicitis frequently is asymptomatic, but some women complain of an abnormal vaginal discharge and intermenstrual vaginal bleeding (e.g., after sexual intercourse).

c. Because cervicitis might be a sign of upper genital-tract infection (endometritis), women with a new episode of cervicitis should be assessed for signs of pelvic inflammatory disease (PID) and should be tested for *C. trachomatis* and for *N. gonorrhoeae* with NAAT; such testing can be performed on either vaginal, cervical, or urine samples.

Women with cervicitis also should be evaluated for the presence of BV and trichomoniasis. Because the sensitivity of microscopy to detect *T. vaginalis* is relatively low (approximately 50%), symptomatic women with cervicitis and negative microscopy for trichomonads should receive further testing.

d. Azithromycin 1 g orally in a single dose or doxycycline 100 mg orally twice a day for 7 days.

4. Chlamydia

a. *C. trachomatis* is an obligate intracellular organism found worldwide.

b. Asymptomatic infection is common among both men and women. Several sequelae can result from *C. trachomatis* infection in women, the most serious of which include PID, ectopic pregnancy, and infertility. Some women who receive a diagnosis of uncomplicated cervical infection already have subclinical upper reproductive-tract infection.

c. *C. trachomatis* urogenital infection can be diagnosed in women by testing first-catch urine or collecting swab specimens from the endocervix or vagina. Diagnosis of

C. trachomatis urethral infection in men can be made by testing a urethral swab or first-catch urine specimen. NAATs are the most sensitive tests for these specimens and therefore are recommended for detecting *C. trachomatis* infection. Rectal and oropharyngeal *C. trachomatis* infection in persons engaging in receptive anal or oral intercourse can be diagnosed by testing at the anatomic site of exposure.

    d. Recommended regimens: azithromycin 1 g orally in a single dose or doxycycline 100 mg orally twice a day for 7 days.

       Alternative regimens: erythromycin base 500 mg orally four times a day for 7 days or erythromycin ethylsuccinate 800 mg orally four times a day for 7 days or levofloxacin 500 mg orally once daily for 7 days or ofloxacin 300 mg orally twice a day for 7 days.

       Recommended regimens in pregnancy: azithromycin 1 g orally in a single dose.

       Alternative regimens in pregnancy: amoxicillin 500 mg orally three times a day for 7 days or erythromycin base 500 mg orally four times a day for 7 days or erythromycin base 250 mg orally four times a day for 14 days or erythromycin ethylsuccinate 800 mg orally four times a day for 7 days or erythromycin ethylsuccinate 400 mg orally four times a day for 14 days.

5. Gonorrhea

    a. *N. gonorrheae*, a gram-negative diplococcus.

    b. Urethral infections caused by *N. gonorrhoeae* among men can produce symptoms that cause them to seek curative treatment soon enough to prevent sequelae, but often not soon enough to prevent transmission to others. Among women, gonococcal infections are commonly asymptomatic or might not produce recognizable symptoms until complications (e.g., PID) have occurred. PID can result in tubal scarring that can lead to infertility and ectopic pregnancy.

    c. Culture and NAAT are available for the detection of genitourinary infection with *N. gonorrhoeae*; culture requires endocervical (women) or urethral (men) swab specimens. NAAT allows for the widest variety of US Food and Drug Administration (FDA)-cleared specimen types, including endocervical swabs, vaginal swabs, urethral swabs (men), and urine (from both men and women). Culture is available for detection of rectal, oropharyngeal, and conjunctival gonococcal infection, but NAAT is not FDA-cleared for use with these specimens. Because of its high specificity (>99%) and sensitivity (>95%), a gram stain of urethral secretions that demonstrates polymorphonuclear leukocytes with intracellular gram-negative diplococci can be considered diagnostic for infection with *N. gonorrhoeae* in symptomatic men. However, because of lower sensitivity, a negative gram stain should not be considered sufficient for ruling out infection in asymptomatic men.

       Detection of infection using gram stain of endocervical, pharyngeal, and rectal specimens also is insufficient and is not recommended.

    d. Recommended regimen for uncomplicated gonococcal infections of the cervix, urethra, and rectum: ceftriaxone 250 mg IM in a single dose plus azithromycin 1g orally in a single dose.

       Alternative regimens for uncomplicated gonococcal infections of the cervix, urethra, and rectum: if ceftriaxone is not available, cefixime 400 mg orally in a single dose plus azithromycin 1 g orally in a single dose.

       Uncomplicated gonococcal infections of the pharynx: ceftriaxone 250 mg IM in a single dose plus azithromycin 1 g orally in a single dose.

       Gonococcal conjunctivitis: ceftriaxone 1 g IM in a single dose plus azithromycin 1 g orally in a single dose.

       Recommended regimen for arthritis and arthritis-dermatitis syndrome: ceftriaxone 1 g IM or intravenous (IV) every 24 hours plus azithromycin 1 g orally in a single dose.

Alternative regimens for arthritis and arthritis-dermatitis syndrome: cefotaxime 1 g IV every 8 hours or ceftizoxime 1 g IV every 8 hours plus azithromycin 1 g orally in a single dose.

Gonococcal meningitis and endocarditis: ceftriaxone 1 to 2 g IV every 12 to 24 hours plus azithromycin 1 g orally in a single dose.

Diseases Characterized By Vaginal Discharge

1. General Management of Vaginitis
   a. The three diseases most frequently associated with vaginal discharge are BV (replacement of the vaginal flora by an overgrowth of anaerobic bacteria including *Prevotella* spp., *Mobiluncus* spp., *Gardnerella vaginalis*, *Ureaplasma*, *Mycoplasma*, and numerous fastidious or uncultivated anaerobes), *T. vaginalis*, and candidiasis. Although vulvovaginal candidiasis (VVC) is usually not transmitted sexually, it is included in this section because it is frequently diagnosed in women who have vaginal symptoms or are being evaluated for STDs.
   b. Usually a vaginal discharge or vulvar itching, possibly malodorous. Occasionally mucopurulent cervicitis (*C. trachomatis* or *N. gonorrhoeae*) may produce a vaginal discharge.
   c. The cause of vaginal symptoms might be determined by pH, a potassium hydroxide (KOH) test, and microscopic examination of fresh samples of the discharge. The pH of the vaginal secretions can be determined by narrow-range pH paper; an elevated pH (i.e., ≥4.5) is common with BV or trichomoniasis. Because pH testing is not highly specific, discharge should be further examined microscopically by first diluting one sample in one or two drops of 0.9% normal saline solution on one slide and a second sample in 10% KOH solution (samples that emit an amine odor immediately upon application of KOH suggest BV or trichomoniasis). Coverslips are then placed on the slides, which are then examined under a microscope at low and high power. The saline-solution specimen might show motile trichomonads or "clue cells" (i.e., epithelial cells with borders obscured by small bacteria), which are characteristic of BV. The KOH specimen typically is used to identify hyphae or blastospores seen with candidiasis. However, the absence of trichomonads in saline or fungal elements in KOH samples does not rule out these infections, because the sensitivity of microscopy is approximately 50% compared with NAAT (trichomoniasis) or culture (yeast). The presence of white blood cells (WBCs) without evidence of trichomonads or yeast may also suggest cervicitis.
   d. Pathogen-dependent.
2. Bacterial Vaginosis
   a. BV is a polymicrobial clinical syndrome resulting from replacement of the normal hydrogen peroxide–producing *Lactobacillus* spp. in the vagina with high concentrations of anaerobic bacteria (e.g., *Prevotella* spp. and *Mobiluncus* spp.), *G. vaginalis*, *Ureaplasma*, *Mycoplasma*, and numerous fastidious or uncultivated anaerobes.
   b. BV is the most prevalent cause of vaginal discharge or malodor; however, most women with BV are asymptomatic.
   c. BV can be diagnosed using clinical criteria (i.e., Amsel's diagnostic criteria) or gram stain. A gram stain (considered the gold standard laboratory method for diagnosing BV) is used to determine the relative concentration of lactobacilli (i.e., long grampositive rods), gram-negative and gram-variable rods and cocci (i.e., *G. vaginalis*, *Prevotella*, *Porphyromonas*, and peptostreptococci), and curved gram-negative rods (i.e., *Mobiluncus*) characteristic of BV. Clinical criteria require three of the following symptoms or signs: (1) homogeneous, thin, white discharge that smoothly coats the vaginal walls; (2) clue cells (e.g., vaginal epithelial cells studded with adherent coccobacilli) on microscopic

examination; (3) pH of vaginal fluid over 4.5; (4) a fishy odor of vaginal discharge before or after addition of 10% KOH (i.e., the whiff test). Detection of three of these criteria has been correlated with results by gram stain. Other tests, including Affirm VP III (Becton Dickinson, Sparks, MD), a DNA hybridization probe test for high concentrations of *G. vaginalis*, and the OSOM BV Blue test (Sekisui Diagnostics, Framingham, MA), which detects vaginal fluid sialidase activity, have acceptable performance characteristics compared with gram stain. Although a prolineaminopeptidase card test is available for the detection of elevated pH and trimethylamine, it has low sensitivity and specificity and therefore is not recommended. PCR has been used in research settings for the detection of a variety of organisms associated with BV, but evaluation of its clinical utility is still underway. Detection of specific organisms might be predictive of BV by PCR. Additional validation is needed before these tests can be recommended to diagnose BV. Culture of *G. vaginalis* is not recommended as a diagnostic tool because it is not specific. Cervical Pap tests have no clinical utility for the diagnosis of BV because of their low sensitivity and specificity.

   d. Treatment is recommended for women with symptoms.

   Recommended regimens: metronidazole 500 mg orally twice a day for 7 days or metronidazole gel 0.75%, one full applicator (5 g) intravaginally, once a day for 5 days or clindamycin cream 2%, one full applicator (5 g) intravaginally at bedtime for 7 days.

   Alternative regimens: tinidazole 2 g orally once daily for 2 days or tinidazole 1 g orally once daily for 5 days or clindamycin 300 mg orally twice daily for 7 days or clindamycin ovules 100 mg intravaginally once at bedtime for 3 days.

   Note that clindamycin ovules use an oleaginous base that might weaken latex or rubber products (e.g., condoms and vaginal contraceptive diaphragms). Use of such products within 72 hours following treatment with clindamycin ovules is not recommended.

3. Trichomoniasis

   a. *T. vaginalis*, a protozoan.

   b. Some infected men have symptoms of urethritis, epididymitis, or prostatitis, and some infected women have vaginal discharge that might be diffuse, malodorous, or yellow-green with or without vulvar irritation. However, most infected persons (70%–85%) have minimal or no symptoms, and untreated infections might last for months to years.

   c. The use of highly sensitive and specific tests is recommended for detecting *T. vaginalis*. Among women, NAAT is highly sensitive, often detecting three to five times more *T. vaginalis* infections than wet-mount microscopy, a method with poor sensitivity (51%–65%). Culture was considered the gold standard method for diagnosing *T. vaginalis* infection before molecular detection methods became available. Culture has a sensitivity of 75% to 96% and a specificity of up to 100%. In women, vaginal secretions are the preferred specimen type for culture, as urine culture is less sensitive. In men, culture specimens require a urethral swab, urine sediment, and/or semen.

   To improve yield, multiple specimens from men can be used to inoculate a single culture. The most common method for *T. vaginalis* diagnosis might be microscopic evaluation of wet preparations of genital secretions because of convenience and relatively low cost. Unfortunately, the sensitivity of wet mount is low (51%–65%) in vaginal specimens and lower in specimens from men (e.g., urethral specimens, urine sediment, and semen). Clinicians using wet mounts should attempt to evaluate slides immediately because sensitivity declines as evaluation is delayed, decreasing by up to 20% within 1 hour after collection. When highly sensitive (e.g., NAAT) testing on specimens is not feasible, a testing algorithm (e.g., wet mount first, followed by NAAT if negative) can improve diagnostic sensitivity in persons with an initial negative result by wet mount.

    d. Recommended regimen: metronidazole 2 g orally in a single dose or tinidazole 2 g orally in a single dose.

      Alternative regimen: metronidazole 500 mg orally twice a day for 7 days.

      Women with HIV infection: metronidazole 500 mg orally twice daily for 7 days.

4. Vulvovaginal Candidiasis

    a. VVC usually is caused by *Candida albicans* but can occasionally be caused by other *Candida* spp. or yeasts.

    b. Typical symptoms of VVC include pruritus, vaginal soreness, dyspareunia, external dysuria, and abnormal vaginal discharge. None of these symptoms is specific for VVC. An estimated 75% of women will have at least one episode of VVC, and 40% to 45% will have two or more episodes.

    c. A diagnosis of candida vaginitis is suggested clinically by the presence of external dysuria and vulvar pruritus, pain, swelling, and redness. Signs include vulvar edema, fissures, excoriations, and thick curdy vaginal discharge. The diagnosis can be made in a woman who has signs and symptoms of vaginitis when either (1) a wet preparation (saline, 10% KOH) or gram stain of vaginal discharge demonstrates budding yeasts, hyphae, or pseudohyphae or (2) a culture or other test yields a positive result for a yeast species. Candida vaginitis is associated with a normal vaginal pH (<4.5). Use of 10% KOH in wet preparations improves the visualization of yeast and mycelia by disrupting cellular material that might obscure the yeast or pseudohyphae. Examination of a wet mount with KOH preparation should be performed for all women with symptoms or signs of VVC, and women with a positive result should be treated. For those with negative wet mounts but existing signs or symptoms, vaginal cultures for candida should be considered. If candida cultures cannot be performed for these women, empiric treatment can be considered.

    d. Intravaginal agents: clotrimazole 1% cream 5 g intravaginally daily for 7 to 14 days or clotrimazole 2% cream 5 g intravaginally daily for 3 days or miconazole 2% cream 5 g intravaginally daily for 7 days or miconazole 4% cream 5 g intravaginally daily for 3 days or miconazole 100 mg vaginal suppository, one suppository daily for 7 days or miconazole 200 mg vaginal suppository, one suppository for 3 days or miconazole 1200 mg vaginal suppository, one suppository for 1 day or tioconazole 6.5% ointment 5 g intravaginally in a single application or butoconazole 2% cream (single dose bioadhesive product), 5 g intravaginally in a single application or terconazole 0.4% cream 5 g intravaginally daily for 7 days or terconazole 0.8% cream 5 g intravaginally daily for 3 days or terconazole 80 mg vaginal suppository, one suppository daily for 3 days.

      Oral agent: fluconazole 150 mg orally in a single dose.

Pelvic Inflammatory Disease

    a. Sexually transmitted organisms, especially *N. gonorrhoeae* and *C. trachomatis*, are implicated in many cases. Recent studies suggest that the proportion of PID cases attributable to *N. gonorrhoeae* or *C. trachomatis* is declining; of women who received a diagnosis of acute PID, less than 50% test positive for either of these organisms. Microorganisms that comprise the vaginal flora (e.g., anaerobes, *G. vaginalis*, *Haemophilus influenzae*, enteric gram-negative rods, and *Streptococcus agalactiae*) have been associated with PID. In addition, cytomegalovirus (CMV), *M. hominis*, *U. urealyticum*, and *M. genitalium* might be associated with some PID cases. Newer data suggest that *M. genitalium* might play a role in the pathogenesis of PID and might be associated with milder symptoms, although one study failed to demonstrate a significant increase in PID following detection of *M. genitalium* in the lower genital tract.

b. PID comprises a spectrum of inflammatory disorders of the upper female genital tract, including any combination of endometritis, salpingitis, tuboovarian abscess, and pelvic peritonitis. Acute PID is difficult to diagnose because of the wide variation in symptoms and signs associated with this condition. Many women with PID have subtle or nonspecific symptoms or are asymptomatic.

c. Presumptive treatment for PID should be initiated in sexually active young women and other women at risk for STDs if they are experiencing pelvic or lower abdominal pain, if no cause for the illness other than PID can be identified, and if one or more of the following minimum clinical criteria are present on pelvic examination:
- cervical motion tenderness
- uterine tenderness
- adnexal tenderness.

One or more of the following additional criteria can be used to enhance the specificity of the minimum clinical criteria and support a diagnosis of PID:
- oral temperature >101°F (>38.3°C)
- abnormal cervical mucopurulent discharge or cervical friability
- presence of abundant numbers of WBCs on saline microscopy of vaginal fluid
- elevated erythrocyte sedimentation rate
- elevated C-reactive protein
- laboratory documentation of cervical infection with *N. gonorrhoeae* or *C. trachomatis.*

If the cervical discharge appears normal and no WBCs are observed on the wet prep of vaginal fluid, the diagnosis of PID is unlikely, and alternative causes of pain should be considered.

The most specific criteria for diagnosing PID include:
- endometrial biopsy with histopathologic evidence of endometritis
- transvaginal sonography or magnetic resonance imaging techniques showing thickened, fluid-filled tubes with or without free pelvic fluid or tuboovarian complex, or Doppler studies suggesting pelvic infection (e.g., tubal hyperemia)
- laparoscopic findings consistent with PID.

d. The decision of whether hospitalization is necessary should be based on provider judgment and whether the woman meets any of the following suggested criteria:
- surgical emergencies (e.g., appendicitis) cannot be excluded
- tuboovarian abscess
- pregnancy
- severe illness, nausea and vomiting, or high fever
- unable to follow or tolerate an outpatient oral regimen
- no clinical response to oral antimicrobial therapy.

Parenteral regimens: cefotetan 2 g IV every 12 hours plus doxycycline 100 mg orally or IV every 12 hours or cefoxitin 2 g IV every 6 hours plus doxycycline 100 mg orally or IV every 12 hours or clindamycin 900 mg IV every 8 hours plus gentamicin loading dose IV or IM (2 mg/kg), followed by a maintenance dose (1.5 mg/kg) every 8 hours. Single daily dosing (3–5 mg/kg) can be substituted.

Alternative parenteral regimen: ampicillin/sulbactam 3 g IV every 6 hours plus doxycycline 100 mg orally or IV every 12 hours

Intramuscular/oral regimens: ceftriaxone 250 mg IM in a single dose plus doxycycline 100 mg orally twice a day for 14 days with or without metronidazole 500 mg orally twice a day for 14 days or cefoxitin 2 g IM in a single dose and probenecid, 1 g orally administered concurrently in a single dose plus doxycycline 100 mg orally twice a day for 14 days with or without metronidazole 500 mg orally twice a day for 14 days or other parenteral third-generation cephalosporin (e.g., ceftizoxime or cefotaxime) plus doxycycline 100 mg orally twice a day for 14 days with or without metronidazole 500 mg orally twice a day for 14 days.

Note that the recommended third-generation cephalosporins are limited in the coverage of anaerobes. Therefore, until it is known that extended anaerobic coverage is not important for treatment of acute PID, the addition of metronidazole to treatment regimens with third-generation cephalosporins should be considered.

Epididymitis

a. Among sexually active men aged under 35 years, acute epididymitis is most frequently caused by *C. trachomatis* or *N. gonorrhoeae*. Acute epididymitis caused by sexually transmitted enteric organisms (e.g., *Escherichia coli*) also occurs among men who are the insertive partner during anal intercourse. In men aged 35 years and over who do not report insertive anal intercourse, sexually transmitted acute epididymitis is less common. In this group, the epididymis usually becomes infected in the setting of bacteriuria secondary to bladder outlet obstruction (e.g., benign prostatic hyperplasia).

b. Acute epididymitis is a clinical syndrome consisting of pain, swelling, and inflammation of the epididymis that lasts less than 6 weeks. Sometimes the testis is also involved—a condition referred to as epididymo-orchitis. A high index of suspicion for spermatic cord (testicular) torsion must be maintained in men who present with a sudden onset of symptoms associated with epididymitis, as this condition is a surgical emergency.

c. All suspected cases of acute epididymitis should be evaluated for objective evidence of inflammation by one of the following point-of-care tests.

- Gram or methylene blue or gentian violet stain (MB/GV) of urethral secretions demonstrating 2 or more WBC per oil immersion field. These stains are preferred point-of-care diagnostic tests for evaluating urethritis because they are highly sensitive and specific for documenting both urethral inflammation and the presence or absence of gonococcal infection. Gonococcal infection is established by documenting the presence of WBC-containing intracellular gram-negative or purple diplococci on urethral gram stain or MB/GV smear, respectively.
- Positive leukocyte esterase test on first-void urine.
- Microscopic examination of sediment from a spun first-void urine demonstrating ≥10 WBC per high power field.

  All suspected cases of acute epididymitis should be tested for *C. trachomatis* and for *N. gonorrhoeae* by NAAT. Urine is the preferred specimen for NAAT testing in men. Urine cultures for chlamydia and gonococcal epididymitis are insensitive and are not recommended. Urine bacterial culture might have a higher yield in men with sexually transmitted enteric infections and in older men with acute epididymitis caused by genitourinary bacteriuria.

d. Acute epididymitis most likely caused by sexually transmitted chlamydia and gonorrhea: ceftriaxone 250 mg IM in a single dose plus doxycycline 100 mg orally twice a day for 10 days.

   Acute epididymitis most likely caused by sexually transmitted chlamydia and gonorrhea and enteric organisms (men who practice insertive anal sex): ceftriaxone 250 mg IM in a single dose plus levofloxacin 500 mg orally once a day for 10 days or ofloxacin 300 mg orally twice a day for 10 days.

   Acute epididymitis most likely caused by enteric organisms: levofloxacin 500 mg orally once daily for 10 days or ofloxacin 300 mg orally twice a day for 10 days.

Human Papilloma Virus (Genital Warts, Plantar Warts, Cervical Warts)

a. Approximately 100 types of human papillomavirus (HPV) infection have been identified, at least 40 of which can infect the genital area.

   Most HPV infections are self-limited and are asymptomatic or unrecognized. Most sexually active persons become infected with HPV at least once in their lifetime. Oncogenic, high-risk HPV infection (e.g., HPV types 16 and 18) causes most cervical, penile, vulvar, vaginal, anal, and oropharyngeal cancers and precancers, whereas nononcogenic, low-risk HPV infection (e.g., HPV types 6 and 11) causes genital warts and recurrent respiratory papillomatosis.

b. Anogenital warts are usually asymptomatic, but depending on the size and anatomic location, they can be painful or pruritic. They are usually flat, papular, or pedunculated growths on the genital mucosa. Anogenital warts occur commonly at certain anatomic sites, including around the vaginal introitus, under the foreskin of the uncircumcised penis, and on the shaft of the circumcised penis. Warts can also occur at multiple sites in the anogenital epithelium or within the anogenital tract (e.g., cervix, vagina, urethra, perineum, perianal skin, anus, and scrotum). Intraanal warts are observed predominantly in persons who have had receptive anal intercourse, but they also can occur in men and women who have not had a history of anal sexual contact.

c. Diagnosis of anogenital warts is usually made by visual inspection. The diagnosis of anogenital warts can be confirmed by biopsy, which is indicated if lesions are atypical (e.g., pigmented, indurated, affixed to underlying tissue, bleeding, or ulcerated lesions).

d. External anogenital warts (i.e., penis, groin, scrotum, vulva, perineum, external anus, and perianus)

   Patient-applied: imiquimod 3.75% or 5% cream (might weaken condoms and vaginal diaphragms) or Podofilox 0.5% solution or gel or sinecatechins 15% ointment (might weaken condoms and vaginal diaphragms).

   Provider-administered: cryotherapy with liquid nitrogen or cryoprobe or surgical removal either by tangential scissor excision, tangential shave excision, curettage, laser, or electrosurgery or trichloroacetic acid (TCA) or bichloroacetic acid (BCA) 80% to 90% solution.

   Note that many persons with external anal warts also have intraanal warts. Thus, persons with external anal warts might benefit from an inspection of the anal canal by digital examination, standard anoscopy, or high-resolution anoscopy.

   Urethral meatus warts: cryotherapy with liquid nitrogen or surgical removal.

   Vaginal warts: cryotherapy with liquid nitrogen or surgical removal or TCA or BCA 80% to 90% solution. (The use of a cryoprobe in the vagina is not recommended because of the risk for vaginal perforation and fistula formation.)

   Cervical warts: cryotherapy with liquid nitrogen or surgical removal or TCA or BCA 80% to 90% solution. (Management of cervical warts should include consultation with a specialist; for women who have exophytic cervical warts, a biopsy evaluation to exclude high-grade squamous intraepithelial lesion (SIL) must be performed before treatment is initiated.)

   Intraanal warts: cryotherapy with liquid nitrogen or surgical removal or TCA or BCA 80% to 90% solution. (Management of intraanal warts should include consultation with a specialist.)

Resources for Further Learning

Centers for Disease Control and Prevention. *Sexually Transmitted Diseases Treatment Guidelines.* CDC; 2015. Available at: https://www.cdc.gov/std/tg2015/default.htm. Accessed September 3, 2020.

Bites and Stings

Nathan Kinder

Bites

REPTILES

A. Snakes
1. Overview: Snake venom often has both hemotoxic and neurotoxic properties, but one usually predominates over another according to the species. Of all snakebites, 25% to 50% are "dry bites" and cause no envenomation.[1,2] Children tend to have more severe envenomations because of the dose of venom relative to weight and body surface area. The antivenin dose is the same for children and adults. Be cognizant of the quantity of fluids used in administration of antivenin to children (typical initial pediatric fluid bolus is 20 mL/kg).[3,4]
    a. Universal care of bites:
        i. Monitor airway, breathing, circulation (ABCs) and provide supportive care (i.e., pain control, fluids, anxiolytics, etc.).
        ii. Assess for progression of swelling or symptoms (remove all restrictive clothing immediately).
        iii. Do not suction wound, tourniquet, incise, place ice packs, or provide electric shock.
        iv. Do limit activity such as walking to a minimum if possible and immobilize the affected area.
        v. Evacuate to the nearest hospital as soon as possible (preferably one with antivenin).
        vi. Do not risk further envenomation to identify snake species.
        vii. Do not hesitate to consult Poison Control or a toxicologist for guidance.
        Specific signs and symptoms and treatments based on species will be discussed below.
2. *Crotalidae* (pit vipers, i.e., water moccasin, rattlesnake, copperhead, bushmaster, lance-heads, temple vipers, jumping vipers)
    a. Found in parts of Europe and Asia and both North and South America
    b. Identified by slit-like pupils, triangular head, and a "pit" located behind the nose
    c. Hemotoxic effects, and swelling/localized pain is marked
    d. Elevate extremity and monitor compartment pressures (fasciotomies in snake bites are controversial and should only be undertaken in extreme circumstances or in consultation with a surgeon)

e. ABCs, intravenous (IV) access, monitor
f. Severity of envenomation is graded based on six areas: respiratory, cardiovascular, local wound, hematologic, gastrointestinal, central nervous system. The severity and quantity of symptoms are a direct correlation with need for antivenin (i.e., a minimal score correlates with few symptoms and does not require treatment but a moderate to severe score correlates with significant symptoms and lab derangements and needs antivenin).
g. Laboratory tests (Complete blood count [CBC], Comprehensive metabolic panel [CMP], Creatine phosphokinase [CPK], coagulation studies, etc.)
h. Administer specific or polyvalent antivenin (Crotalidae Polyvalent Immune Fab or FabAV) as soon as possible preferably within 6 hours (FabAv is known in the US by the registered name *CroFab*)
  i. FabAV administration is 4 to 6 vials in 250 mLs of normal saline IV over 1 hour.
  ii. Monitor closely for allergic or anaphylaxis symptoms.
  iii. Repeat 4 to 6 vials/dose IV until localized swelling halts progression and/or coagulation tests normalize.
  iv. Patient may need 2 vials IV q 6 hours for 18+ hours.[5]
i. Other antivenins exist and have specific administration instructions (follow instructions on the packaging insert).
j. There is a risk of immediate hypersensitivity (anaphylaxis occurs within minutes to hours) and delayed hypersensitivity (serum sickness occurs from 1 to 12 days; mean 7 days) with antivenin (total risk ~15%).[6–9]
  i. Overall rare events and should not preclude lifesaving intervention
  ii. Pretreatment with antihistamines or steroids has no benefit.
  iii. Skin testing of antivenin is not recommended before administration.

3. *Elapidae* (i.e., coral snakes, kraits, cobras, mambas, asps)
a. Found in most tropical and subtropical regions of the world except Europe
b. Typically identified by long/slender bodies with smooth scales, round pupils, and heads that seem indistinct from the rest of the body
c. Primarily neurotoxic effects with local necrosis
d. More insidious symptom onset than with the Crotalidae species
e. Paralysis is the most deadly feature and usually begins with ptosis and then progresses to eventually involve muscles of respiration leading to death if no intervention.
f. ABCs, IV access, monitor, and supportive care
g. Antivenin if available and signs of severe systemic symptoms (can survive with supportive care alone with adequate respiratory support)
h. Anticholinesterase drugs have been used successfully to aid treatment of elapids snake bites as neurotoxic symptoms closely resemble myasthenia gravis.
i. Pretreat with glycopyrrolate 0.1 mg IV or atropine 0.6 mg IV
j. Neostigmine 0.5–2.5 mg IV q 1 hour or as a continuous infusion (based on symptom severity)[10]

4. Hydrophilidae: sea snakes
a. Neurotoxic and myotoxic
b. Generalized myalgias: can be severe and last for months if untreated
c. Myotoxic effects include the release of myoglobin and potassium resulting in renal failure or life-threatening potassium levels.
d. May require ventilator support
e. ABCs, IV access, monitor, and supportive care
f. Antivenin if available and severe symptoms
Note that Antivenin has some risk of anaphylaxis or severe reactions. Weigh the risk versus benefit carefully in each patient. Anaphylaxis is not a reason to terminate

treatment as the antivenin is the antidote needed for resolution. Slow the infusion and treat symptoms of anaphylaxis and shock appropriately.
B. Lizards
Most lizards produce localized pain and swelling only. The Gila Monster Lizard and the closely related Mexican Beaded Lizard can cause systemic symptoms such as nausea, vomiting, sweating, fever, generalized weakness, and even some difficulty breathing but rarely death.
1. Monitor lizards
   a. Native to Africa, Asia, and the Indo-Pacific regions but can now be found all over the world as pets
   b. Size ranges from 20 cm to 3 m (7.9 in to 10 ft)
   c. Can be aggressive if provoked
   d. No antivenin exists. Symptomatic care only. See later
2. Komodo dragons
   a. Native to Indonesia
   b. Can grow to sizes of up to 3 m or 10 ft
   c. Some reported fatalities but usually caused by injuries/trauma and not because of envenomations
   d. No antivenin exists. Symptomatic care only.
3. Gila Monster
   a. Found in the Southwestern United States and Northern Mexico
   b. Size approaches 60 cm or 2 ft
   c. Does produce a potent neurotoxic venom but only small amounts are excreted during a bite and therefore very rarely fatal
   d. Symptomatic care. No antivenin available.
4. Mexican Beaded Lizard
   a. Native to Mexico and Guatemala
   b. Adults range from 57 to 91 cm (22–36 in)
   c. Venom is hemotoxic in nature and therefore coagulation studies should be followed to resolution.
   d. Symptomatic care only. No antivenin.
5. Prehospital care
   a. Many lizards are known for clamping onto the victim with great force and not letting go.
   b. It is important to try to pry the animal away without causing more damage to the victim.
   c. Techniques include using a stick or a metal bar to pry the animal's mouth open and away from the victim.
   d. After the lizard is removed, bandage the area if bleeding and monitor ABCs.
   e. Do not tourniquet or try to suction the wound.
6. Signs and symptoms
   a. Mostly local pain and swelling
   b. Can have systemic symptoms such as nausea, vomiting, lightheadedness, hypertension, and rarely breathing difficulty
7. Treatment
   a. No commercially available antivenin exists
   b. Supportive care
   c. IV, monitor, ABCs
   d. Local wound care
   e. Monitor for signs of infection
   f. Antibiotics (amoxicillin/clavulanate 875 mg twice a day for 7–10 days or clindamycin 300 mg four times a day for 7–10 days or doxycycline 100 mg twice a day for

7–10 days) reserved for secondary infection or high-risk wounds (highly contaminated wounds, neurovascular compromise, deep penetrating wounds [especially in distal extremities], associated cellulitis, significant medical comorbidities such as diabetes, delayed presentation of >12 hours for extremity wounds or >24 hours on the face, or an immunocompromised state).[11]

    g. Remove foreign bodies; x-rays or ultrasound may aide in the identification of foreign bodies (i.e., teeth, dirt, and debris).

C. Crocodiles and Alligators

  1. Technically classified in separate biological families but will be discussed together as the medical treatment remains the same

  2. Found in warm wet climates of the Americas, Africa, Asia, and Australia

  3. Can be aggressive and are responsible for many human deaths every year

  4. Bites can cause significant trauma and death is usually secondary to wounds or blood loss.

  5. Treatment should focus on the following:

    a. Supportive care to include trauma resuscitation

    b. IV, monitor, ABCs

    c. Local wound care for minor bites or scratches

    d. Remove foreign bodies; x-rays or ultrasound may aide in the identification of foreign bodies (i.e., teeth, dirt, and debris)

    e. Routine antibiotics are not warranted but can be considered for secondary infection, someone who will not have follow-up care, or high-risk wounds (highly contaminated wounds, neurovascular compromise, deep penetrating wounds [especially in distal extremities], associated cellulitis, significant medical comorbidities such as diabetes, delayed presentation of >12 hours for extremity wounds or >24 hours on the face, or an immunocompromised state).[11]

    f. Antibiotics could include the following: amoxicillin/clavulanate 875 mg twice a day for 7–10 days or clindamycin 300 mg four times a day for 7–10 days or doxycycline 100 mg twice a day for 7-10 days.

SPIDERS

A. Widow Spiders (*Lactrodectus* species): most common is the black widow spider of North America but also includes the Australian red-back spider, the brown widow spider, and the "button" spider of South America

  1. Found in every continent except Antarctica and other areas prone to extreme hot or cold climates (high concentration in North America and Australia)

  2. Typically found in dark spaces close to the ground such as wood piles, sheds, and cluttered basements/garages

  3. Classic appearance of North American female black widow spider is a black spider with red "hourglass" on abdomen

  4. Venom can cause symptoms ranging from mild local pain to severe generalized muscle pain, abdominal cramping, vomiting, headache, and abnormal vital signs.

  5. Symptomatic care should include ABCs, monitor, updated tetanus, and pain control.

  6. There is an antivenin available, but given the risk of anaphylaxis or other adverse outcomes, the risk versus benefits should be weighed and discussed with patient before administration.

  7. Envenomation is rarely fatal and therefore antivenin is justified only for severe symptoms.

  8. Narcotic pain medications as well as benzodiazepines are helpful (i.e., morphine 0.1 mg/kg IV q 2 hours; hydrocodone/Tylenol 5/325 mg 1–2 tabs PO q 4–6 hours; diazepam 2–10 mg IV q 4 hours or diazepam 5 mg PO q 8 hours).

9. Calcium gluconate is not beneficial.[12]
10. Antibiotics not necessary
  B. Brown Recluse (*Loxosceles reclusa*)
    1. Small brown spider with dark brown "fiddle" or "violin" on back
    2. Typically found in the Central to Southeastern United States and discovered in undisturbed locations like sheds, wood piles, basement corners, closets, and so on.
    3. Bite causes minimal pain initially progressing to severe pain from about 2 to 8 hours after bite.
    4. Most bites require no treatment, but a small percentage can become necrotic.
    5. Necrosis leads to ulceration which can progress over several days.
    6. Eventually the lesion heals with secondary intention, with minimal to no scarring most of the time.
    7. Systemic effects include malaise, nausea, and fevers.
    8. Rarely do life-threatening conditions such as disseminated intravascular coagulopathy, renal failure, rhabdomyolysis, angioedema, or death occur.
    9. Supportive care to include monitor, pain medication, local wound care, and tetanus is usually sufficient. Antibiotics are usually reserved for superimposed bacterial infections only.
    10. Concern for systemic involvement should prompt laboratory studies to evaluate for renal function, hemolysis, and rhabdomyolysis.
    11. Various other treatments have been suggested with varying but limited success. These include such treatments as: steroids, dapsone, surgical debridement, antibiotics, nitroglycerin patches, and colchicine. Owing to lack of good evidence, these therapies are not routinely recommended outside of expert consultation.

MAMMALS

  A. Cautions/Special Considerations
    1. Bites on extremities (especially hands and feet) have a higher risk of infection.
    2. Wound cultures are not necessary for noninfected wounds.
    3. X-rays to assess for foreign bodies (ultrasound can also be helpful)
    4. Perform full range of motion of the injured area to assess for hidden injuries.
    5. *Pasteurella multocida*, *Capnocytophaga*, anaerobes, *Staphylococcus* species, and *Streptococcus* species are the most common bacteria isolated from mammalian bite wounds.
    6. Most common wounds are from dogs and cats. Dog bites tend to have crushed/macerated tissue, whereas cat bites can look inconspicuous but tend to have deep seed bacteria leading to higher rate of infection, complications, and delayed diagnosis.
    7. Rabies is nearly 100% fatal if contracted (most have saliva contact on broken skin or mucous membranes, scratches, or bites to transmit rabies).
    8. The wild animals typically associated with rabies are foxes, bats, raccoons, skunks, and coyotes.
    9. Bat contact or questionable exposure warrants rabies vaccination/rabies immunoglobulin.
    10. High-risk wounds include crush injuries, puncture wounds, bites of the hands and feet, cat and human bites, greater than 12 hours since bite (or 24 hours on the face).
  B. Management/Treatment
    1. Clean wounds with povidone iodine or benzalkonium solution along with pressure irrigation.
    2. Update tetanus as necessary.
    3. If patient has not completed the initial tetanus vaccine series (a three-shot series typically completed as a child in the form of the DTaP vaccination) then a tetanus vaccination and tetanus immunoglobulin (TIG; 500 units IM) should be given. The tetanus

immunoglobulin should be partially administered at the wound site and the rest administered at a different site than the tetanus vaccination (TDAP or TD 0.5 mL IM).[13]
4. Prophylactic antibiotics (amoxicillin/clavulanate 875 mg twice a day for 7–10 days or clindamycin 300 mg four times a day for 7–10 days or doxycycline 100 mg twice a day for 7–10 days) are controversial and therefore should only be used for high-risk wounds such as highly contaminated wounds, neurovascular compromise, deep penetrating wounds (especially in distal extremities), associated cellulitis, significant medical comorbidities such as diabetes, delayed presentation of more than 12 hours for extremity wounds or more than 24 hours on the face, or an immunocompromised state.[11]
5. Most wounds will/should heal by secondary intention because of the risk of a deep seeded infection worsening in a closed wound. (Do not use tissue adhesives for this reason.)
6. Rabies vaccine can be given prophylactically in a three-shot series before traveling to a high-risk area or in a four-shot series in conjunction with human rabies immune globulin (HRIG) after potential rabies exposure.
   a. IM vaccination given on day of exposure (day 0) and then days 3, 7, and 14 after exposure (if immunocompromised then another vaccination is given on day 28 and preexposure prophylaxis series is day 0, 7, and 21 or 28. Booster doses based on rabies antibody titer level every 2 years.
   b. If a previously vaccinated person is exposed to rabies then the postexposure prophylaxis is given on day 0 and 3.
   c. Vaccine should be given as soon as possible after the incident and is still effective even if started several days after exposure.
      i. HRIG is given for high-risk wounds or exposures (i.e., rabies endemic area, unprovoked animal attacks, bizarre animal behavior, unknown vaccination status of animal, etc.) to those who have not been previously vaccinated against rabies.
      ii. Dose is 20 units/kg IM.
      iii. Infiltrate as much as possible around the wound/bite.
      iv. The rest of the HRIG is given at the most proximal site away from the wound.
      v. Never give the rabies vaccine and HRIG in the same location.
      vi. Previously vaccinated persons should not receive HRIG even if previous vaccination was some years ago.[14]

Stings

A. Insects
   1. *Hymenoptera* (bees, wasps, hornets, yellow jackets, ants, etc.)
      a. ABCs, IV access, monitor
      b. Remove stinger/venom sac if present (use a dull edge such as a credit card to scrape along the skin)
      c. Supportive care to include: ice to the affected area, elevation to limit swelling, pain medication, antihistamine administration, and update tetanus
      d. Severe cases (anaphylaxis) may include hives, tongue/lip swelling, wheezing, decreased level of consciousness, hypotension, throat swelling, and so on.
         i. Epinephrine IM initially but may need IV doses/infusion (epinephrine 1:1000 0.01 mg/kg IM, maximum dose of 0.5 mg; IV infusion of 0.1–1 mcg/kg per minute titrated to effect)
         ii. H1 and H2 blockers (i.e., diphenhydramine 25–50 mg IV; ranitidine 50 mg IV)
         iii. Steroids (i.e., methylprednisolone 1–2 mg/kg per day IV)
         iv. Monitor/manage airway (do not hesitate to intubate early in anaphylaxis to protect the airway)

v. Bronchodilators as needed for wheezing and respiratory distress (i.e., albuterol 2.5–5 mg nebulized or continuous nebulizer treatment if severe)

2. Centipede, millipede, caterpillar
   a. Rarely, if ever, fatal
   b. Symptomatic care is usually sufficient (ice, pain medication, antihistamines, steroid creams, etc.).
   c. Centipede bites can be as painful as a bee sting.
   d. Millipede secretions can be irritating, especially if rubbed into eyes (flush eyes frequently if this occurs).
   e. Caterpillars: irritating hairs usually with localized symptoms (can attempt to remove hairs with tape for symptom relief but not required)
   f. Anaphylaxis is very rare but potentially fatal (treat appropriately; see Hymenoptera for explanation of anaphylaxis treatment).

B. Scorpions: Deathstalker, Fat-tail, Emperor, Indian Red, and Blue Scorpions
   1. Found in every continent except Antarctica but typically prefer habitats between 68°F and 99°F (20°C–37°C)
   2. Nocturnal creatures that can be found using ultraviolet "black lights" owing to fluorescent chemicals within the cuticle portion of the exoskeleton
   3. Can be aggressive if provoked
   4. Signs and symptoms of envenomation
      a. Neurotoxic venom
      b. Can be fatal
      c. Bites graded on a scale of I to IV
         i. Grade I: local pain and paresthesias
         ii. Grade II: local and remote pain and paresthesias
         iii. Grade III: cranial nerve dysfunction (dysphagia, drooling, abnormal eye movements, slurred speech, etc.) or somatic skeletal muscular dysfunction (muscle fasciculations, jerking of extremities, restlessness, etc.)
         iv. Grade IV: cranial nerve and skeletal muscle symptoms. Also can have hyperthermia, rhabdomyolysis, wheezing, bronchospasm, respiratory failure.[15]
      d. Children have more severe symptoms because of venom versus body surface area ratio (can see pathologic hypertension from adrenergic release).
   5. Management and treatment
      a. ABCs, monitor, tetanus, labs generally reserved for grade III to IV envenomations, supportive care
      b. Pain control: depending on severity of symptoms
         i. Oral pain control for minor symptoms
         ii. If using IV narcotics, use short-acting forms such as fentanyl (0.5–2 mcg/kg IV) owing to less histamine release.
         iii. Severe extremity stings can be managed with a regional block.
         iv. Benzodiazepines (i.e., diazepam 2–10 mg IV) for pain/muscle spasm (caution when using antivenin as the patient may become oversedated once the symptoms of envenomation are subsiding)
      c. Antivenin
         i. Only suggested for grade III or IV envenomations
         ii. Several different types and manufacturers (check local resources)
         iii. Give in conjunction with poison control if available (In the United States call 1(800) 222-1222.)
         iv. Some risk of anaphylaxis: risk versus benefit and prepare for complications
         v. Children require the same amount of antivenin as the envenomation is the same amount (caution with the amount of fluid used for children).

vi. *Centruroides* species antivenin most commonly used in the United States and Mexico

vii. Administer two to three vials in 50 mL of normal saline IV over 10 minutes.

viii. Continue to give single vials diluted in normal saline solution every 30 to 60 minutes for up to five doses or until resolution of symptoms. (Each dose is administered over 10 minutes.)

Marine Envenomations

General treatments include tetanus, hot water bath (40°C–45°C), and removing all foreign bodies. Antibiotics are reserved for infection or high-risk wounds (i.e., ciprofloxacin, doxycycline, trimethoprim/sulfamethoxazole). Coverage should include *Vibrio* species as well as typical *Staphylococcus* and *Streptococcus* species.

  A. Coelenterates (Portuguese Man-of-War, Jellyfish, Box-Jellyfish, Coral, and Anemones)

1. Hot water bath (40°C–45°C) for 30 to 60 minutes to relieve pain
2. Jellyfish stings should be rinsed with 5% acetic acid (vinegar) or isopropyl alcohol 40% to 70% (do not rub area or rinse with fresh water as this will cause nematocysts to discharge and worsen symptoms).
3. Lacerations caused by coral are prone to infection.
4. Only supportive care unless infected
5. Update tetanus if necessary (tetanus toxoid TD 0.5 mL IM)
6. The Box-Jellyfish or Sea Wasp (*Chironex fleckeri*) sting is deadly
   a. Most deadly species found in the Indo-Pacific region but subspecies have been found in the Atlantic Ocean and Mediterranean Sea.
   b. They are nearly transparent and have a characteristic box shape measuring up to 20 cm (7.9 in) each side and long tentacles measuring up to 3 m (9.8 ft).
   c. Can cause respiratory paralysis, shock, muscle spasm, and death within 2 to 5 minutes in severe envenomations
   d. Envenomation causes death by allowing large amounts of potassium to leak from cells leading to cardiovascular collapse.
   e. ABCs, monitor, respiratory support, tetanus
   f. Acetic acid 5% immediately to wound before removal of tentacles to neutralize nematocysts
   g. An antivenin does exist and should be given rapidly to increase chance of survival.
   h. Antivenin dose and administration is one ampule (20,000 units) diluted in 20 cc of normal saline given IV over 20 minutes or give three ampules IM once (at three different sites). Repeat IV doses until symptoms improve or maximum dose of 60,000 units achieved.[16]

  B. Echinoderms (Starfish, Sea Urchins, and Sea Cucumbers)

1. Hot water immersion provides good pain relief (40°C–45°C or 104°F–113°F).
2. Local anesthetic or even regional nerve blocks may be needed in severe pain.
3. Remove all retained foreign bodies (x-ray or ultrasound may help in diagnosis).
4. Symptomatic care
5. Local irritation can be treated with steroid creams or calamine lotion.
6. Sea cucumber stings may benefit from acetic acid 5% or isopropyl alcohol 40% to 70%.

  C. Vertebrates (Stonefish, Catfish, Stingrays, Lionfish, Weever Fish, etc.)

1. Hot water baths seem to help with pain (temperatures around 45°C or 113°F or as hot as can be reasonably tolerated by the patient).
2. Remove all foreign bodies (the barbs of stingrays can be particularly difficult to remove and sometimes require surgical removal if indicated by location or predicted difficult of removal).

3. There are some rare cases of death from penetrating stingray stings.
4. Most vertebrates only cause local pain and swelling.
5. Antibiotics are reserved for secondary infections or high-risk wounds such as a deep penetrating wound (especially on the distal extremities), immunocompromised host, very dirty wounds, and so on.
6. Allow wounds to heal by secondary intention because of the risk of closing a wound in an area with potentially deep seeded bacteria.
7. Antivenin only exists for stonefish envenomations and is only used in severe cases such as respiratory distress, severe pain, cardiovascular compromise, and so on.
   a. Antivenin developed to specifically combat the neurotoxic effects
   b. Dose is one ampule IM per two barbs puncture wounds with maximum administration of three ampules IM total.[17]
   c. No absolute contraindications for administration but monitor closely for signs and symptoms of anaphylaxis
D. Mollusks (Blue-Ringed Octopus, Cone Snail)
   1. Cone snails
      a. Typically found in the Indo-Pacific but have been identified off the coast of California, South Africa, and the Mediterranean region.
      b. Snails inhabit beautifully decorated shells, which can be problematic as people try to collect the shells.
      c. The snails inject a neurotoxic venom in defense or when hunting other sea creatures.
      d. No antivenin exists.
      e. Treatment revolves around symptomatic care and early ventilatory support. Even in severe envenomations, chances of survival are good with proper respiratory care.
      f. The venom also has some anticoagulant properties and therefore coagulation studies should be checked and followed until resolution.
   2. Blue-ringed octopus
      a. Typically found in the coral reefs and tidal pools of the Indo-Pacific region of the world
      b. Only 12 to 20 cm (5–8 inches) in length and characterized by multiple blue rings on the body which flash as a warning to intruders when the octopus is provoked
      c. Envenomations are extremely dangerous because of the activity of the deadly compound tetrodotoxin.
      d. Tetrodotoxin is a powerful neurotoxin that causes sodium channel blockade leading to muscle paralysis.
      e. Symptoms start rapidly and can lead to total body flaccid paralysis, respiratory arrest, and subsequent death within minutes.
      f. Mainstay of treatment is symptomatic care and ventilatory support until the effects of the toxin subside and are excreted from the body.

References

1. Theakston RD, Warrell DA, Griffiths E. Report of a WHO workshop on the standardization and control of antivenoms. *Toxicon.* 2003;41(5):541–557. doi:10.1006/s0041-0101(02)00393-8.
2. Tintinalli JE, Stapczynski JS, Ma OJ, et al. *Tintinalli's emergency medicine: A coprehensive study guide.* 7th ed. McGraw-Hill; 2011:1354.
3. Thomas NJ, Carcillo JA. Hypovolemic shock in pediatrics patients. *New Horiz.* 1998;6(2):120.
4. Offerman SR, Bush SP, Moynihan JA, et al. Crotaline Fab antivenom for the treatment of children with rattlesnake envenomation. *Pediactrics.* 2002;110:968.
5. Lavonas EJ, Ruha A-M, Banner W, et al. Unified treatment algorithm for the management of crotaline snakebite in the United States: Results of an evidence-informed consensus workshop. *BMC Emerg Med.* 2011;11:2.

6. Ruha A-M, Curry SC, Beuhler M. Initial postmarketing experience with Crotalidae Polyvalent Immune Rab for treatment of rattlesnake envenomation. *Ann Emerg Med.* 2002;39:609.

7. Pizon AF, Riley BD, LoVecchio F, et al. Safety and efficacy of Crotalidae Polyvalent Immune Fab in pediatric crotaline envenomation. *Acad Emerg Med.* 2007;14:373.

8. Corneille MG, Larson S, Stewart RM, et al. A large single-center experience with treatment of patients with crotalid envenomations: outcomes with and evolution of antivenin therapy. *Am J Surg.* 2006;192:848.

9. Tintinalli JE, Stapczynski JS, Ma OJ, et al. *Tintinalli's emergency medicine: A coprehensive study guide.* 7th ed. McGraw-Hill; 2011:1356.

10. Ahmed SM, Ahmed M, Mahajan J, et al. Emergency treatment of a snake bite: Pearls from literature. *J Emerg Trauma Shock.* 2008;1(2):97–105 Jul-Dec.

11. Tintinalli JE, Stapczynski JS, Ma OJ, et al. *Tintinalli's emergency medicine: A coprehensive study guide.* 7th ed. McGraw-Hill; 2011:1360.

12. Clark RF, Wethern-Kestner S, Vance MV, et al. Clinical presentation and treatment of black widow spider envenomation: a review of 163 cases. *Ann Emerg Med.* 1992;21:782.

13. Tintinalli JE, Stapczynski JS, Ma OJ, et al. *Tintinalli's emergency medicine: A coprehensive study guide.* 7th ed. McGraw-Hill; 2011:357.

14. Tintinalli JE, Stapczynski JS, Ma OJ, et al. *Tintinalli's emergency medicine: A coprehensive study guide.* 7th ed. McGraw-Hill; 2011:1053.

15. Isbister GK, Bawaskar HS. Scorpion envenomation. *N Engl J Med.* 2014;371:457–463.

16. Andreosso A, Smout MJ, Seymour JE. Dose and time dependence of box jellyfish antivenom. *J Venom Anim Toxins Incl Trop Dis.* 2014;20:34.

17. Currie BJ. Marine antivenoms. *J Toxicol Clin Toxicol.* 2003;41(3):301–308. doi:10.1081/clt-120021115.

CHAPTER 8

Global Toxicology

Joseph K. Maddry ■ Chetan U. Kharod

General Principles

Within developed countries, regulatory and engineering controls have largely limited the population's exposure to many fatal pesticides and industrial toxins; however, worldwide, poisoning accounts for substantial morbidity and mortality. Global medicine presents the challenge of providing care to unique poisonings with limited resources. Fortunately, most poisonings are successfully managed using basic principles.

Activated charcoal: For exposures occurring because of the ingestion of a poison, gastrointestinal decontamination may provide benefit. Activated charcoal adsorbs some poisons; however, this therapy is not without risk. Given the high frequency of vomiting with toxic ingestions there is the potential for aspiration of activated charcoal resulting in significant pulmonary damage and death. Therefore, activated charcoal should not be given to patients who are sedated or have the potential to become sedated, unless their airway is protected via endotracheal intubation. Activated charcoal should also not be given for ingestions for which no significant toxicity is anticipated. Although some clinicians report that activated charcoal provides no benefit if given over an hour after the overdose, there is evidence clearly demonstrating that overdose may result in delayed gastric emptying and increase the duration from ingestion that activated charcoal is potentially beneficial. Activated charcoal is not expected to provide significant adsorption of most caustics, hydrocarbons, metals, or alcohols.

Syrup of ipecac: Syrup of ipecac has not demonstrated benefit, can cause significant harm, and is not recommended in the treatment of overdose.

The majority of toxicology deaths can be prevented through standard supportive care. This includes airway management, ventilator support, intravenous (IV) fluids and vasopressors for hypotension, and benzodiazepines for seizures and agitation. Of note, benzodiazepines are the preferred medication for poison-induced seizures and are preferred over phenytoin and other anticonvulsants.

Pesticides

Eliminating exposure is the most effective means of decreasing poisoning morbidity and mortality. When possible, clinicians should advocate for eliminating access to these toxins while maintaining balance with the potential benefits pesticides may provide (e.g., controlling disease vectors, decreasing malnutrition by increasing crop production).

Insecticides

ORGANIC PHOSPHORUS COMPOUNDS AND CARBAMATES

Worldwide, anticholinesterase insecticides are one of the leading causes of acute poisoning deaths. Organic phosphorous compounds (OPs) inhibit the enzyme acetylcholinesterase, resulting in excessive stimulation of the postsynaptic cholinergic and nicotinic receptors.

The excessive stimulation of cholinergic receptors results in a toxidrome of symptoms that can be memorized using the acronym SLUDGE and the killer "B"s:

Salivation
Lacrimation
Urination
Defecation
Increased Gastric motility
Emesis
Bradycardia
Bronchospasm
Bronchorrhea
Seizure

Symptoms resulting from the excessive stimulation of nicotinic receptors include muscle fasciculation, weakness, and paralysis.

Death results from excessive bronchorrhea and decreased respiratory muscle strength, resulting in respiratory failure.

Treatment consists of the administration of intramuscular (IM) or IV atropine. Atropine blocks the postsynaptic acetylcholine receptors thereby decreasing the SLUDGE and the symptoms of the killer "B"s, but has no effect upon the nicotinic receptors. Doses for inhalational exposure typically range from 1 to 6 mg IV/IM in adults. For ingestions or organophosphates, patients may require significantly higher doses.

Pralidoxime and other oximes are used to chemically remove the OP from acetylcholinesterase. Of note, some organophosphates (particularly chemical warfare agents) undergo "aging," which is the development of a permanent covalent bond between the organophosphate and acetylcholine. Therefore, for pralidoxime to have an effect, it must be administered before aging. Although pralidoxime use is widely accepted for exposure to chemical warfare organophosphates, studies have demonstrated conflicting evidence regarding its use for pesticide exposures. There is therefore no consensus on whether pralidoxime should be used for organophosphate ingestion.

For respiratory depression resulting from excessive stimulation of the nicotinic muscle receptors, endotracheal intubation and mechanical ventilation is the treatment of choice.

Intermediate syndrome: Approximately 2 to 4 days following exposure, patients may develop proximal motor weakness. Early recognition is necessary to avoid the potentially fatal rapid onset of respiratory muscle weakness. These symptoms last for 1 to 3 weeks and do not respond to atropine or oximes. Treatment consists of mechanical ventilation support.

TABLE 8.1 ■ Other Insecticides

Agent	Mechanism of Action	Clinical Manifestations	Management
Organic chlorine pesticides	Hyperexcitability of the central nervous system via multiple mechanisms.	Nausea, vomiting, headache, parasthesias, tremor, seizures, hyperthermia, respiratory failure, death.	Airway management, skin decontamination with soap and water, benzodiazepines for seizures.
Pyrethrins and pyrethroids	Bind to voltage-sensitive sodium channels in the open state, causing prolonged depolarization.	Paresthesias, vomiting, fasciculations, altered mental status, seizures, acute lung injury.	Skin decontamination with soap and water, consider activated charcoal for ingestions, benzodiazepines for tremor and seizures.
N,N-deithyl-3-methylbenzamide (DEET)	Unknown.	Although rare, severe exposure may result in encephalopathy, ataxia, convulsions, respiratory failure, hypotension, and death.	Skin decontamination with soap and water, consider activated charcoal for ingestions, benzodiazepines for tremor and seizures.

Organophosphate-induced delayed neuropathy (OPIDN): Some cholinesterase inhibitors may cause a delayed peripheral neuropathy causing a frequently permanent dysfunction of the long nerves of the legs.

Carbamate pesticides produce toxicity via the same mechanism as organophosphates; however, carbamates are less toxic because of decreased penetration into the central nervous system and a shorter duration of effect (<24 hours). Carbamates do not undergo aging and pralidoxime should not be used for carbamate poisonings.

Additional insecticides are shown in Table 8.1.

Herbicides

PARAQUAT AND DIQUAT

Paraquat and diquat are dipyridiyl herbicides, used worldwide given their efficacy and low cost. They are extremely potent toxins that may result in multisystem organ damage when absorbed through the skin, inhaled, or ingested. Ingestion of 10 to 20 mL of 20% paraquat solution may result in death.

Dipyridyls produce reactive free radicals via nicotinamide adenosine dinucleotide phosphate (NAPDH)-dependent reduction and oxidation cycling, resulting in lipid peroxidation inducing cell death. Paraquat is concentrated in the pulmonary alveolar cells, resulting in significant and frequently fatal pulmonary damage. Diquat is not taken up into pulmonary alveolar cells and does not cause pulmonary toxicity. Both paraquat and diquat cause renal, hepatic, and cardiovascular failure.

Symptoms of dipyridyl ingestion include oral pain/swelling, nausea, vomiting, and abdominal pain. Ingestion of 20 to 40 mg/kg of paraquat leads to death days to weeks after the ingestion via progressive pulmonary fibrosis. Larger ingestions of 20 to 40 mg/kg of paraquat lead to gastrointestinal injury, myonecrosis, shock, and death within hours to days. Diquat ingestion results in similar symptoms without the pulmonary fibrosis.

TABLE 8.2 ■ Other Herbicides

Agent	Mechanism of Action	Clinical Manifestations	Management
Glyphosate	Toxicity is frequently attributed to the surfactant the glyphosate is dissolved in.	Gastrointestinal symptoms, respiratory distress, hypotension, altered mental status, and oliguria.	Symptomatic and supportive care, skin decontamination with soap and water.
2,4-D and chlorophenoxy herbicides	Cell membrane damage, uncoupling of oxidative phosphorylation, and disruption of acetyl coenzyme A.	Vomiting, abdominal pain, diarrhea, tachycardia, muscle weakness, rhabdomyolysis, hepatitis, renal failure, metabolic acidosis, seizure, coma.	Skin decontamination with soap and water, consider activated charcoal for ingestions, benzodiazepines for tremor and seizures. Monitor the patient for at least 6–12 h after ingestion owing to the potential for delayed symptom onset.
Glufosinate and bialaphos	Inhibits glutamate decarboxylase resulting in decreased gamma-aminobutyric acid (GABA).	Initially nausea and vomiting with delayed central nervous system (CNS) symptoms 4–8 h after ingestion. CNS symptoms include sedation, confusion, respiratory depression, seizure, and coma.	Symptomatic and supportive care, consider activated charcoal for ingestions, endotracheal intubation for sedation and respiratory depression, benzodiazepines for tremor and seizures. Monitor the patient for at least 12 h after ingestion.
Nitrophenolic herbicides (dinitrophenol and substituted nitrophenolic compounds)	Uncoupling of oxidative phosphorylation.	Malaise, rash, headache, dyspnea, diaphoresis, hyperthermia, death, delayed onset cataracts.	No specific antidote, paralysis using a nondepolarizing neuromuscular blocker may decrease hyperthermia, sedation with benzodiazepines or barbiturates.

Treatment: Symptomatic and supportive care should be employed. Given the potential for supplemental oxygen to increase redox cycling in pulmonary alveolar cells, it should only be used for clinically significant hypoxia. There is no specific antidote for dipyridyl exposure. Skin should be washed thoroughly with soap and water. Activated charcoal (100 g in adults; 1.5 g/kg in children) should be administered as soon as possible followed by a second dose 1 to 2 hours later. If activated charcoal is unavailable, fuller's earth (a superabsorbent form of aluminum silicate) can be used as an alternative. Although multiple other therapies have been used, none have proven effective.

Additional herbicides are shown in Table 8.2.

OTHER PESTICIDES

See Table 8.3 for descriptions of other pesticides.

TABLE 8.3 ■ Other Pesticides

Agent	Mechanism of Action	Clinical Manifestations	Management
Barium	Competitive blocking of cellular potassium channels leading to intracellular potassium sequestration and severe hypokalemia.	Vomiting, abdominal pain, diarrhea, tachycardia, muscle weakness resulting in respiratory depression, lactic acidosis, seizure, ventricular dysrhythmias, death.	Symptomatic and supportive care. Endotracheal intubation for sedation and respiratory depression. Administer potassium chloride for hypokalemia (large doses may be required). Magnesium sulfate or sodium sulfate (adults, 30 g; pediatrics, 250 mg/kg) orally to precipitate ingested barium. Monitor the patient for cardiac dysrhythmias for at least 6–8 h.
Sodium monofluoroacetate and fluoroacetamide	Metabolized to fluorocitrate which blocks the Krebs cycle resulting in systemic cellular poisoning.	Vomiting, diarrhea, tachycardia, renal failure, hypocalcemia, lactic acidosis, confusion, seizure, coma, respiratory arrest, ventricular dysrhythmias, death.	Symptomatic and supportive care. Given the time necessary for the body to convert the pesticide into fluorocitrate, patients should be monitored for 36–48 h. Ethanol may theoretically provide benefit by increasing blood acetate levels which decreases the conversion to fluorocitrate (recommend two standard alcoholic drinks per hour or IV ethanol infusion with a blood alcohol concentration target of 100 g/dL).
Yellow phosphorus	Highly corrosive and a general cellular poison. Causes cardiovascular collapse following ingestion. Spontaneously combusts in air at room temperature to a highly irritating fume.	Inhalation: Mucous membrane irritation, cough, wheezing, chemical pneumonitis, pulmonary edema. Ingestion: Gastrointestinal burns and hemorrhage, vomiting, abdominal pain, diarrhea, "smoking stools," headache, delirium, shock, seizures, coma, arrhythmias, metabolic derangements, hepatic failure, renal failure, death.	Symptomatic and supportive care. Whole bowel irrigation for ingestions. DO NOT INDUCE VOMITING. Aggressive IV fluid replacement. Rescuers must wear appropriate protective gear and the patient's stool should be placed in a sealed container to avoid exposure to toxic fumes. Contaminated skin should be irrigated with soap and water and covered with moist dressing to prevent spontaneous combustion of yellow phosphorus.
Strychnine	Competitively antagonizes the inhibitory neurotransmitter glycine in the spinal cord.	Muscular stiffness and painful cramps; generalized muscle contractions leading to rhabdomyolysis, renal failure, and respiratory arrest. Muscle contractions exacerbated by noise, touch, and other sensations.	Benzodiazepines and analgesics for mild muscle contractions. Paralysis with a nondepolarizing neuromuscular blocker and mechanical ventilation for more severe symptoms.

Heavy Metals

LEAD

Lead exposure can occur through drinking water, lead piping, lead-based paint ingestion, mining, folk remedies, contaminated foods, children's products, lead-glazed ceramics, firearm ranges, and huffing of leaded gasoline. A recent outbreak of lead poisoning occurred in Nigeria resulting in severe toxicity and multiple deaths. Many of the exposures were pediatric and from families mining the local soil for gold.

Mechanism of Action

Lead binds to sulfhydryl, phosphate, and carboxy ligands, thereby inactivating or altering multiple enzymes. The enzyme alteration results in the impairment of cellular and mitochondrial membranes, neurotransmitter synthesis/function, heme synthesis, cellular redox, and nucleotide metabolism.

Clinical Presentation

Large acute ingestion: abdominal pain, anemia (hemolytic), toxic hepatitis, and encephalopathy.

Subacute/chronic exposure:

1. Constitutional: Fatigue, malaise, irritability, anorexia, weight loss, arthralgias, myalgias.
2. Gastrointestinal: Abdominal pain (lead colic), nausea, constipation.
3. Central nervous system: Depending upon the severity of exposure, symptoms range from mild (impaired concentration, headache, tremor, decreased coordination) to severe (encephalopathy with agitated delirium, lethargy, convulsions, death). Chronic low-level exposures in children lead to decreased intelligence and impaired neurobehavioral development.
4. Cardiovascular effects: Hypertension.
5. Peripheral motor neuropathy: Severe extensor muscle weakness, particularly in the upper extremities (wrist drop).
6. Hematologic: Normochromic or microcytic anemia, possibly with basophilic stippling.
7. Nephrotoxic: Acute tubular dysfunction and chronic interstitial fibrosis. Hyperuricemia and gout.
   Repeated, intentional leaded gasoline inhalation (huffing): Ataxia, myoclonic jerking, hyperreflexia, delirium, and convulsions.

Diagnosis

Given the nature of global medicine, the diagnosis of lead poisoning may need to be made based upon clinical symptoms and a source of exposure. When available, whole-blood lead level is the most accurate indication of lead exposure. Of note, the blood samples must be obtained and stored in lead-free syringes/tubes/stoppers, to avoid falsely elevated values. Although not providing a specific level, opaque transverse metaphyseal bands at the growth plates on a pediatric x-ray ("lead lines") may indicate lead exposure.

Treatment

Minimizing future lead exposure is the most prudent means to ensure the health of the patient and population at risk. This can be challenging in some environments as lead may be an inherent risk associated with the population's primary financial income. Global health providers should attempt to develop a trusting relationship with the population's leaders and mothers while advising them of the risks of lead and how to minimize exposure. Minimizing exposure is especially important in children who are particularly susceptible to lead's deleterious effects.

Beyond standard symptomatic and supportive care, chelation therapy is indicated in specific circumstances. It should be noted that although chelation therapy has been associated with improvement of symptoms and decreased mortality, controlled trials are lacking and treatment guidelines are based upon empiric data. Depending on the severity of toxicity, potential chelation therapies include dimercaprol (British anti-lewisite, BAL), edetate calcium disodium (calcium EDTA), and succimer (meso 2,3-dimercaptosuccinic acid [DMSA]). Owing to the complexity of dosing regimens and significant adverse effects related to chelation, we recommend consulting a toxicologist when considering this therapy. Within the United States, a toxicologist can be reached by calling a Poison Control Center (1-800-222-1222).

ARSENIC

Arsenic is found in the soil (potentially resulting in groundwater contamination), folk remedies, and various industrial and commercial products.

Mechanism of Action

Arsenic exerts its effects via induction of oxidative stress, inactivation or alteration of enzymes, alteration of gene expression, and other mechanisms resulting in impairment of numerous organ systems.

Clinical Presentation

Acute Exposure

Acute exposure typically occurs via ingestion. This ingestion may be accidental, intentional (suicide), or deliberate poisoning (homicide). A massive ingestion results in a constellation of symptoms over the next hours to weeks. Symptoms include:
1. Gastrointestinal: Nausea, vomiting, diarrhea, abdominal pain, and hemorrhagic gastroenteritis.
2. Central nervous system: Lethargy, agitation, delirium, and seizures may occur in severe exposures.
3. Cardiovascular effects: Third spacing of fluids, tachycardia, shock, QT interval prolongation, torsade de pointes, and death.
4. Peripheral motor neuropathy: Sensorimotor axonal peripheral neuropathy potentially progressing to paralysis may occur 1 to 5 weeks following exposure.
5. Hematologic: Pancytopenia 1 to 2 weeks after ingestion. Basophilic stippling may occur.
6. Dermatologic: Desquamation (particularly of palms and soles), diffuse maculopapular rash, and herpetic lesions 1 to 6 weeks following the acute ingestion. Transverse white striae may appear on the nails months after the exposure.

Chronic Exposure
1. Fatigue, malaise, gastroenteritis, leukopenia, anemia, sensory peripheral neuropathy, liver enzyme elevation, portal hypertension, and peripheral vascular insufficiency may occur. Epidemiologic studies demonstrate an association between chronic arsenic exposures and increased risk of hypertension, cardiovascular disease, and diabetes mellitus. Weight loss, arthralgias, and myalgias have been reported.
2. Dermatologic: After years of exposure to arsenic, patients may develop spotted pigmentation of the torso and extremities and hyperkeratotic changes on the palms and soles. Arsenic also leads to increased risk of squamous cell carcinoma, Bowen's disease, and basal cell carcinoma.
3. Non-cutaneous cancer: Chronic inhalation increases the risk of lung cancer. Chronic ingestion can cause lung and bladder cancer.

Diagnosis

Arsenic poisoning may need to be diagnosed based upon clinical symptoms and a source of exposure. Laboratory testing should not delay treatment when a large, life-threating poisoning is suspected. When available, a 24-hour urinary arsenic level is the most accurate indication of exposure. Because seafood frequently contains nontoxic organoarsenicals that will result in a nonclinically significant elevation of the urine arsenic levels, arsenic speciation should be performed by the laboratory. If arsenic speciation is not available, the urine should be collected after a 1-week abstinence from seafood

Treatment

Because of the high mortality associated with acute arsenic poisoning, aggressive therapy is required. This includes maintaining potassium, magnesium, and calcium levels to minimize QT prolongation. Hypoglycemia and dehydration should be treated as necessary. Because metals do not bind well to activated charcoal, whole bowel irrigation should be administered if any radiopaque material is seen on x-ray of the abdomen. Chelation should be initiated as soon as possible and before laboratory confirmation to decrease morbidity and mortality. Potential chelation therapies include unithiol (2,-dimercaptopropanesulfonic acid [DMPS]), dimercaprol (BAL), and succimer (DMSA). BAL is administered parenterally, therefore it is used initially until the patient is able to tolerate per os (PO) and their gastrointestinal tract is cleared of arsenic, at which point the patient can be transitioned to succimer. Owing to the complexity of dosing regimens and significant adverse effects related to chelation, we recommend consulting a toxicologist when considering this therapy. Within the United States, a toxicologist can be reached by calling a Poison Control Center (1-800-222-1222).

For chronic exposures, minimizing further exposure is the most prudent means to ensure the health of the patient and the population at risk. This may require relocating wells to avoid exposure through drinking water. Depending on the severity of toxicity, potential chelation therapies include unithiol (DMPS), dimercaprol (BAL), and succimer (DMSA).

Antimalarials

QUININE

Quinine is an older antimalarial occasionally still used in regions with chloroquine-resistant malaria. The minimum toxic dose in human adults is 3 to 4 grams.

Mechanism of Action

Quinine is a type Ia antiarrhythmic resulting in sodium channel blockade, decreased myocardial contractility, decreased cardiac conduction, and prolonged cardiac repolarization. Quinine also causes direct toxicity to the retina.

Clinical Presentation

Mild toxicity includes nausea, vomiting, tinnitus, hearing loss, vertigo, headache, and alterations in vision. Severe toxicity causes ataxia, confusion, obtundation, convulsions, coma, respiratory arrest, QRS widening, QT prolongation, and fatal dysrhythmias.

Quinine's retinal toxicity can cause blurred vision, decreased color perception, visual field constriction, and blindness. Visual effects may improve with time; however, permanent impairment frequently occurs.

Treatment

Provide symptomatic and supportive care. Administer activated charcoal if appropriate. Monitor for significant electrocardiogram (EKG) changes for 6 hours. Treat QRS widening greater than 100 ms with IV sodium bicarbonate (1–2 mEq/kg by rapid IV bolus, repeat as necessary as long as serum

TABLE 8.4 ■ Other Antimalarials

Agent	Mechanism of Action	Clinical Manifestations	Management
Primaquine	Causes oxidative stress potentially resulting in methemoglobinemia and hemolysis in normal individuals.	Symptoms of hypoxia: Dyspnea, chest pain, ischemic electrocardiogram (EKG) changes, chocolate-colored blood (methemoglobinemia), pulse oximetry of approximately 85% secondary to colorimetric interpretation of methemoglobinemia, hemolysis on blood samples.	Symptomatic and supportive care. Activated charcoal for oral overdoses. Methylene blue for methemoglobinemia. Exchange transfusion for massive hemolysis.
Halofantrine	Cardiac potassium channel impairment.	QTc prolongation, Torsade de pointes, ventricular fibrillation, hypotension, syncope.	Activated charcoal. Magnesium and atropine/isoproterenol/overdrive pacing for QTc prolongation and torsade de pointes.
Dapsone	Causes oxidative stress potentially resulting in methemoglobinemia and sulfhemaglobinemia in normal individuals. Acute or delayed hemolysis.	Symptoms of hypoxia: Dyspnea, chest pain, ischemic EKG changes, chocolate-colored blood (methemoglobinemia), pulse oximetry near 85% secondary to colorimetric interpretation of methemoglobinemia, hemolysis on blood samples.	Symptomatic and supportive care. Activated charcoal for oral overdoses. Methylene blue for methemoglobinemia. Exchange transfusion for massive hemolysis.

pH remains below 7.55). Avoid class Ia and Ic antiarrhythmics. Although older literature recommended stellate ganglion block for blindness, this practice is not effective and is potentially harmful.

CHLOROQUINE, HYDROXYCHLOROQUINE, AND AMODIAQUINE

Although chloroquine, hydroxychloroquine, and amodiaquine have cardiac toxicity similar to quinine, they are less potent and do not possess the retinal toxicity. Clinical presentation and treatment are also similar (see quinine). A specific protocol using early intubation, diazepam 2 mg/kg over 30 minutes and then 1 to 2 mg/kg per day for 2 to 4 days combined with epinephrine (0.2 micrograms/kg per minute with 5% dextrose in water), titrated to maintain a systolic blood pressure over 100 mmHg, improved survival. Serum potassium should be monitored and replaced as necessary.

See Table 8.4 for additional antimalarials.

Antituberculous Medications

ISONIAZID

Isoniazid (INH) is commonly used in the treatment of tuberculosis, a disease which results in an enormous global health burden.

TABLE 8.5 ■ **Other Antituberculosis Medications**

Agent	Mechanism of Action	Clinical Manifestations	Management
Rifamycins	Inhibition of RNA synthesis and disruption of protein synthesis leading to cell death.	Nausea, vomiting, diarrhea, abdominal pain, flushing, facial edema, obtundation, muscle weakness, death.	Symptomatic and supportive care. Activated charcoal.
Ethambutol	Unknown.	Nausea, abdominal pain, confusion, visual hallucinations, optic neuropathy, death.	Symptomatic and supportive care Activated charcoal.

Mechanism of Action

INH interferes with the synthesis of the primary inhibitory neurotransmitter gamma-aminobutyric acid (GABA) via multiple mechanisms.

Clinical Presentation

Acute Toxicity. The classic presentation of acute INH overdose consists of seizures refractory to conventional therapy, severe metabolic acidosis, and coma. Seizures may occur with doses greater than 20 mg/kg. Vomiting, slurred speech, dizziness, and tachycardia may occur before seizure onset. The coma is frequently protracted, lasting 24 to 36 hours. Additional findings include hypotension, renal failure, and hyperglycemia.

Chronic Toxicity. Chronic therapeutic INH use may cause hepatocellular necrosis, peripheral neuropathy, and optic neuritis. The neuropathy is primarily sensory, in a stocking-glove distribution.

Treatment

Acute Toxicity. The antidote for INH-induced seizures is pyridoxine in conjunction with benzodiazepines. The dose of pyridoxine is 1 g IV per gram of INH ingestion. An initial empiric dose of pyridoxine of 70 mg/kg IV (max dose of 5 g) is recommended in ingestions of unknown quantity. A sodium bicarbonate drip may be used for a pH under 7.0. Asymptomatic patients should be observed for 6 hours.

Chronic Toxicity. Hepatitis resulting in an aminotransferase elevation greater than two to three times the baseline necessitates the termination of INH therapy. Peripheral neuropathy can be prevented or treated with oral pyridoxine at a dose of 50 mg/d in adults.

See Table 8.5 for additional antituberculosis medications.

Marine Food Poisoning

Symptoms attributed to seafood ingestion may be biological organisms such as *Vibrio parahaemolyticus* (esp. crustaceans, shrimp), *V. cholerae* (esp. crabs, mollusks), *Salmonella typhi* (mollusks), *Campylobacter jejuni* (clams), hepatitis A virus (mollusks, esp. clams and oysters), and Norwalk agent (oysters, other mollusks). Alternatively, contamination with chemicals such as mercury may cause adverse health effects. Specific poisons may be found in various sea life. Dinoflagellates are single-celled aquatic organisms, some of which can produce toxins. Ingestion of vertebrate fish and shellfish contaminated with toxin-producing dinoflagellates can result in poisoning.

CIGUATERA POISONING

Ciguatera poisoning occurs following the ingestion of vertebrate fish contaminated with ciguatoxin from dinoflagellates. Ciguatera poisoning is one of the most common fishborne poisonings and commonly occurs with the ingestion of large saltwater fish, typically in more tropical locations (e.g., barracuda, sea bass, parrot fish, red snapper, grouper, amberjack, kingfish, and sturgeon). Ciguatoxin is heat stable and tasteless. Certain toxins have specific tests (i.e., enzyme-linked immunosorbent assay [ELISA] assays are available to test fish flesh for ciguatera toxin), but provide little clinical value in the management of the poisoned patient.

Mechanism of Action

Ciguatoxin binds to voltage-sensitive sodium channels increasing sodium channel permeability and ultimately opening sodium channels.

Clinical Presentation

The majority of patients experience symptoms 2 to 6 hours after ingestion but these can be delayed for as long as 24 hours. Symptoms include diaphoresis, nausea, vomiting, profuse diarrhea, and neurologic symptoms. Classic neurologic symptoms include the sensation of loose, painful teeth; tingling and numbness of the lips, tongue, and throat; a metallic taste; reversal of temperature discriminations (hot things feel cold and cold things feel hot); ataxia; and weakness. Myalgias and arthralgias are also common. Death is rare, but when reported is due to seizures or paralysis.

Treatment

Treatment is supportive, to include IV fluid and vasopressors if necessary. Although mannitol has been reported to improve neurologic symptoms, a randomized controlled trial showed no benefit compared with IV saline.

SCOMBROID POISONING

Scombroid poisoning occurs following the ingestion of fish contaminated with histidine. Histidine is produced when bacteria that possess the enzyme histidine decarboxylase act on warm, freshly killed fish, converting histidine to histamine. Histamine is a heat-stable toxin but refrigerating or freezing the fish shortly after being caught will prevent its production. The fish most reported to result in scombroid poisoning include mahi mahi, amber jack, tuna, albacore, bonito, and mackerel.

Mechanism of Action

Histamine binds to histamine receptors, mimicking an allergic reaction.

Clinical Presentation

Patients sometimes report noticing a peppery taste when eating the fish. This is followed by numbness, tingling, or a burning sensation in the mouth minutes to hours later. A diffuse erythema of the face, neck, and torso may occur. Rarely, more severe allergy symptoms occur to include pruritus, urticarial, angioedema, and bronchospasm.

Treatment

Treatment is similar to that of allergic reaction. Antihistamines (diphenhydramine) and H_2-receptor antagonists (cimetidine or ranitidine) alleviate symptoms. Inhaled beta 2-adrenergic agonists and epinephrine can be used for bronchospasm.

TETRODON POISONING

Tetrodotoxin is found in various puffer-like fish (including the Japanese delicacy *fugu*), gastropod mollusks, horseshoe crab eggs, newts, and salamanders. Poisoning occurs following the ingestion of the fish. The blue-ringed octopus administers tetrodotoxin via its bite, resulting in the death of unsuspecting humans interacting with the attractive octopus.

Mechanism of Action

Tetrodotoxin inhibits sodium channels, resulting in neurotoxicity.

Clinical Presentation

Symptoms occur within minutes and include headache, diaphoresis, paresthesias, dysphagia, dysarthria, vomiting, and abdominal pain. Symptoms may progress to weakness, loss of coordination, fasciculations, and ascending paralysis, occurring in 4 to 24 hours. In severe cases, hypotension may occur. Death is caused by respiratory paralysis and can occur in up to 50% of cases.

Treatment

Treatment is supportive, including the administration of activated charcoal to prevent absorption, airway protection via endotracheal intubation if necessary, and mechanical ventilation.

SHELLFISH POISONING

Ingestion of oysters, clams, mussels, and scallops contaminated with dinoflagellates can result in toxicity. Syndromes include neurotoxic, paralytic, and amnestic shellfish poisoning (Table 8.6).

TABLE 8.6 ■ Shellfish Poisoning

Syndrome	Toxin/Mechanism of Action	Clinical Manifestations	Management
Neurotoxic shellfish poisoning	Brevetoxin/increased sodium channel permeability.	Bronchospasm, temperature reversal sensation, nausea, vomiting, diarrhea, paresthesias.	Symptomatic and supportive care.
Paralytic shellfish poisoning	Saxitoxin/decreased sodium channel permeability.	Nausea, vomiting, diarrhea, paresthesias, respiratory depression.	Symptomatic and supportive care. Respiratory support.
Amnestic shellfish poisoning	Domoic acid/ glutamate analog.	Nausea, vomiting, diarrhea, paresthesias, respiratory depression, amnesia.	Symptomatic and supportive care. Respiratory support.

CHAPTER 9

Environmental Diseases and Injuries

Lina Maria Sanchez Rubio ■ Rocio del Pilar Garzón Ayala ■ Alexandra Mejía Delgado ■ María Alejandra Corzo Zamora ■ Diego Leonel Malpica Hincapie

Environmental Diseases

In the following pages the most common environmental diseases will be presented. They will be divided according to the causative factor.

BASIC PHYSICS DEFINITIONS

Definitions below will be mentioned during the whole chapter; for that reason, it is important to emphasize how to understand the basics of some environmental diseases, especially those related to high altitude, flight, and diving.[1,2]

1. Dalton's Law: This law states that the total pressure of a mixture of gas is equal to the sum of the partial pressure of each gas in the mixture. It explains hypoxia.

$$\text{Total pressure} = P_1 + P_2 + P_3 + \cdots + P_n$$

2. Boyle's Law: This states that at constant temperature, the volume of a gas is inversely proportional to the pressure to which it is subjected. It explains the trapped gases phenomenon.

$$\left(P_1 / P_2\right) = \left(V_2 / V_1\right)$$

3. Henry's Law: This law states that the amount of gas dissolved in solution varies directly with the pressure of that gas over the solution. It explains the nitrogen movement in decompression sickness (DCS).

$$\left(P_1 / P_2\right) = \left(A_1 / A_2\right)$$

4. Graham's Law: Known as the law of gaseous diffusion, this law states that "A gas will diffuse from an area of high concentration to an area of low concentration."

TABLE 9.1 ■ **Classification of Altitudes**

Altitude	Range in Meters Over Sea Level	Range in Feet Over Sea Level
Sea level	0–1000	0–3280
Low altitude	1000–2000	3280–6561
Intermediate altitude	2000–3000	6561–9842
High altitude	3000–5000	9842–16,404
Extreme high altitude	5000–8848	16,404–29,028

Data from Gore CJ, Clark SA, Saunders PU. Nonhematological mechanisms of improved sea-level performance after hypoxic exposure. *Med Sci Sports Exerc.* 2007;39(9):1600–1609.

HIGH-ALTITUDE MEDICINE

In high-altitude medicine, it is necessary to know how altitude is divided to explain the different expected physiologic findings in each range. Although in the literature it is possible to find different classifications, for the purposes of this subject, the classification proposed by Gore et al.[3] will be used (see Table 9.1).

Exposure to high altitude can cause the exposed subject to experience a wide range of signs and symptoms that may be determined by the altitude, the subject's fitness, previous medical conditions, and previous acclimatization. Related conditions at different ranges of altitude are known as high-altitude illnesses.

1. Acute mountain sickness (AMS)
   a. Definition: condition that affects individuals who ascend rapidly to high altitude.
   b. Signs and symptoms:
      i. Symptoms may be present between 6 and 24 hours after ascending.
      ii. Symptoms: headache, anorexia, nausea, vomiting, fatigue, lightheadedness, sleep disturbance.
      iii. Signs: During the physical examination, it is possible not to find signs, and the diagnosis is based on clinical history. However, it is possible to find peripheral edema, crackles in the chest, and early speech impairment.[4,5]
   c. Treatment: most cases of AMS get better within 24 to 48 hours without treatment. However, some may progress to acute pulmonary edema or cerebral edema, and treatment depends on symptoms and clinical features (Table 9.2).[4]
2. High altitude cerebral edema (HACE)
   a. Definition: severe presentation of AMS that affects neurologic function. It may affect unacclimatized individuals that ascend over 3000 m.
   b. Signs and symptoms[6]
      i. Symptoms: Usually, symptoms of HACE are preceded by AMS symptoms, and they are present within 24 to 36 hours. Symptoms include headache, nausea, vomiting, photophobia, loss of appetite, irritability, bizarre and irrational behavior, and blurred vision.
      ii. Signs: ataxia, irrationality, hallucinations, clouding consciousness, brisk deep-tendon reflexes, diplopia, tachycardia, and cyanosis.
   c. Treatment: descend to lower altitudes as soon as possible; supply oxygen; dexamethasone 8 mg initial doses followed by 4 mg every 6 hours.[7]
3. High-altitude pulmonary edema (HAPE)
   a. Definition: severe presentation of AMS that affects respiratory function. It can affect unacclimatized individuals that ascend over 2000 to 7000 m.[8]

TABLE 9.2 ■ Treatment in Acute Mountain Illness

Procedure	Dose	Reference
High-Altitude Headache		
Stop ascent/rest		[12]
Paracetamol	500–1000 mg	[13]
Ibuprofen	400–600 mg	[14]
Oxygen	2–4 L/m (night)	[15]
Cerebral Edema		
Immediate descend	300–500 m	
Acetazolamide	125–250 mg every 8–12 h	[16]
Dexamethasone	4 mg every 6 h orally	[17]
Portable hyperbaric chamber	193 mbar during 1 h	[18]
Acute Mountain Sickness (AMS)		
Mild AMS		
Stop ascent/rest	24 h	[12]
Paracetamol	1 g every 6 h	[15]
Ibuprofen	400 mg every 8 h	[14,15]
Acetazolamide	125–500 mg every 12 h	[15]
Moderate/Severe AMS		
Descend	300–500 m	[15]
Paracetamol	1 g every 6 h	[14,15]
Ibuprofen	400 mg	[14,15]
Dexamethasone	4 mg PO, IM, IV	[17,18]
Oxygen	1–2 L/m	[15,18]
Portable hyperbaric chamber	193 mbar during 1 h	[15,18]

IM, Intramuscularly; *IV*, intravenously.
Please verify drugs avaliability in your country or equivalents.

    b. Symptoms and signs: The subject usually presents with symptoms of AMS and may then present with symptoms of HAPE.[9,10]

        i. Symptoms: shortness of breath, lethargy, chest pain, dry cough, nocturnal dyspnea, hemoptysis, insomnia, dizziness.

        ii. Signs: tachycardia, tachypnea, crackles at lung bases, cyanosis, respiratory distress, orthopnea, bubbling respirations, coma.

    c. Treatment: descend as soon as possible; supply oxygen; dexamethasone initial doses 8 mg, and then 4 mg every 6 hours; nifedipine 20 mg slow release.

  4. Other medical conditions at high altitude

    a. Neurovascular disorders

      At high altitude, some neurologic signs unrelated to AMS, HAPE, or HACE have been reported, some of which are transient. This range of conditions has been associated with

---

BOX 9.1 ■ Neurovascular Disorders Not Included in Acute Mountain Sickness

Transient ischemic attacks and strokes
Cerebrovascular attack
Migraine
Cerebral venous thrombosis
Subarachnoid hemorrhage
Seizures, epileptic fits
High-altitude syncope
Transient global amnesia
Delirium at high altitude
Cranial nerves palsies
Ophthalmological problems
Possible coagulation problems

Basnyat B, Wu TY and Certsch JH. Neurological conditions at altitude that fall outside the definition of altitude illness. *High Alt Med Biol*. 2004;5:171–179.

a vascular origin (spasm, thrombosis, embolus, or hemorrhage); whereas others may be neurologic disorders or of unknown origin. Basnyat et al.[11] list neurovascular disorders that are not included in AMS (Box 9.1).

b. Dry eye syndrome: a common finding in climbers and trekkers. Its origin is a reduced production of tears with altitude where dry air, windy conditions, and glare are present.[12]

   i. Symptoms: irritation of eyes, light sensitivity, blurred vision, and burning sensation.

   ii. Prevention: use of goggles with protection Ultraviolet A (UVA)-Ultraviolet B (UVB); tear-substitute eye drops.

Heat Stress and Illness

Definition: temperature-related illnesses encompassing a broad spectrum of symptoms that can lead to death if not treated correctly. Heatstroke affects people trapped in hot conditions with little or no air circulation; it mostly affects those with medical conditions, those using pharmacological treatments, or those unaware of the physiologic effects of heat.[19]

High temperatures are thought to cause at least 70,000 deaths/year in Europe, with an average mortality of 40 people every year in the United Kingdom and 200 each year in the United States from heatstroke.[19,20]

Risk factors: A broad spectrum of factors increase the probability of heat illness[21–23]:

- Ambient temperature above 35°C and relative humidity over 60%
- Overweight and obesity
- Sleep deprivation
- Overexertion syndrome
- Medical conditions
- Fever
- History of cardiovascular disease
- Seizures
- Drug abuse
- Medication
- Beta-blockers
- Angiotensin converting enzyme (ACE) inhibitors
- Furosemide—hydrochlorothiazide
- Antihistamines
- Antispasmodics
- Alpha-agonists

- Stimulants
- Burns
- Muscular exertion
- Dehydration

1. Heat stroke

   a. Definition: condition produced when heat exchange mechanisms fail to dissipate heat, and abnormal mental status and neurologic function impairment begin to set in. This is a medical emergency, and treatment must be given immediately to prevent death, using different cooling measures.[19,24–27]

   b. Signs and symptoms[20,23]:

     i. Increase in core body temperature above 40.5°C

     ii. Altered mental status and loss of motor coordination

     iii. Increase in respiratory, pulse, and heart rate

     iv. Slowly decreasing sweating capacity

     v. Arterial pressure drop

   c. Treatment

     i. Cooling measures[27,28–30]

     ii. Secure airway, oxygen, and administer only intravenous (IV) fluids (2 L of normal saline solution, children 20 mL/kg with an initial bolus).

     iii. Use cold packs on neck, chest, axillae, abdomen, and inguinal region.

     iv. Use benzodiazepines if needed to sedate patient (midazolam 0.2 mg/kg intramuscular [IM]).

     v. Wet the patient with ambient-temperature water and ventilate for cooling.

     vi. Treat shivering with chlorpromazine or midazolam to prevent muscle heat production.

     vii. Core body temperature must be checked regularly, making sure cooling efforts are maintained until a body temperature of 38°C is reached.

     viii. Evacuate patient via air or land.

2. Heat exhaustion

   a. Definition: condition presented when core body temperature is below 38°C. Patient presents with nonspecific symptoms such as headache, weakness, malaise, nausea and/or vomiting.[31,32]

   b. Diagnosis

     i. Clinical diagnosis supported by nonspecific symptoms, and core body temperature is mildly elevated.

     ii. Rapid heart and respiration rate

     iii. Orthostatic hypotension

     iv. Sweating

     v. Normal mental status, and neurologic examination is normal

   c. Treatment

     i. Decrease heat gain, moving patient to the shade and well-ventilated area

     ii. Remove clothing to improve heat loss

     iii. Administer at least 1 to 3 L of oral fluids initially.

     iv. Place cool packs on the neck, chest wall, abdomen, and axillae and ventilate the patient, being careful not to leave ice packs in direct contact with skin for too long, to avoid frostbite.

     v. Evacuation or inpatient treatment often not necessary.

3. Heat edema

   a. Definition: condition produced by increases in hydrostatic pressure along with a hyperhemodynamic physiologic start of heat stress that produces peripheral edema in a hot environment in unacclimatized patients.[20,33–34]

    b. Diagnosis:
        i. Edema with or without fovea might be present, especially in lower extremities
        ii. Facial edema
    c. Treatment
        i. This is a self-limited condition and supportive physical measures may be given to provide comfort
        ii. Do not administer any diuretics.

4. Miliaria rubra
    a. Definition: skin reaction produced after being exposed to warm and humid climates. It produces epidermis desquamation that may last 7 days.[20,34]
    b. Diagnosis
        i. Eczema
        ii. Pruritus
        iii. Erythematous papules
        iv. Desquamation of the skin from 7 to 10 days
    c. Treatment
        i. Dry and cool the affected skin
        ii. Antihistamines (fexofenadine 180 mg/day)

5. Heat syncope
    a. Definition: loss of consciousness produced by lengthy sun exposure either standing or with physical activity[19,20,34]
    b. Diagnosis
        i. Syncope when risk factors are present (ambient temperature >35°C, humidity >60%)
    c. Treatment
        i. Patient must be treated following the initial CAB approach (Compressions-Airway-Breathing)
        ii. Assess traumatic lesions secondary to syncope
        iii. Make sure Trendelenburg position is adopted
        iv. Cool the patient
        v. Administer at least 1 to 2 L of hydration fluids
        vi. If the patient does not recover, must be deferred for treatment because of heatstroke potential or other causes of loss of consciousness

6. Heat cramps
    a. Definition: When exposed long enough to heat, dehydration sets in and electrolyte imbalance may lead to heat cramps. Those who are not acclimatized to heat or profuse sweaters may experience them.[20,31,34]
    b. Diagnosis
        i. Spasmodic muscle cramps
        ii. Pain
        iii. Recurrence may be triggered by manipulation of the muscle.
    c. Treatment
        i. Move patient to a cooler environment
        ii. Rehydration using balanced electrolyte solutions
        iii. Stretching the muscles involved

7. Dehydration and hyponatremia
    a. Definition: Hyponatremia is set when serum sodium is less than 130 mEq/L. It can be confused with water intoxication from drinking large amounts of hypoosmolar fluids. Also, it is easily confused with heat illness in which the core body temperature is increased; in hyponatremia, body temperature is usually normal.[20,34]

b. Diagnosis[20,32,34]
  i. Weakness
  ii. Painful muscle spasmodic cramps
  iii. Hyporexia
  iv. Nausea and vomiting
  v. Altered mental status
  vi. Core body temperature usually below 38°C
  vii. Seizures
  viii. Serum sodium level below 130 mEq/L (to confirm diagnosis)
c. Treatment and prevention
  i. If intolerant to drinking oral fluids, IV line must be placed with normal saline solution 500 to 1000 mL/h
  ii. If not vomiting, oral rehydration solutions can be given.
d. Prevention: Wet bulb globe temperature (WBGT) must be calculated considering humidity and ambient temperature. Normal thermometers are not predictors of heat illness because these are not capable of measuring humidity. An alternative to WBGT equipment in the field is to use a psychrometer.[20,35]
e. Acclimatization: takes different times in each individual, with a range of 10 to 14 days. The rate of physiologic change depends on body composition, ambient temperature, and preexisting medical conditions.[19,20,35]
  i. Benefits of acclimatization include lower heart rate, increase in blood flows, sweat production, increase in plasma proteins (preventing edema), reduced core temperature, fluid and sodium loss, and improved renal reabsorption of sodium and water by means of aldosterone adequate equilibrium.[19,20,35]
  ii. Sweat rate improves heat loss, and changes appear from day 1 to day 5, increasing from 0.5 to 3 L/h coupled with exercise improves acclimatization, but this implies fluid intake must be enough for this mechanism to be effective.[36,37]

Solar Radiation

ACUTE SUNBURN

1. Definition: Sunburn is an acute cutaneous inflammatory reaction that follows excessive exposure of the skin to ultraviolet radiation (UVR) from the sun. Long-term adverse health effects of repeated exposure to UVR are well described, and its classification comes from superficial or first-degree burns. The main injury responsible for sunburn is direct damage to DNA by UVR, resulting in inflammation and apoptosis of skin cells; this inflammation causes vasodilation of cutaneous blood vessels.[29]
2. Diagnosis: The acute inflammatory response is greatest 12 to 24 hours after exposure. The representative erythema usually occurs 3 to 4 hours after exposure, with peak levels at 24 hours, and resolves over 4 to 7 days, usually with skin scaling and peeling.
  a. Warmth
  b. Tenderness
  c. Edema
  d. Blistering (severe cases)
  e. Pain
3. Treatment: Most sunburns, while painful, are not life threatening, and treatment is primarily symptomatic. Nonsteroidal antiinflammatory drugs (NSAIDs) may relieve pain and inflammation, especially when given early. Cool soaks with water or aluminum acetate solution also provide temporary relief. Additionally, fluid replacement (oral or IV) for severe erythema or concomitant fluid loss.[38]

PHOTO PROTECTION

1. Sunscreens: Most healthcare providers and the American Academy of Dermatology recommend:
   a. Use a sunscreen with an SPF of 30 or greater on exposed skin.
   b. Use a sunscreen that protects against both UVA and UVB radiation.
   c. You may need a higher SPF if you are fair-skinned, if you will be in the sun for a long time, or if you anticipate intense sun exposure.[32,39]
2. Clothing
   In addition to sunscreen, clothing can be an excellent form of sun protection. The most important determinant is tightness of the weave. Consider covering exposed skin with a wide-brimmed hat, long-sleeved shirt, and long pants. A hat made of tightly woven material can provide shade for the face, ears, and back of the neck. Clothing made from tightly woven dark fabrics tends to provide greater protection than light-colored fabrics. Some manufacturers have sun-protective clothing with SPF.[40,41] Some countries, such as Australia, have standards dealing with solar UVR protection, namely the Sunscreen Standard (AS2604) and the Sunglass Standard (AS1067). With these standards, there is the ability to impose substantial penalties for noncompliance.[42]
3. Sunglasses
   Many studies indicate that long-term exposure to short-wavelength visible light, UV radiation, and lower wavelength visible light may be hazardous and cause increased risk of certain ocular pathologies such as cataracts and maculopathy, which are a concern for military and civilian aircrews. Pilots may be exposed to solar radiation for long periods of flight where UV radiation is known to be significantly greater than at sea level. Aircraft windshields should have a standard for optical transmission, particularly for short-wavelength radiation. Any sunglasses used must follow national quality standards.[43] However, a substantial number of commercially available sunglasses are being manufactured without apparent regard for these potential hazards.[44] Aircrew have to wear certificated sunglasses that ensure protection from UVA and UVB radiation.

Scuba Diving Disorders

Scuba diving implies that the body is exposed to a high-pressure environment. Associated disorders can be divided into two categories[45]: (1) conditions derived from gas expansion according to Boyle's Law and (2) liberation of a gas phase from tissues following Henry's Law.

EAR AND SINUS BAROTRAUMA

1. Definition: Described as the most common injury for divers (30%), it is defined as tissue injury as a consequence of a failure in equalizing pressure in gas-filled spaces (middle ear and paranasal sinuses). Ear barotrauma is present mainly during ascent when the Eustachian tube cannot equalize pressure, whereas sinus barotrauma is caused by a blockage of the sinus ostium.[46]
2. Diagnosis: main symptom is pain. Facial pain with epistaxis is common for sinus barotrauma, whereas ear pain is common for ear barotrauma; sometimes vertigo and conductive hearing loss are present.[47]
3. Clinical findings:
   a. Ear barotrauma: injection of the tympanic membrane, hemotympanum, and/or ruptured tympanic membrane
   b. Sinus barotrauma: mucosal edema, facial pain
4. Treatment: decongestants, analgesics and antiinflamatory drugs

PULMONARY OVER-INFLATION SYNDROMES

1. Definition: syndrome that is produced by the expansion of gas during ascent (Boyle's Law) derived from breathing additional gas, during scuba diving. It appears when the inhaled gas is not exhaled during ascent, thus mechanical forces can disrupt lung parenchyma.[48]
2. Signs and symptoms[49]
   a. Mild features
      i. Symptoms: hemoptysis and dyspnea
      ii. Signs: tachypnea, pneumomediastinum or pneumothorax, gas embolism
   b. Severe features: (<4%): collapse, loss of consciousness, hemiparesis, confusion, loss of coordination, apnea, and cardiac arrest

DECOMPRESSION SICKNESS IN SCUBA

1. Definition: syndrome produced by gas liberation (nitrogen) from tissues to blood by a reduction in barometric pressure (Henry's Law). Released nitrogen forms bubbles that depending on their localization produce a range of signs and symptoms that are described below.[50,51]
2. Bends: This is the most common symptom and the earliest. Bends is defined by pain, mainly in the large joints. It affects hips, elbows, and knees mainly; however, pain can be present in other joints. Bends occurs within 6 hours after exposure, but it can be found 12 to 24 hours after.[50,51]
3. Chokes: Also known as cardiovascular DCS, this is caused by high venous gas embolism in the pulmonary artery. Symptoms include cough, shortness of breath, substernal chest pain, and sometimes collapse.[50,51]
4. Skin bends: Also known as creeps, skin bends are caused by transcutaneous passage of nitrogen bubbles. Cutis marmorata (diffuse/blotchy rash) is another form of skin DCS. It is caused by extravasated blood from cutaneous vessels derived from endothelium injury caused by bubbles, and it may disappear after 12 hours.[50,51]
5. Lymphatic DCS: This appears when a bubble blocks lymphatic vessels. Its symptoms include lymphedema of the affected area.[50,51]
6. Neurological DCS: The wide range of symptoms of this condition makes diagnosis difficult. Symptoms depend on the area affected by the bubbles. Headache, paresthesias, paralysis, vertigo, loss of consciousness may be found.[50,51]
7. Treatment: recompression in hyperbaric chamber breathing 100% oxygen; endovenous liquids.[50,51]

A summary of Scuba diving disorders and their primary treatment is presented[44] in Table 9.3, and a comparison of diving and altitude DCS is seen in Table 9.4.

Aerospace Medicine

This is a specialty of medicine that integrates components of physiology, emergency medicine, preventive and occupational health, that works for promoting the health of pilots, aircrews, or people involved in aviation activities and spaceflight. The specialty strives to treat and to prevent conditions owing to the aeronautical or space environment. This specialty applies medical knowledge to the human factors in aviation and is thus a critical component of aviation safety.[58,59]

HYPOXIA

1. Description: hypoxia is defined as a reduction of the partial pressure of oxygen that is delivered to the tissues; as a consequence, a malfunction begins of the metabolism for providing energy from oxidation of complex chemical materials to simpler compounds. Arterial oxygen values below 90% are considered low.[1,60–62] Humans are susceptible to oxygen-level

TABLE 9.3 ■ Scuba diving Disorders and Primary Treatment

Diving Condition	Clinical Feature	Clinical Findings	Treatment	Reference
Ear barotrauma	Acute ear pain Vertigo Conductive hearing loss	Tympanic membrane changes according to severity of barotrauma with or without rupture	Slow equalization on descent Decongestants analgesics Antibiotic according to clinical findings	52,53
Sinus barotrauma	Acute facial pain epistaxis	Facial pain Mucosal edema	Decongestants analgesics Antibiotic according to clinical findings	53
Pulmonary barotrauma	Substernal pain Coughing Swallowing Severe cases: apnea unconsciousness Cardiac arrest	Pneumomediastinum Subcutaneous emphysema Pneumopericardium Pneumothorax Hamman's sign	Oxygen 100% Recompression hyperbaric chamber	54,55
Bends	Marked fatigue Joint pain	Pain in rest that increase with movement	Oxygen 100% Alert emergency rescue service Recompression hyperbaric chamber	56
Creeps or skin bends	Cutaneous itching	Cutis marmorata Irregular erythematous, pruritic rash	Oxygen 100% Oral fluid administration (500–1000 mL) Alert emergency rescue service	56,57
Neurological and cardiovascular decompression sickness	Paresthesia paresis Shortness of breath Impaired vision Dizziness Nausea Chest pain Impaired consciousness Loss of consciousness	Numbness Dizziness weakness gait abnormality hypoesthesia Vital signs instability	Oxygen 100% Fluid replacement intravenously Alert emergency rescue service Recompression hyperbaric chamber immediately	52,56

deficiency, which decreases body functions, with particular effects shown in the neurologic tissue.[1,60-62]

2. Types: Hypoxia is generally divided into four types[1,60,61]

  a. Hypoxic or anemic hypoxia is caused by a decrease in the oxygen available to the body. Example: flying in an unpressurized cabin.[63-65]

TABLE 9.4 ■ **Major Differences Between Diving and Altitude Decompression Sickness**

Altitude Decompression Sickness (DCS)	Diving DCS
1. Decompression starts from a ground-level tissue N_2 saturated state.	1. Upward excursions from saturation diving are rare.
2. Breathing gas is usually high in O_2 to prevent hypoxia and promote denitrogenation.	2. Breathing gas mixtures are usually high in inert gas because of oxygen toxicity concerns.
3. The time of decompressed exposure to altitude is limited.	3. The time at surface pressure following decompression is not limited.
4. Permission of denitrogenation (preoxygenation) reduces DCS risk.	4. The concept of preoxygenation is generally not applicable.
5. DCS usually occurs during the mission.	5. DCS risk is usually greatest after mission completion.
6. Symptoms are usually mild and limited to joint pain.	6. Neurologic symptoms are common.
7. Recompression to ground level is therapeutic and universal.	7. Therapeutic chamber recompression is time limited and sometimes hazardous.
8. Tissue PN_2 decreases with altitude exposure to very low levels.	8. Tissue PN_2 increases with hyperbaric exposure to very high levels.
9. Metabolic gases become progressively more important as altitude increases.	9. Inert gases dominate.
10. There are very few documented chronic sequelae.	10. Chronic bone necrosis and neurologic damage have been documented.

PN₂, Nitrogen pressure.
From Pilmanis AA, Webb JT. Fifty years of decompression sickness research at Brooks AFB, TX: 1960–2010. *Aviat Space Environ Med*. 2011;82:A1–A25.

b. Hypemic hypoxia is caused by a reduction in the oxygen-carrying capacity of the blood for any reason. Example: When hemoglobin is saturated by gases for which it has a higher affinity, the most common of which is carbon monoxide. Carbon monoxide is found at levels of 6% to 8% in the blood of a heavy smoker, and such individuals may become significantly hypoxic at altitudes below 10,000 feet.

c. Stagnant hypoxia caused by a reduction in total cardiac output, pooling of the blood, or restriction of blood flow. Examples: Heart failure, shock, continuous positive pressure breathing, and G forces in flight can create stagnant hypoxia. Local stagnant hypoxia can occur with tight and restrictive clothing or, in the cerebral circulation, in association with vasoconstriction as a result of respiratory alkalosis provoked by hyperventilation.

d. Histotoxic hypoxia refers to poisoning of the respiratory cytochrome system by chemicals such as cyanide or carbon monoxide, but it can also be caused by the effects of alcohol.

The most serious single physiologic hazard during flight at altitudes is hypobaric hypoxia,[62–65] because on ascent, according to Dalton's Law, as barometric pressure descends, the oxygen partial pressure falls, and thus the molecular content of oxygen in the lung. Variation in arterial blood gases values of subjects exposed to altitude is presented in Table 9.5.

3. Stages

Stages of hypoxia are shown in Table 9.6.

TABLE 9.5 ■ Typical Values for Arterial Blood Gases of Resting Subjects Acutely Exposed to Altitude

	Arterial Blood Gases			
Altitude (Feet)	Oxygen Tension (mmHg)	Carbon Dioxide Tension (mmHg)	Oxygen Concentration (mL (STPD)/100 mL blood)	Oxygen Saturation Hemoglobin (%)
Breathing Air				
0	95	40	20.5	97
8,000	56	38	18.8	93
12,000	43	35	16.9	84
15,000	37	30	15.7	78
18,000	32	28	14.5	72
20,000	29	26	13.2	66
Breathing 100% Oxygen				
33,000	95	40	20.5	97
40,000	45	38	16.9	84
43,000	36	30	15.4	76

STPD, Standard temperature and pressure, dry.
From Gradwell DP. Hypoxia and hyperventilation. In: Rainford DJ, Gradwell DP, eds. *Ernsting's Aviation Medicine.* 4th ed. London: Hodder Arnold; 2006. pp48.

TABLE 9.6 ■ Stages of Hypoxia

Stage	Altitude Breathing Air	Altitude Breathing 100% Oxygen	Arterial Oxygen Saturation %	Physiological Effects of Hypoxia
Indifferent	Sea level to 10,000 feet	FL 340–FL 390	98–87	Decrease in night vision as low as 5000 feet
Compensatory	10,000–15,000 feet	FL 390–FL 425	87–80	Drowsiness, poor judgment, impaired coordination, impaired efficiency
Disturbance	15,000 feet–FL 200	FL 425–FL 448	80–65	Impaired flight control, impaired handwriting, impaired speech, decreased coordination
Critical	FL 200–FL 230	FL 448–FL 455	65–60	Circulatory failure, central nervous system failure, convulsions, cardiovascular collapse, death

FL, Flight level.
Adapted from Reinhart RO. *Basic Flight Physiology.* 3rd ed New York: McGraw-Hill; 2008. pp55.

4. Symptoms: Individuals may present with different symptoms[63–65]
   a. Cyanosis
   b. Air hunger
   c. Increase in heart rate
   d. Increase in respiratory rate and hyperventilation
   e. Changes in peripheral vision
   f. Visual acuity impairment
   g. Difficulty in visual accommodation
   h. Diminished night vision
   i. Headache
   j. Nausea
   k. Fatigue or feeling sleepy
   l. Impairment of mental performance
   m. Motor skills and reasoning abilities deteriorate
   n. Poor response to verbal command
   o. Forgetfulness
   p. Poor task completion
   q. Muscular coordination impairment
   r. Personality changes
   s. Loss of muscular control
   t. Reaction time decreased
   u. Overconfidence
   v. Tingling in fingers and toes
   w. Loss of consciousness
   x. Personality changes
   y. Loss of memory

   Many of these are subjective, and most symptoms are not an exact measure of how hypoxic the pilot is; the result is that, in many cases, the pilot may become seriously hypoxic without appreciating that there is a problem.[1,60–65]

5. Factors influencing tolerance to hypoxia[1,60,61]
   a. Tolerance to hypoxia varies from individual to individual and from time to time.[1,60,61]
   b. Acclimatization: continual exposure to high altitudes and varies with the level of the hemoglobin and the oxygen carrying capacity of the blood.
   c. Absolute altitude
   d. Rate of ascent
   e. Duration of exposure
   f. Physical activity during exposure
   g. Self-imposed factors such as alcohol, smoke, fatigue
   h. Cold
   i. Physical fitness
   j. Inherent tolerance
   k. Emotionality

6. Treatment of hypoxia
   a. Provide 100% oxygen as immediate measure, which is the essential step; getting the airplane or cabin altitude below 10,000 feet is mandatory. This is a valid cause for declaring an emergency to air traffic controllers.[1,60,61]

7. Time of useful consciousness or "effective performance"
   a. The period of time a pilot has from the time oxygen becomes less available until the time when they lose their ability to take action, their mental and physical efficiency, and their alertness (Table 9.7).[1,60,61]

TABLE 9.7 ■ **Effective Performance Time at Altitude**

Altitude	Time of Useful Consciousness
FL 180	20–30 min
FL 220	5–10 min
FL 250	3–5 min
FL 280	2.5–3 min
FL 300	1–3 min
FL 350	30–60 s
FL 400	15–20 s
FL 430	9–15 s
FL 500 and above	6–9 s

FL, Flight level
From Pickard JS, Gradwell DP. Respiratory physiology and protection against hypoxia. In: *Fundamentals of aerospace medicine*. 4th ed: Lipppincott Williams and Wilkins; pp34.

  b. The variation is a reflection of the influence of many factors. This period is shorter (almost half) when hypoxia is induced by rapid decompression rather than by slow ascent.[66]
8. Prevention[61,67]
  a. Paramount is to avoid situations that can cause it, such as ascent to altitudes without supplementary oxygen, maintaining high-altitude flying for a prolonged time, failure of personal breathing equipment to supply oxygen at an adequate concentration and/or pressure, or decompression of the pressure cabin at high altitude.
    i. Perform proper PRICE (P: Pressure, R: Regulator, I: Indicator, C: Connectors, E: Other emergency systems) check and maintain oxygen discipline
    ii. Maintain a high level of suspicion when flight is over 5000 feet
    iii. Altitude chamber training of early recognition of symptoms
    iv. Avoid self-imposed factors (smoke cessation, fitness)
9. Education and training
  The best option for providing education is altitude chamber training.[64,65,68]

HYPERVENTILATION

1. Description: Hyperventilation may be described as an excessive respiratory rate, which results in exhaling high levels of carbon dioxide during respiration that can disable the patient. It may be voluntary or involuntary. Carbon dioxide, the most potent stimulus to respiration, is blown off in excessive amounts. The $PaCO_2$ falls, and respiratory alkalosis develops. The cerebral vessels become constricted.[1,60,61] In pilots, the most common precipitating causes are anxiety, fear, excessive concentration on a flight procedure, and as a reaction to pain or illness.[69]
2. Symptoms[1,60,69]
  a. Rapid breathing
  b. Dizziness

      c. Neuromuscular irritability
      d. Paresthesia of face and extremities
      e. Carpopedal spasm
      f. Feeling of dizziness
      g. Coldness and tingling around the lips
      h. Nausea
      i. Unconsciousness
      j. Tetany
  3. Treatment
      a. If one considers the symptoms of hypoxia and hyperventilation, it will be seen that they are remarkably similar. As it is imperative in the air that no mistake is made, the treatment for both is to breathe 100% oxygen and to reduce the rate and depth of respiration. With the breath held, the carbon dioxide levels build up once more and the symptoms disappear in reverse order.[60,61,67]

BAROTRAUMA

  1. i. According to Boyle's Law, the volume of a gas is inversely proportional to the pressured applied upon it; therefore, during ascent in flight, the pressure outside the aircraft decreases and the air contained in the body cavities can expand. Also, during descent, the pressure outside the aircraft increases, and volume of air contained in the body cavities is reduced, creating a relative negative pressure that requires equalizing pressure in the body cavities with the ambient air pressure.[1,70,71]
      ii. Some barotraumas of concern in aerospace medicine are conditions that describe the varying degrees of injury or inflammation that result when the air-filling body cavities are exposed to an uncompensated change in ambient pressure.[72-75]
  2. Physiopathology and diagnosis
      a. Barotitis
         i. The middle air or tympanic cavity is an air-filled space within the petrous pyramid of the temporal bone, lined by mucoperiosteum. It is separated from the outer ear by tympanic membrane and communicates with nasopharynx through the Eustachian tube.
         ii. During ascent, the gas within the tympanic cavity expands, pushes the tympanic membrane laterally, and leads to the Eustachian tube to open passively into the nasopharynx, allowing gas to escape, equalizing pressures between tympanic cavity and atmosphere.
         iii. During descent, the gas within the middle ear decreases, causes a relative negative pressure, pushes the tympanic membrane medially, requiring the active opening of the Eustachian tube (through swallowing, yawning, jaw movement, and in specific cases, Valsalva manoeuvre) to allow air passage into the tympanic cavity.
         iv. If this process is affected, pressure changes are not equalized, and may lead to inadequate ventilation of the middle ear, injury and inflammation, changes in tympanic membrane, fullness, serous exudate, hemorrhages, severe pain, vertigo, rupture of the tympanic membrane, and conductive hearing loss.
         v. This medical condition is described as otic barotrauma or barotitis.[1,70-72]
      b. Barosinusitis
         i. The paranasal sinuses are also air-filled spaces within the bones of the face, lined by respiratory mucosa, that connect to the nasal cavity through openings named sinus ostia.
         ii. During ascent, the ambient pressure decreases; the gas contained within paranasal sinuses is expanded against the rigid sinus walls, increasing intrasinus pressure,

which in normal condition is released passively through the sinus ostia into the nasal cavity, equalizing pressure with atmosphere.

   iii. During descent, the gas within the sinus decreases, creating a relative negative pressure that requires gas passage into the sinus to compensate pressures.

   iv. When this process is affected, pressure changes are not equalized and may lead to inadequate ventilation, edema, inflamation, mucosal injuries, severe pain, and hemorrage.

   v. This medical condition is described as sinus barotrauma or barosinusitis.[70,71,74]

  c. Barodontalgia

   i. Toothache can occur mainly during ascent by expansion of gas in teeth with inadequate filling, cavities, or abscesses.[75]

  d. Gastrointestinal tract

   i. The gas inside normal gastrointestinal tract expands during flight ascent, and usually can be released through the mouth and the anus. When people have difficulties venting this gas, they may manifest symptoms as abdominal discomfort and pain. Also, gas expansion may produce respiratory compromise and severe pain may cause vasovagal syncope.[70-71]

3. Prevention and treatment[70–75]

  a. Barotitis and barosinusitis

   i. Avoid flying with cold, inflammation, infection, or any recent medical condition of the upper respiratory tract.

   ii. Emphasize to aircrew and passengers about the importance of control of predisposing medical conditions (like severe allergic rhinitis) prior to flight.

   iii. Aircrew instruction about operational and physiological procedures to prevention

   iv. Could be required treatment with descongestants, analgesics, and antiinflamatory drugs.

   v. Some cases may require otolaryngology evaluation and eventually surgical treatment in recurrent problems.

  b. Barodontalgia

   i. Adequate dental health promotion, prevention, and treatment

  c. Gastrointestinal

   i. Avoid chewing gum, carbonated beverages, or food that can produce gas. Release any gastrointestinal gas through belching or flatus.

DECOMPRESSION SICKNESS IN AVIATION

1. Description[70,71,76,77]

  a. DCS in altitude is a condition caused by gas liberation in the form of bubbles from tissues to blood, which is produced according Henry's Law by exposure to low pressure, as when humans reach altitude in flight. It may manifest with several signs and symptoms in different body organs and systems.

  b. Altitude DCS may develop during exposure to reduced atmospheric pressure, high-altitude flight, depressurization of aircraft. It has also been described during depressurization in altitude chamber training.

  c. Nitrogen at ground-level pressure keeps saturated tissues and blood, but at altitude during decompression becomes supersaturated, forming bubbles primarily shaped by nitrogen, and also some carbon dioxide, oxygen, and water vapor.

  d. It has been studied that the signs and symptoms of DCS result from interaction of the bubbles with the body tissues, blood, arteries, and veins that can lead to local tissue dysfunction, compressive effects on peripheral nerves, blockage of vessels, local ischemic changes, and biochemical and hematologic responses.

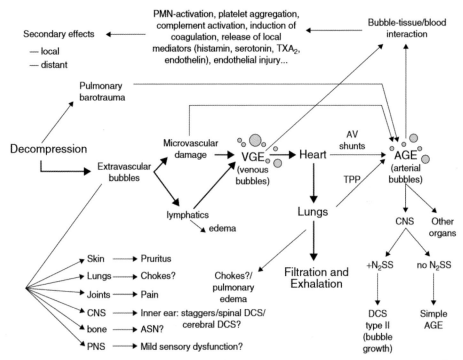

Fig. 9.1 Synopsis of the putative pathophysiological pathways of bubbles in decompression sickness. *AGE*, Arterial gas emboli; *ASN*, aseptic bone; *AV*, arteriovenous; *CNS*, central nervous system; *DCS type II*, serious neurologic (cerebral) decompression sickness; *N2SS*, nitrogen supersaturation; *PMN*, neutrophilic leucocytes; *TPP*, transpulmonary passage; *TXA2*, thromboxane A2; *VGE*, venous gas emboli. (From Stepanek J, Webb JT. Physiology of decompressive stress. In: Davis JR, Johnson R, Stepanek J, Fogarty JA, eds. *Fundamentals of Aerospace Medicine*. 4th ed. Philadelphia, PA: Lippincott Williams and Wilkins; 2008:60.)

    e. Stepanek and Webb outlined a synopsis of the pathophysiological pathways of bubbles in DCS that may affect different body organs and systems (Fig. 9.1).

  2. Diagnosis and treatment

    a. Signs and symptoms[70,71,76–78]

      The DCS signs and symptoms mainly reported from research studies in aviation and hypobaric chamber are:

      i. Musculoeskeletal symptoms as pain are one of the more frequently reported—mainly in joints, less often in muscles. Respiratory symptoms are characterized by cough, dyspnea, and substernal chest pain. Neurologic symptoms include headache, visual disturbances, sensory and motor deficits, dizziness, vertigo, sweating, nausea, numbness, paresthesia, weakness, paralysis, convulsions, fatigue, and personality changes. Skin symptoms such as hot or cold sensation, pruritus, urticaria, erythema, tingling, and mottled skin (cutis marmorata). A few cases can present as circulatory collapse and conscious impairment.

      ii. Pilmanis and Webb described some similarities and differences between diving and altitude DCS of important consideration in prevention and treatment (Table 9.4).

    b. Treatment[70,71,76,77]

      i. In flight, is recommended keep breathing 100% oxygen, descend to ground level and, declare a physiological emergency.

      ii. In most cases, altitude DCS will be resolved during descent or when ground level is reached, while breathing 100% oxygen.

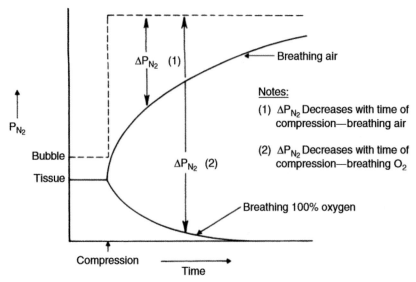

Fig. 9.2 Bubble nitrogen gradients when breathing pure oxygen. P_{N_2}, Nitrogen pressure. (From Stepanek J, Webb JT. Physiology of decompressive stress. In: Davis JR, Johnson R, Stepanek J, Fogarty JA, eds. *Fundamentals of Aerospace Medicine.* 4th ed. Philadelphia, PA: Lippincott Williams and Wilkins; 2008:70.)

      iii. At ground level, it is important to do a complete physical examination, including neurological evaluation, continue breathing 100% oxygen for 2 hours, reduce activity, ensure hydration and keep observation.

      iv. If symptoms persist, continue breathing 100% oxygen, supply endovenous liquids, and recompression hyperbaric therapy must be considered.

  3. Prevention[76,77,79-82]

    a. Predisposing factors

      i. Although further research is required, several predisposing factors to altitude DCS have been studied with variable scientific evidence, such as altitude level around or above 18,000 feet, longer time of exposure, rapid rate of ascent, previous exposures to altitude, flying following diving, exercise, dehydration, obesity, age, gender, hypoxia, and temperature.

    Protection measures:

    b. The main measures recommended are

      i. Aircraft pressurization below 10,000 feet.

      ii. Denitrogenation breathing 100% oxygen during 30 minutes before flying.

      iii. Identify predisposing factors that can be controlled.

      iv. Also, continuing education of pilots and physicians in recognition of signs and symptoms of DCS, health and fitness promotion, qualifying for aeromedical certification standards, and encouraging research are important.

NOISE AND VIBRATION

  1. Vibration

    a. Description

      i. Vibration is defined as an oscillatory motion in dynamic systems like the human body in aerospace operations. It is described in terms of frequency, amplitude, resonance, direction, spectrum, and duration.[83,84]

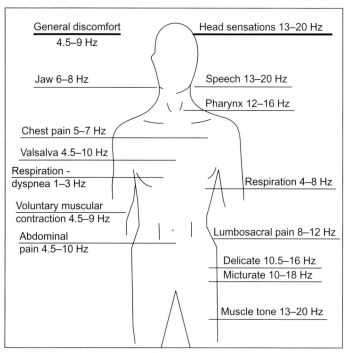

Fig. 9.3 Symptoms for frequencies between 2 and 20 Hz at tolerance levels. (Magid EB, Coermann RR, Ziegenruecker GH. Human tolerance to whole body sinusoidal vibration. *Aerospace Med*. 1960;31:915–924. From Smith SD, Goodman JR, Grosveld FW. Vibration and acoustics. In: Davis JR, Johnson R, Stepanek J, Fogarty JA, eds. *Fundamentals of Aerospace Medicine*. 4th ed. Philadelphia, PA: Lippincott Williams and Wilkins; 2008:118.)

    ii. Vibration can be transferred to the humans by contact or airborne transmission and can lead to physiological and psychological effects that vary according to vibration characteristics and conditions of exposure.

  b. Sources

    i. In aviation, the sources of vibration are related mainly to engines and structure of the aircraft (fixed-wing and rotatory-wing), and also with environment conditions (terrain, atmospheric turbulence, sound pressure).

    Aircraft maintenance plants and workstations, auxiliary equipment, and support vehicles must also be considered.[83–85]

  c. Health-related issues[83,86–88]

    i. Some authors have pointed out that acute exposures to vibration, primarily in the frequency range of 1 to 20 cycles per second (cps) or hertz (Hz), have not resulted in harm or injury (Fig. 9.3).[83]

    ii. On the other hand, long-term exposure to vibration has been linked to several medical conditions.[83–94]

    iii. Various symptoms that have been associated with vibration exposure, including headache, fatigue, back pain, cough, dyspnea, chest pain, giddiness, hypopharyngeal discomfort, cutaneous flushing, and tingling. Additionally, research studies have described the effects of vibration on different organs and systems such as vision, cardiovascular, respiratory, nervous, gastrointestinal and musculoskeletal. Also, vibration is identified affecting neurocognitive function and motor performance.[83–94]

    iv. Some research studies have described the vibroacoustic disease (VAD) as an emerging pathology, caused by excessive exposure to low frequency noise (LFN), identified in aircraft technicians, pilots, cabin crewmembers, ship machinists, restaurant workers, disk-jockeys, and also in several populations exposed to environmental LFN. The authors of these studies describe that VAD can be the cause of several signs and symptoms such as thickening of cardiovascular structures, headache, nose bleeds, bronchitis, depression, aggressiveness, tendency for isolation, cognitive impairment, asthenovegetative and neurotic syndromes, neurological changes, and malignancies.[85–87,91–94]

  d. Prevention[83–86]

    i. As strategies to mitigate vibration health effects are described the control measures on sources, related mainly to design and maintenance engineering.

    ii. Also, it is necessary to implement prevention programs that include monitoring and analysis of vibration sources, workers' education, recommendations about exposure times and protection, promotion of fitness and health, and periodic evaluations of potential sign and symptoms.

    iii. It is essential to promote research from different disciplines.

2. Noise

  a. Description[83,95–97]

    i. Sound is defined as a wave motion transmitted through an elastic medium, such as gas, liquid, or solid, as a form of physical energy that can be heard. The air is the most common transmission medium in humans.

    ii. Noise is a sound perceived as unpleasant, unwanted, or annoying, usually considered a subjective concept.

    iii. The control of noise level and exposure time is very important in aerospace medicine because it affects health and performance.

    iv. In addition to vibration, sound has significant physical properties: frequency, amplitude, and duration. All of them provide valuable information to understand potential risk of ear injuries and other medical issues.

    v. Hearing frequency is measured in cycles per second (cps) or hertz (Hz). The range of human hearing is between 20 and 20000 Hz, and the most sensitive region for understanding speech is from 500 to 4000 Hz.

    vi. The amplitude of a sound wave determines its intensity and perception. It is measured in decibels (dB), the unit of sound pressure level (SPL).
      The range of normal hearing threshold is between 0 and 20 dB, measured by audiometry.

    vii. Duration is related to exposure time.

  b. Sources

    i. There are several external and internal noise sources, mainly related to the type of aircraft (jet, helicopter, military), engines, pressurizing systems, air conditioners, fans, pumps, and other kinds of equipment and machinery. Equally important is the noise generated by aerodynamic flow across the aircraft structure. Also, high levels of noise are identified at or near the aviation facilities such as airports, aircraft maintenance plants, and workstations.[83,87,95,96]

    ii. SPLs in decibels caused by some common sources can be seen in Table 9.8.

  c. Health-related issues

    i. In the aerospace sector, noise is recognized as one of the most harmful environmental problems and has been linked to physiological and psychological responses identified as auditory and non-auditory health effects.[99–102]

TABLE 9.8 ■ Sound Pressure Levels in Decibels Caused by Some Common Sources

Source	SPL (dB)
Threshold of Hearing	
Quietest audible sound for persons with excellent hearing under laboratory conditions	0
Quietest Audible Sound for Persons Under Normal Conditions	
Virtual silence (audiometric test room)	10
Rustling leaves	20
Noticeably Quiet—Voice, Soft Whisper	
Quiet whisper (1 m)	30
Home (quiet room)	40
Moderate	
Quiet street (whispered speech)	50
Loud—Unusual Background, Voice Conversation 1 m	
Conversation at 1 m	60
Loud—Voice Conversation 0.3 m	
Inside a car Passenger car 80 km/h (15 m) Vacuum cleaner (3 m) Freight train (30 m)	70
Loud singing	75
Loud—Intolerable for Phone Use	
Automobile (10 m) Maximum sound up to 8 h (OSHA criteria—hearing conservation program) Pneumatic tools (15 m) Buses, diesel trucks, motorcycles (15 m) Road with busy traffic	80
Motorcycle (10 m)	88
Food blender (1 m) Maximum sound up to 8 h (OSHA criteria—engineering or administrative noise controls) Jackhammer (15 m) Bulldozer (15 m) Noisy factory Newspaper press	90
Subway (inside)	94
Very Loud	
Diesel truck (10 m) Motor horns at distance of 7 m	100

(Continued)

TABLE 9.8 ■ Sound Pressure Levels in Decibels Caused by Some Common Sources—cont.

Source	SPL (dB)
Lawn mower (1 m)	107
Pneumatic riveter (1 m)	115
Threshold of Discomfort	
Large aircraft (150 m overhead)	110
Chainsaw (1 m) Very noisy work—boilermakers workshop, etc.	117
Deafening, Human Pain Limit	
Amplified hard rock (2 m) Siren (30 m) Pneumatic chipper	120
Jet plane (30 m) Artillery fire (3 m)	130
Upper limit for unprotected ear for impulses	140
Short Exposure Can Cause Hearing Loss	
Military jet take-off (30 m)	150
Large military weapons	180

OHSA, Occupational Health and Safety Administration; *SPL*, sound pressure level.
From Engineering ToolBox. Sound Pressure. Available in http://www.engineeringtoolbox.com/sound-pressure-d_711.html.

   d. Auditory health effects[83,96,97,102]
      i. Noise exposure might cause temporal or permanent hearing damage, which manifests as hearing loss.
      ii. Hearing levels greater than 25 dB are considered abnormal and constitute hearing loss.
      iii. Hearing loss is classified as conductive, sensorineural, or mixed.
      iv. Conductive hearing loss is caused by impairment of outer or middle ear, which may have medical or surgical treatment, and usually manifests as air conduction reduction of hearing sensitivity, measured by audiometry.
      v. Sensorineural hearing loss is caused by inner ear impairment, usually shows an air and bone conduction loss of sensitivity in high frequencies, and often appears as an audiometric "notch" pattern in the 4000 or 6000 Hz region that can progress to lower frequencies, and generally does not respond to medical or surgical treatment.
      vi. Mixed hearing loss is a combination of conductive and sesorineural.
      vii. Hearing losses greater than 35 to 40 dB in the speech frequency range affect communication.
      viii. Noise-induced hearing loss is shown as a sensorineural hearing loss; it is one of the most common occupational illnesses in aviation workers and has been extensively researched.[83,95,103–106]
      ix. The comparison between sensorineural hearing loss and conductive hearing loss audiograms is shown in Fig. 9.4.

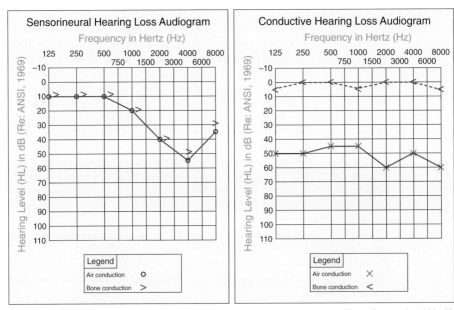

Fig. 9.4 Sensorineural hearing loss versus conductive hearing loss audiograms. (From Occupational Health and Safety Administration. Section III: Chapter 5 noise. Washington, DC. Available at https://www.osha.gov/dts/osta/otm/new_noise/index.html#whatisnoise.)

TABLE 9.9 ■ **Extended Workshifts and Action Level Reduction**

Exposure Time (h)	Action Level (dBA)
8	85
9	84.2
10	83.4
12	82.1
16	80

From Occupational Safety and Health Administration. Section III: Chapter 5 noise. Washington, DC. Available at https://www.osha.gov/dts/osta/otm/new_noise/index.html#whatisnoise.

x. It has been studied and documented that health effects increase when workers are exposed to noise levels greater than 85 dB, and extended shifts longer than 8 hours.[95]

xi. Action level for hearing conservation, based on shift duration, for works working longer than an 8 hours shift, is shown in Table 9.9.

xii. Tinnitus is a sound perception, usually disturbing and not attributable to an external source.[100]

xiii. Acoustic trauma is a permanent sensorineural hearing loss, as a consequence of a single and sudden exposure to high noise levels such as gunshot or explosion.[97]

xiv. Pain or discomfort in the ears and tympanic membrane rupture have been reported in some cases.

    e. Non-auditory health effects[102,105]:

       i. Although further research studies need to be done, significant evidence has been reported about non-auditory physiological and psychological effects of noise. These include: reduced visual acuity, chest wall vibrations, muscle tension, respiratory rhythm changes, vertigo, disorientation, nausea, and vomiting. Also, noise exposure has been associated with cardiovascular disease, cardiovascular risk factors, stroke, hypertension, sleep disturbances, psychological ill health, negative effect on cognitive skills, learning problems, annoyance, irritability, stress, fatigue, and increase in the risk of accidents.[83,96,102,105]

      ii. All of the auditory and non-auditory health effects have implications to occupational and public health.[94,95,98,99,101,103,104] In aerospace medicine, operational performance, workload, concentration, communication, ability to understand speech, radio transmissions, and accurate assessment of warning tones in the cockpit can have a significant impact on flight safety.[83,96,103,104,106]

    f. Prevention[83,93,94,99,107]

       i. Although further studies and analysis are still required for non-auditory health effects associated with noise exposure, noise-induced hearing loss is an occupational disease widely recognized as preventable. Furthermore, prevention is the only option to preserve hearing if we understand that noise-induced hearing loss does not have treatment.

      ii. Also, many of the strategies proposed for hearing loss prevention can contribute to reduce other health-related problems.

      iii. Some of the most important recommendations, are: control measures on noise sources, related mainly to design and maintenance engineering.

      iv. Implementing of prevention programs that include continuing education, noise monitoring, periodic audiometric evaluation, personal protective equipment such as hearing protection devices (earplugs, earmuffs, helmets), sound insulation, noise level and exposure times guidelines, reduction of unnecessary noise exposure in and out of work environment, and promoting fitness and health.

      v. Finally, policies and regulations about environmental noise and public health must be constantly updated through further multidisciplinary research.

References

1. Reinhart RO. *Basic Flight Physiology*. 3rd ed. New York: McGraw-Hill; 2008.
2. Gradwell DP. The earth's atmosphere. In: Gradwell DP, Rainford DJ, eds. *Ernsting's Aviation and Space Medicine*. 5th ed. London: CRC Press Taylor & Francis Group; 2016.
3. Gore CJ, Clark SA, Saunders PU. Nonhematological mechanisms of improved sea-level performance after hypoxic exposure. *Med Sci Sports Exerc*. 2007;39:1600–1609.
4. Hackett PH, Rennie D, Levine HD. The incidence, importance, and prophylaxis of acute mountain sickness. *Lancet*. 1976;2:1149–1154.
5. Cymerman A, Lieberman P, Hochstadt J, Rock PB, Butterfield GE, Moore LG. Speech motor control and acute mountain sickness. *Aviat Space Environ Med*. 2002;73:766–772.
6. Roach RC, Maes D, Sandoval D, et al. Exercise exacerbates acute mountain sickness at simulated high altitude. *J Appl Physiol*. 2000;88:581–585.
7. Ferrazzini G, Maggiorini M, Kriemler S, Bärtsch P, Oelz O. Successful treatment of acute mountain sickness with dexamethasone. *BMJ*. 1987;294:1380–1382.
8. Smedley T, Grocott M. Acute high-altitude illness: a clinically orientated review. *Br J Pain*. 2013;7:85–94.
9. Peter B, Mairbaurl H, Maggiorini M, Swenson ER. Physiological aspects of high-altitude pulmonary edema. *J Appl Physiol*. 2005;98:1101–1110.
10. Rupp T, Jubeau M, Millet GY, et al. The effect of hypoxemia and exercise on acute mountain sickness symptoms. *J Appl Physiol*. 2013;114:180–185.

11. Basnyat B, Wu TY, Certsch JH. Neurological conditions at altitude that fall outside the definition of altitude illness. *High Alt Med Biol.* 2004;5:171–179.
12. Barry PW, Pollard AJ. Altitude Illness. *BMJ.* 2003;326:915–919.
13. Queiroz LP, Rapoport AM. High-altitude headache. *Curr Pain Headache Rep.* 2007;11:293–6.20.
14. Harris NS, Wenzel RP, Thomas SH. High altitude headache: efficacy of acetaminophen vs. ibuprofen in a randomized, controlled trial. *J Emerg Med.* 2003;24:383–387.
15. Imray C, Wright A, Subudhi A, Roach R. Acute mountain sickness: pathophysiology, prevention, and treatment. *Prog Cardiovasc Dis.* 2010;52:467–484.
16. Grissom CK, Roach RC, Sarnquist FH, Hackett PH. Acetazolamide in the treatment of acute mountain sickness: clinical efficacy and effect on gas exchange. *Ann Intern Med.* 1992;116:461–465.
17. Hackett PH, Roach RC, Wood RA, Foutch RG, Meehan RT, Rennie D, et al. Dexamethasone for prevention and treatment of acute mountain sickness. *Aviat Space Environ Med.* 1988;59:950–954.
18. Bärtsch P, Merki B, Hofstetter D, Maggiorini M, Kayser B, Oelz O. Treatment of acute mountain sickness by simulated descent: a randomised controlled trial. *Br Med J.* 1993;306:1098–1101.
19. Johnson C, Dallimore J, Dhillon S, et al. Hot, dry environments: deserts. In: Jonhson C, Anderson S, Dallimore J, Imary C, Winser s, Moore J, Warrell D, eds. Oxford Handbook of Expedition and Wilderness Medicine. 2nd ed. New York: Oxford University Press; 2015:745–767.
20. O'Brien KK, Leon LR, Kenfick RW, O'Connor F. Clinical management of heat-related illnesses. In: Aurbach PS, Cushing T, Harris NS, eds. Auerbach's Wilderness Medicine. 7th ed. Philadelphia: Elsevier; 2017:67–274.
21. Sloan BK, Kraft EM, Clark D, Schmeissing SW, Byrne BC, Rusyniak DE. On-site treatment of exertional heat stroke. *Am J Sports Medicine.* 2015;43:823–829.
22. Leon LR, Bouchama A. Heat stroke. Compr. Physiol. 2015;5:61–647.
23. Yeo TP. Heat stroke: A comprehensive review. AACN Clin Issues. 2004;15:280–293.
24. Casa DJ, Armstrong LE, Kenny GP, O'Connor FG, Huggins RA. Exertional heat stroke: new concepts regarding cause and care. *Curr Sports Med Rep.* 2012;11:115–123.
25. Adams T, Stacey E, Stacey S, Martin D. Exertional heat stroke. *Brit J Hosp Med.* 2012;73:72–78.
26. Hadad E, Rav-Acha M, Heled Y, Epstein Y, Moran DS. Heat stroke: a review of cooling methods. *Sports Med.* 2004;34:501–511.
27. Epstein Y, Yanovich R. Heatstroke. *N Engl J Med.* 2019;380:2449–2459.
28. Mittal SK, Gupta RK. Heat stroke. *Indian Pediatr.* 1986;23(Suppl):155–160.
29. Clowes Jr GH, O'Donnell Jr TF. Heat stroke. *N Engl J Med.* 1974;291:564–567.
30. Boname JR, Wilhite WC, Jr. The acute treatment of heat stroke. *South Med J.* 1967;60:885–887.
31. National Athletic Trainers Association, Korey Stringer Institute. Tips for exercising safely in the heat: steer clear of heat cramps, heat exhaustion, and heat stroke with key information. NASN Sch Nurse. 2011;26:230–232.
32. Glazer JL. Management of heatstroke and heat exhaustion. *Am Fam Physician.* 2005;71:2133–2140.
33. Kim SH, Jo SN, Myung HN, Jang JY. The effect of pre-existing medical conditions on heat stroke during hot weather in South Korea. *Environ Res.* 2014;133:246–252.
34. Forgey WW. Wilderness Medicine: Beyond First Aid. 6th ed. Guilford, CT: FalconGuides; 2012.
35. Bledsoe GH, Manyak MJ, Townes DA. Expedition and Wilderness Medicine. New York: Cambridge University Press; 2009.
36. DeMartini JK, Casa DJ, Belval LN, et al. Environmental conditions and the occurrence of exertional heat illnesses and exertional heat stroke at the Falmouth Road Race. *J Ath Train.* 2014;49:478–485.
37. Jardine DS. Heat illness and heat stroke. *Pediatr Rev.* 2007;28:249–258.
38. Kramer DA, Shayne P. Sun-induced disorders. In: Schwartz GR, ed. Principles and Practice of Emergency Medicine. 4th ed. Baltimore, MD: Lippincott Williams &Wilkins; 1999:1581.
39. Linos E, Katz KA, Colditz GA. Skin Cancer—The Importance of Prevention. *JAMA Intern Med.* 2016;176(10):1435–1436. doi:10.1001/jamainternmed.2016.5008.
40. Bielinski K, Bielinski N. UV radiation transmittance: regular clothing versus sun-protective clothing. Cutis. 2014;94:135–138.
41. Ghazi S, Couteau C, Coiffard LJ. What level of protection can be obtained using sun protective clothing? Determining effectiveness using an in vitro method. *Int J Pharm.* 2010;397:144–146.
42. Roy CR, Gies PH, McLennan A. Sun protective clothing: 5 years of experience in Australia. *Recent Results Cancer Res.* 2002;160:26–34.

43. Chorley AC, Evans BJ, Benwell MJ. Civilian pilot exposure to ultraviolet and blue light and pilot use of sunglasses. *Aviat Space Environ Med*. 2011;82:895–900.
44. Fishman GA. Ocular phototoxicity: guidelines for selecting sunglasses. *Surv Ophthalmol*. 1986;31(3): 119–124.
45. Lee Y, Ye B. Underwater and hyperbaric medicine as a branch of occupational and environmental medicine. *Ann Occup Environ Med*. 2013;25:39.
46. Hunter SE, Farmer JC. Ear and sinus problems in diving. In: Bove AA, Davis JC, eds. Diving Medicine. 4th ed. Philadelphia, PA: Saunders; 2004:431–459.
47. Cheshire WP. Headache and facial pain in scuba divers. *Curr Pain Headache Rep*. 2004;8:315–320.
48. Vann RD. Mechanisms and risks of decompression. In: Bove AA, Davis JC, eds. Diving Medicine. 4th ed. Philadelphia, PA: Saunders; 2004:127–164.
49. Lynch JH, Bove A. Diving medicine: a review of current evidence. *J Am Board Fam Med*. 2009;22: 399–407.
50. Neuman T. Arterial gas embolism and decompression sickness. *News Physiol Sci*. 2002;17:77–81.
51. Neuman T. Pulmonary barotrauma. In: Bove AA, ed. Diving Medicine. 3rd ed. Philadelphia: Saunders; 1997:176–183.
52. Kay E. Doc's diving medicine. Prevention of middle ear barotrauma. Available at: http://faculty.washington.edu/ekay/.
53. Lynch JH, Bove A. Diving medicine: a review of current evidence. *JABFM*. 2009;22(4):399–407.
54. Harker CP, Neuman TS, Olson LK, Jacoby I, Santos A. Theroentgenographic findings associated with air embolism in sport scuba divers. *J Emerg Med*. 1993;11:443–449.
55. Bove AA. Diving medicine. *Am J Respir Crit Care Med*. 2014. doi:10.1164/rccm.201309-1662CI.
56. Eichhorn L, Leyk D. Diving medicine in clinical practice. *Dtsch Arztebl Int*. 2015;112:147–158. doi:10.3238/arztebl.2015.0147.
57. Vasileios K. Cutis marmorata in decompression sickness. *N Engl J Med*. 2010;362:2.
58. International Civil Aviation Organization. What is Aviation medicine? Available in https://www.icao.int/safety/aviation-medicine/pages/desc.aspx.
59. Aerospace Medical Association. Aerospace Medicine. Available in https://www.asma.org/about-asma/careers/aerospace-medicine.
60. Gradwell DP. Hypoxia and hyperventilation. In: Rainford DJ, Gradwell DP, eds. Ernsting's Aviation Medicine. 5th ed. London: CRC Press Taylor & Francis Group; 2016.
61. Pickard JS, Gradwell DP. Respiratory physiology and protection against hypoxia. In: Davis JR, Johnson R, Stepanek J, Fogarty JA, eds. Fundamentals of Aerospace Medicine. 4th ed. Philadelphia: Lipppincott Williams and Wilkins; 2008.
62. Cable GG. In-flight hypoxia incidents in military aircraft: causes and implication for training. *Aviat Space Environ Med*. 2003;74:169–172.
63. Tu MY, Chiang KT, Cheng CC, Li FL, Wen YH, Lin SH, et al. Comparison of hypobaric hypoxia symptoms between a recalled exposure and a current exposure. PLoS ONE. 2020;15(9):e0239194. https://doi.org/10.1371/journal.pone.0239194.
64. Beer JMA, Shender BS, Chauvin D, Dart TS, Fischer J. Cognitive deterioration in moderate and severe hypobaric hypoxia conditions. *Aerosp Med Hum Perform*. 2017;88(7):617–626.
65. Asmaro D, Mayall J, Ferguson S. Cognition at altitude: impairment in executive and memory processes under hypoxic conditions. *Aviat Space Environ Med*. 2013;84(11):1159–1165.
66. Yoneda I, Tomada M, Takumaru O, Sato T, Watanabe Y. Time of useful consciousness determination in aircrew members with reference to prior altitude chamber experience and age. *Aviat Space Environ Med*. 1999;71:72–76.
67. Gradwell DP, Macmillan AJF. Oxygen systems, pressure cabin and clothing. In: Gradwell DP, Rainford DJ, eds. Ernsting's Aviation and Space Medicine. 5th ed. London: CRC Press Taylor & Francis Group; 2016.
68. Bouak F, Vartanian O, Hofer K, Cheung B. Acute mild hypoxic hypoxia effects on cognitive and simulated aircraft pilot performance. *Aerosp Med Hum Perform*. 2018;89(6):526–535.
69. Shahala H, Khademi A. Hyperventilation in military aviation and diving. *Ann. Milit. Health Sci. Res*. 2012;10:339–343.
70. Stepanek J, Webb JT. Physiology of decompressive stress. In: Davis JR, Johnson R, Stepanek J, Fogarty JA, eds. Fundamentals of Aerospace Medicine. 4th ed. Philadelphia: Lipppincott Williams and Wilkins; 2008.

71. Macmillan AJF. Principles of the pressure cabin and the effects of pressure change on body cavities contain gas. In: Rainford DJ, Gradwell DP, eds. Ernsting's Aviation Medicine. 4th ed. London: Hodder Arnold; 2006.

72. Ryan P, Treble A, Patel N, Jufas N. Prevention of otic barotrauma in aviation: a systematic review. *Otology and Neurotology*. 2018;39:539–549.

73. Mitchell-Innes A, Young E, Vasijevic A, Rashid M. Air travellers' awareness of the preventability of otic barotrauma. *Journal of Laringology and Otology*. 2014;128:494–498.

74. Vaezeafshar R, Psaltis AJ, Rao VK, et al. Barosinusitis: comprehensive review and proposed new classification system. *Allergy & Rhinology*. 2017;8(3).

75. Zadic Y, Zapnick L, Goldstein L. In-flight barodontalgia: analysis of 29 cases in military aircrew. *Aviat Space Environ Med*. 2007;78:593–596.

76. Pilmanis AA, Webb JT. Fifty years of decompression sickness research at Brooks AFB, TX: 1960 – 2010. *Aviat Space Environ Med*. 2011;82:A1–A25.

77. Green RD, Leich DR. Twenty years of treating decompression sickness. *Aviat Space Environ Med*. 1987;58:362–366.

78. Auten JD, Kuhne MA, Walker HM, Porter HO. Neurologic decompression sickness following cabin pressure fluctuations at high altitude. *Aviat Space Environ Med*. 2010;81:427–430.

79. Vann RD, Denoble P, Emmerman MN, Corson KS. Flying after diving. *Aviat Space Environ Med*. 1993;64:801–807.

80. Sulaiman ZN, Pilmanis AA, O'Connor RB. Relationship between age and susceptibility to altitude decompression sickness. *Aviat Space Environ Med*. 1997;68:695–698.

81. Bendrick GA, Ainscough NJ, Pilmanis AA. Prevalence of decompression sickness among U-2 pilots. *Aviat Space Environ Med*. 1996;67:199–206.

82. Kennet A. Identifying the subtle presentation of decompression sickness. *Aerosp Med Hum Perform*. 2015;86:1058–1062.

83. Smith SD, Goodman JR, Grosveld FW. Vibration and acoustic. In: Davis JR, Johnson R, Stepanek J, Fogarty JA, eds. Fundamentals of Aerospace Medicine. 4th ed. Philadelphia: Lipppincott Williams and Wilkins; 2008.

84. Rollin Stott JR. Vibration. In: Rainford DJ, Gradwell DP, eds. Ernsting's Aviation Medicine. 4th ed. London: Hodder Arnold; 2006.

85. Castelo Branco NAA, Alves-Pereira M. Vibroacoustic disease. *Noise and Health*. 2004;6:3–20.

86. Castelo Branco NAA, Rodriguez E. The vibroacoustic disease-an emerging pathology. *Aviat Space Environ Med*. 1999;70:A1–A6.

87. Castelo Branco NA. The clinical stages of vibroacoustic disease. *Aviat Space Environ Med*. 1999;70:A32–A39.

88. Mellert V, Baumann I, Fresse N, Weber R. Impact of sound and vibration on health, travel comfort and performance of flight attendants and pilots. *Aerospace Science and Technology*. 2008;12:18–25.

89. De Oliveira CG, Nadal J. Transmissibility of helicopter vibration in the spines of pilots in flight. *Aviat Space Environ Med*. 2005;76:576–580.

90. Harrer KL, Yniguez D, Majar M, Ellenbecker D. Whole body vibration exposure for MH-60s pilots. *Aviat Space Environ Med*. 2005;55:556–557.

91. Martinho Pimenta AJF, Castelo Branco NAA. Neurological aspects of vibroacoustic disease. *Aviat Space Environ Med*. 1999;70:A91–A95.

92. Marciniak W, Rodriguez E, Olszowaka K, Atrov O, et al. Echocardiographic evaluation in 485 aeronautical workers exposed to different noise environments. *Aviat Space Environ Med*. 1999;70:A46–A53.

93. Reis Ferreira JM, Couto AR, Jalles-Tavares N, Castelo Branco MSN, Castelo Branco NAA. Airway flow limitations in patients with vibroacoustic disease. *Aviat Space Environ Med*. 1999;70:A63–A69.

94. Gomes LMP, Martinho Pimenta AJF, Castelo Branco NAA. Effects of occupational exposure to low frequency noise on cognition. *Aviat Space Environ Med*. 1999;70:A115–A118.

95. Occupational Safety and Health Administration. Section III: Chapter 5 Noise. Available in https://www.osha.gov/dts/osta/otm/new_noise/index.html#whatisnoise. Updated: August 15, 2013. Washington D.C.

96. Rood GM, James SH. Noise. In: Rainford DJ, Gradwell DP, eds. Ernsting's Aviation Medicine. 4th ed. London: Hodder Arnold; 2006.

97. Dobie R. Hearing loss. In: Ladou J, Harrisson R, eds. Current Diagnosis & Treatment, Ocupational & Environmental Medicine. 5th ed. New York: McGraw-Hill; 2014.

98. Engineering ToolBox. Sound Pressure. Available in http://www.engineeringtoolbox.com/sound-pres-sure-d_711.html.

99. Basner M, Clark Ch, Hansell A, Hileman JI, Jansen S, Shepherd Sparow V. Aviation noise impact: state of the science. *Noise and Health.* 2017;19:41–50.

100. Sliwi'nska-Kowalska M, Zaborowski K. WHO environmental noise guidelines for the european region: a systematic review on environmental noise and permanent hearing loss and tinnitus. *Int. J. Environ. Res. Public Health.* 2017;14(10):1139. doi:10.3390/ijerph14101139.

101. Zhdanko IM, Zinkin VN, Soldatov SK, Bogomolov AV, Sheshegov PM. Fundamental and applied aspects of preventing adverse effects of aviation noise. *Human Physiology.* 2016;42:705–714.

102. Basner M, Babisch W, Davis A, Brink M, Ch Clark, Jansen S. Auditory and non-auditory effects of noise on health. *The Lancet.* 2014;383:1325–1332.

103. Orsello CA, Moore JE, Reese C. Sensorineural hearing loss incidence among U.S. military aviators between 1997 and 2011. *Aviat Space Environ Med.* 2013;84:975–979.

104. Greenwell BM, Tvaryanas AP, Maupin GM. Risk factors for hearing decrement among U.S. Air Force aviation-related personnel. *Aerosp Med Hum Perform.* 2018;89:80–86.

105. Alves-Pereira M. Noise-induced extra-aural pathology: a review and commentary. *Aviat Space Environ Med.* 1999;79:A7–A21.

106. Dehais F, Causse M, Vachon F, Regis N, Menand E, Tremblain S. Failure to detect critical auditory alerts in cockpit: evidence for inattentional deafness. *Hum. Factors: The Journal of the Human Factors and Ergonomics Society.* 2014;56:631–644.

107. Abel SM, Odell P. Sound attenuation from earmuffs and earplugs in combination: maximum benefits vs missed information. *Aviat Space Environ Med.* 2006;77:899–904.

CHAPTER 10

Public Health and Field Epidemiology

Lucas A. Johnson ■ Andrew Isaac Geller ■ Ellen Yard ■ Juan I. Ubiera

Site Selection/Establishing Camp

Responders to a disaster are rarely afforded the luxury of selecting a site for creating a displaced persons camp. Despite the realities of establishing field operations in disaster-affected areas, responders should strive to organize camps that minimize the transmission of disease and provide a safe haven from conflict. Ideal camps:

- Do not compete for resources with the surrounding community
- Are located an appropriate distance from known insect/animal vectors and other environmental/industrial health risks
- Have access to surface or ground water supplies of adequate quantity and quality
- Have adequate drainage to prevent flooding/standing water
- Are easily accessible by ground transportation
- Are located in areas where geopolitics afford freedom of movement of persons

Overcrowding substantially complicates the ability to maintain an orderly, hygienic environment. A minimum usable surface area of 45 m² per person is recommended when calculating the total footprint required for a camp providing all necessities (shelter, cooking areas, educational facilities, toileting areas, recreation areas, roads and paths, etc.) within the confines of the camp itself.[1] Each individual should be provided a minimum of 3.5 m² of covered space for shelter. Ensuring space between individual structures as well as collections of structures greatly improves opportunities for maintaining a sanitary camp and decreases opportunities for fires.

Water

Ample quantities of safe water are necessary for preservation of health, hygiene, and morale. Unsafe water can transmit a variety of bacterial, viral, protozoan, and parasitic diseases, exacerbating already difficult standards of living. Similarly, insufficient quantities of water available for hygiene activities can be an equally important contributor to many health problems observed in the aftermath of a disaster.[1] Although unique climactic, cultural, and infrastructure considerations affect the quantities of water required by a population affected by a disaster, Sphere standards identify 15 liters per day per person as a key indicator for levels generally considered acceptable for drinking, cooking, and personal hygiene needs.[1] Certain vulnerable subpopulations generate water demands substantially greater than population-accepted levels; field hospitals operating in emergency environments have been documented to require between 150 and 200 liters per patient per day, child feeding centers typically require 30 to 40 liters per child per day.[2]

Untreated water sources require evaluation for potability by personnel with water sanitation experience. Historically, attempts to provide two distinct sources of water (one for potable use and another for nonpotable use) fail because of complicated logistics and end-user misunderstanding. Responders should instead focus efforts on generating a single source of potable water to meet all survival needs (drinking, cooking, and personal hygiene).[2] Whenever possible, responders should ensure the standard of potability is the same for both displaced persons and the neighboring local population to prevent potential conflict.[2]

Contamination of a water supply with fecal coliforms, predominantly *Escherichia coli*, serves as a sentinel indicator of other potentially harmful pathogens. As such, Sphere guidelines recommend treating water if any fecal coliforms are present. Minimum recommended water quality standards are outlined in Table 10.1.

A variety of options exist for substantially improving the safety and potability of water sources in austere environments. Overwhelmingly, chlorination is the preferred method for water disinfection as it has a measurable residual that both continues to kill organisms after initial treatment and can also serve as a sentinel for potential contamination when residual chlorination levels fall below acceptable thresholds. Manufacturer information can provide specific

TABLE 10.1 ■ Sphere Potable Water Standards

Standard	Value	Applicability
Chlorine residual	0.5 mg/L	• Piped supplies • All water supplies at times of risk of diarrheal epidemics
Turbidity	5 nephelometric turbidity units (NTU)	• Piped supplies • All water supplies at times of risk of diarrheal epidemics
Fecal coliforms	None per 100 mL	• At point of delivery

TABLE 10.2 ■ **Options for Treating Water in the Field**

Treatment Method	Strengths	Limitations
Polyethylene terephthalate (PET) bottle solar sterilization	• Inexpensive • Capable of destroying large percentage of pathogens	• Limited production volume • Time intensive • Posttreatment contamination possible • Requires acceptable fresh water source
Iodine	• Inexpensive • Simple technology • Can be performed at household level	• Requires substantial logistics for replenishment of consumables • Requires acceptable fresh water source
Boiling	• Inexpensive • Simple technology • Can be performed at household level	• Limited production volume • Time intensive • Requires reliable fuel source • Posttreatment contamination possible • Requires acceptable fresh water source
Slow sand filtration	• Inexpensive • Simple technology	• Posttreatment contamination possible • Requires acceptable fresh water source • May require finished water distribution system
Chlorination	• Gold standard of water treatment • Residual chlorine continues to kill organisms after initial treatment • Can be performed at household level	• Resource intensive • May require finished water distribution system • Requires substantial logistics for replenishment of consumables
Reverse osmosis	• Can generate potable water from seawater/briny/brackish water	• Expensive • Requires substantial logistics for replenishment of consumables • Requires reliable source of power • Posttreatment contamination possible if not chlorinated
Commercial bottled water	• Does not require finished water distribution system	• Expensive • Requires substantial logistics

dosing recommendations depending upon the product used and volume of water to be treated. Concentration of dissolved solids, pH, and temperature can all affect the volume of chlorine required to safely kill pathogens. Chlorine requires a minimum of 30 minutes of contact time to disinfect water for drinking. Table 10.2 briefly summarizes strengths and limitations of various methods for treating water in the field.

Careful thought must also be given to how water will be distributed to populations. Ideal water delivery should be geographically convenient, located in an area that minimizes the potential exploitation of women and children who are often culturally delegated to perform household water collection, afford procurement without unnecessarily long wait queues, and be sufficiently designed as to minimize standing surface water, which can serve as a vector breeding habitat.[1] Guidelines recommend striving for no more than 250 people per tap, 500 people per hand pump, and 400 people per single-user open well.[1]

Even after proper treatment and delivery of field water, there exists substantial health risk because of the increased likelihood of postdelivery contamination in crowded settings. Sphere guidelines recommend at least two clean water-collecting or storage containers (10–20 L each) per household to minimize postdelivery contamination risk. Additionally, continued surveillance of water at point of use can help identify potential sources or practices jeopardizing treated water.

Food

Food-borne illness imposes a substantial burden of morbidity and mortality in hygiene-challenged settings. Common factors contributing to food-borne illness include food from unsafe sources, poor personal hygiene, inadequate cooking, and inadequate storage. Specific interventions and best practices addressing each of these factors can substantially reduce the likelihood of food-borne illness.

FOOD FROM UNSAFE SOURCES

Assuring a safe food supply begins with procuring food from safe sources. When responding to disasters, a safe food source extends well beyond procuring items with reasonable assurances of pathogen absence from a supplier. Considerations for the ability to safely store food items before preparation, fuel availability to properly cook temperature-sensitive food items, safe storage of prepared food items not immediately consumed, and overall availability and application of hand hygiene substantially affect a food item's safety.

POOR PERSONAL HYGIENE

Inadequate hygiene, particularly hand hygiene, is frequently identified as a factor contributing to outbreaks of food-borne illness. The importance of reinforcing hand hygiene before meal preparation and consumption is critical in field settings.

In settings with centrally prepared messing facilities, food handlers should receive specific training on hand hygiene technique and actions or events throughout the food preparation and serving process that would require repeat hand washing. Food handlers should be free of communicable diseases and should be required to report symptoms of potential illness (vomiting, diarrhea, nausea, jaundice, sore throat with fever, skin lesions). A low threshold for exclusion from food preparation duties should be applied to food handlers to minimize the possibility of food-borne illness resulting from a communicable disease.

INADEQUATE COOKING

Proper cooking temperatures destroy pathogenic organisms and minimize the potential for food-borne illness. Raw animal foods must be cooked to a temperature and for a time period that ensures destruction of common food-borne pathogens. Availability of reliable fuel sources will substantially affect the ability to safely eliminate pathogens in raw foods that require cooking.

INADEQUATE STORAGE

Improper food storage, either before or after preparation, is critical to ensuring a safe food supply. Environmental conditions and the logistic realities of fieldwork impose substantial limitations on the ability to store food safely. Each disaster response situation imposes unique challenges; responders charged with organizing the procurement and provisioning of food items must account for logistic realities when considering what commodities will be made available to displaced persons. Similarly, considerations must be made to prevent contamination of food items after they have been prepared. If not immediately consumed after preparation, a variety of food items require specific holding temperatures to prevent the growth of pathogens. Restricting rations of such items may be warranted to discourage preparation of temperature-sensitive items in excess of what is to be immediately consumed.

Toileting

Methods employed for the disposal of human waste are influenced by material availability, soil conditions, source and location of drinking water, and environmental regulations. Positioning of toileting facilities should reduce or minimize the transmission of disease by vermin, vectors, or direct human contact. In general, field toileting facilities should be located at least 30 m from groundwater sources or food preparation areas.[1] All attempts should be made to create handwashing stations at the exit of any toileting facility; handwashing with soap and water is ideal but hand sanitizer is an acceptable alternative. In the absence of soap, handwashing with water alone or water and a natural abrasive such as sand should still be encouraged.

Two factors are critical when implementing any toileting solutions following a disaster. First, toileting practices presented to a population must be culturally acceptable. The fundamental purpose of established toileting facilities—the prevention of indiscriminate defecation—hinge upon identifying a solution the population served is willing to use. Second, special considerations must be made to ensure toileting facilities are designed and located in ways that do not place vulnerable populations (unaccompanied children, women, and the elderly) at harm. Placing toileting facilities far from other camp activities for the sake of privacy inconveniences inhabitants and unnecessarily isolates potentially exploitable persons, potentially exposing them to harm during a particularly vulnerable activity.

Defecation fields are the crudest of toileting options available and appropriate only in the initial phase of a disaster response; however, their ability to prevent indiscriminate defecation is critical to establishing basic hygiene measures in a new camp. Defecation fields are simply open fields designated and marked for use as open toileting. Typically, defecation fields are used from the back forward, with sections successively closed after use to allow for appropriate decomposition of waste. Hung sheets are sometimes employed as a modest effort to afford some privacy and to indicate to the user sections of the defecation field that remain open for use.

Pit latrines are another simple toileting option; however, their practicality is influenced by soil conditions and water table depth. Hard or rocky soil can make digging pit latrines extremely difficult. A shallow water table can result in contamination of natural water sources and restrict the maximum depth to which a latrine can be dug; the bottom of a pit latrine should be no closer than 1.5 m from the water table.[1] Ideally, pit latrines require periodic treatment with appropriate insecticides to prevent vector breeding. Additionally, latrines fitted with seating should have the means to place a lid over unused seats to further minimize vector breeding. Pit latrines should be closed and filled in with earth once the contents of the latrine reach 1 foot from ground level.

Burn barrels are sometimes used by military forces when establishing field activities. Burn-barrel latrines use 55-gallon drums cut in half to collect and burn human waste. Before use or reuse, a barrel is primed with approximately 3 inches of diesel fuel to ensure more efficient burning of solid waste, while also serving as an insect repellant. The contents of burn barrels are then burned when more than half full. A mixture of four parts diesel to one part gasoline should completely cover the barrel contents. Occasional stirring of the ignited contents is necessary but minimized with use of priming fuel. Successful use of burn barrels requires minimizing the urine content, to burn waste more efficiently and reduce fuel requirements.

As camps mature, transitioning to family- or community-level toileting options reduces the potential for exploitation of vulnerable persons and increases accountability for maintaining sanitary toileting facilities. As such, responders should strive for family toilets with one toilet per 20 people.[1] In situations where public toileting is the only option, approximately three women's facilities are recommended for every one men's facility.[1]

Waste Disposal

Field operations generate large amounts of waste products. Waste products may contain infectious agents such as cholera or typhoid; may attract dogs, birds, other wildlife, and vermin capable of spreading zoonotic disease; and can serve as breeding grounds for many vectors of human disease. As conditions permit, waste should be collected and disposed of in accordance with local, federal, or host nation law. Personnel responsible for the welfare of populations residing in field conditions must be familiar with basic principles of waste management and assure waste management is addressed in the planning stages of any field activity.

SOLID WASTE

Solid waste generated in field environments is disposed via burial, incineration, or commercial hauling. Burial is suitable only for short-term activities involving small numbers of people. Although commercial hauling for off-site disposal is greatly preferable, logistic or geopolitical realities often necessitate incineration of waste on site. Open burn pits are convenient for use when first establishing camps; however, attempts should be made to replace open burn pits with improved incineration techniques as soon as practical because of potential health risks associated with unimproved combustion of solid waste.

LIQUID WASTE

Proper management of liquid waste (gray water) is critical in camp settings, as improperly managed water waste generates mud or standing water, which greatly complicates daily life for camp inhabitants. Standing water also serves as a breeding ground for vectors and an attractant for vermin and other undesirable wildlife.

Waste water generated from field activities must be disposed of in accordance with applicable local, federal, and host nation laws. Use of municipal sanitary sewers is preferred but often unavailable in austere settings. When necessary, soakage pits and evaporation beds may be used to dispose of waste water without attracting vermin or serving as breeding pools for vectors. Soakage pits are simply pits filled with a coarse medium such as crushed gravel into which gray-water liquid waste is disposed. Soakage pits may become clogged or saturated over time, requiring the construction of additional soakage pits. Evaporation beds are contained fields of earth groomed into rows of depressions and ridges, similar to agricultural growing beds. The field is flooded to the top of the ridges and waste water is allowed to penetrate the soil and evaporate. A series of evaporation beds are used on a rotating basis to allow approximately 3 days of evaporation before the next use. To control mosquito populations, the height of evaporation bed ridges must not be constructed so high as to require more than 3 days for water to evaporate completely from the beds.

Vector Control

The existing burden of vector-borne disease already experienced by communities in low-resource settings is further exacerbated by disaster. Climate change further increases the likelihood of tempering environments previously inhospitable to arthropod vectors and spreading vector-borne disease to novel areas.[16] Although select diseases have effective vaccine or chemoprophylaxis measures, such measures are typically unaffordable or unavailable when performing fieldwork. Minimizing exposure to vectors remains the cornerstone of all vector-borne illness prevention.

Minimizing vector exposure begins with avoidance. Locations chosen for habitation in the field should consider the surrounding vector habitat. Whenever possible, sites for human habitation should be open, dry, and positioned away from local settlements, animal pens, or rodent burrows. Habitat denial measures should be taken to minimize vector burden. Camps should be cleared of unnecessary vegetation and waste should be disposed of in an orderly manner. All efforts should be made to minimize standing water and ensure appropriate physical measures are in place to minimize potential anthropogenic vector breeding habitats (i.e., using lids or screens on vessels containing or capable of collecting water).

Both the lifecycle and preferred feeding time of many arthropod vectors follow well-established seasonal, rainfall, and diurnal patterns. Minimizing outdoor exposure during peak biting periods can substantially decrease the likelihood of bites. Physical barriers such as appropriate long-sleeved clothing and use of insect screens or bed nets (if available) can substantially decrease exposure. Chemical repellants further augment bite avoidance; however, their availability is sometimes limited. Permethrin is typically the agent of choice for long-term treatment of clothing, bed nets, and some types of tent fabric.

Animals/Livestock

In addition to serving as sources of food and animal labor for agricultural activities, livestock in many developing countries also represent the net worth of individuals and families. In such environments, owners are extremely reluctant to be separated from animals that represent their financial security. When possible, consideration for providing a nearby secured area to maintain and graze livestock is important when establishing a camp.

Animals serve as important reservoirs or intermediate hosts for a variety of zoonotic diseases and enteric pathogens. As such, animal populations should be located outside of camp areas exclusively for human use and located an appropriate distance from housing, food storage and preparation, and human toileting areas to minimize potential for disease transmission. Animal waste contains a variety of pathogens, and appropriate care should be exercised to ensure animal waste does not contaminate sources of drinking water.

Surveillance

In clinical medicine, clinicians use patient history and physical examination to establish a diagnosis and formulate a plan of treatment. Field epidemiologists establish a community "diagnosis" for public health action by examining indicators to describe community health problems and guide a plan of action.[3] This process is known as public health surveillance (also called epidemiologic surveillance), defined as the ongoing, systematic collection, analysis, interpretation, and dissemination of health data to help guide public health decision-making and action.[4] Public health surveillance serves several critical functions for protecting and promoting the health of populations such as estimating the magnitude of a health problem; determining the geographic distribution of illness; portraying the natural history of disease(s); identifying cases for follow-up or contact tracing; detecting epidemics/defining the problem; generating hypotheses/stimulating research; evaluating control measures; monitoring changes in infectious agents; detecting changes in health practices; and facilitating planning.[5]

Public health surveillance can draw from a variety of data sources, including health surveys, registries of vital events such as births and deaths, medical and laboratory information systems, environmental monitoring systems, research studies, and other resources (Fig. 10.1).[6]

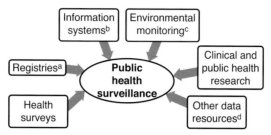

Fig. 10.1   Public health surveillance: data inputs. [a]Vital registration (e.g., births and deaths), cancer registries, and exposure registries. [b]Medical and laboratory records, pharmacy records. [c]Weather, climate, and pollution. [d]Criminal justice information, online databases and search engines, census. (Modified from Thacker, 2012.)[6]

THE SURVEILLANCE CYCLE AND REALITIES OF THE FIELD

Public health surveillance is an ongoing process in which the relevant data are systematically collected and analyzed, and then disseminated to those involved in disease control and public health decision-making, as part of a surveillance "cycle" (Fig. 10.2).[7]

Those deploying to field environments, especially those in resource-limited settings, may find many elements of this ideal surveillance cycle to be missing. Data collection may be inconsistent, substandard, or not exist at all; geographic, technological, and/or financial constraints may constrain collection, interpretation, and/or sharing of relevant health information; and acute stresses to the system (such as natural disasters or a propagating epidemic) may impair surveillance capacity. Even in the absence of an acute strain to the public health infrastructure, surveillance in resource-limited environments may differ from that in industrialized countries in at least three important ways: (1) more must be done with less; (2) strengthening surveillance is more complicated; and (3) sustainability is challenging.[8] Notwithstanding, the field epidemiologist can work with available resources following the same basic steps: identifying and collecting public health data, and communicating this information and its analysis to stakeholders to guide action and further inform data collection efforts. For example, one can use sick call logs as a rapid, readily available data collection resource.

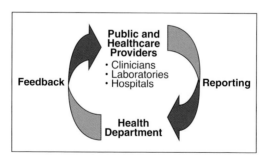

Fig. 10.2   The surveillance cycle: Surveillance information flows from public and healthcare providers, such as clinicians, laboratories, and hospitals and health departments. Feedback flows from health departments back to public and healthcare providers. (From Centers for Disease Control and Prevention (U.S.) Office of Workforce and Career Development. *Principles of Epidemiology in Public Health Practice: An Introduction to Applied Epidemiology and Biostatistics.* 2012. Available at: http://www.cdc.gov/ophss/csels/dsepd/SS1978/SS1978.pdf.)

TABLE 10.3 ■ Types of Information Relevant to Community Health Assessment

- General information
  - History, physical and climatic features of area, community organization, economic development, occupations, and organization of local government
  - Geographic distribution of villages and towns, major roads, important features such as rivers and mountains
- Population
  - Area's population size, age and sex structure, geographic distribution, migration patterns, and growth rate
- Health status, morbidity and mortality patterns
  - Demographic indices for birth and fertility rates and for maternal, infant, child, and overall mortality rates
  - Common causes of morbidity and mortality
  - Underlying health problems such as food availability, housing, water supply, and excreta disposal
- Health services
  - Number and distribution of governmental and nongovernmental facilities, personnel, and programs
  - Adequacy of management support, logistics, and supplies
- Area health programs
  - Pregnancy: antenatal, delivery, and postnatal care
  - Nutrition: growth monitoring and malnutrition
  - Environmental health: water supplies, excreta disposal, and hygiene
  - Communicable disease control: cases diagnosed and control activities

From Vaughan P, Morrow RH. *Manual of Epidemiology for District Health Management*. Geneva: World Health Organization; 1989.

COMMUNITY HEALTH ASSESSMENT

To assess the health of a population or a community, relevant data sources need to be identified for analysis by person, place, and time (descriptive epidemiology) to address questions such as, What are the actual and potential health problems in the community? Where are they occurring? Which populations are at increased risk? Which problems have declined over time? Which ones are increasing or have the potential to increase? How do these patterns relate to the level and distribution of public health services available?[7,9] Various types of information may be relevant (Table 10.3),[3] and ultimately, the decision about what data to collect depends on a host of factors, including what objective(s) are sought, what health information is already available, what resources can be committed to surveillance, and—just as importantly—terms of reference with local, regional, and/or national health authorities.

DISEASE REPORTING AND OUTBREAK DETECTION

Detecting disease outbreaks—the occurrence of more disease cases than expected—is perhaps the best-recognized objective of public health surveillance; notwithstanding, many outbreaks may go undetected, even in environments with robust surveillance.[7] Opportunities to uncover an outbreak include: (1) reviewing routinely collected surveillance data (if any); (2) astute observation of single events or clusters by clinicians, infection control practitioners, or laboratory personnel; and (3) reviewing reports by one or more patients or members of the public.[7] To facilitate early detection of outbreaks, mandatory reporting has been instituted for certain diseases or events. The 2005 International Health Regulations (IHR) framework, the only binding international agreement on disease control, requires countries to report certain diseases and public health events of international concern (PHEICs) to the World Health Organization (WHO).[8,10] Under IHR, WHO

TABLE 10.4 ■ **Reportable Public Health Events to the World Health Organization Under the International Health Regulations**

Always Notifiable	Other Potentially Notifiable Events
• Smallpox • Poliomyelitis attributed to wild-type poliovirus • Human influenza caused by a new subtype • Severe acute respiratory syndrome (SARS)	• May include cholera, pneumonic plague, yellow fever, viral hemorrhagic fever, and West Nile fever, and any others that meet International Health Regulations (IHR) criteria • Other biological, radiological, or chemical events meeting IHR criteria

From U.S. Centers for Disease Control and Prevention (12 May 2017) Frequently Asked Questions about the International Health Regulations (IHR). Available at https://www.cdc.gov/globalhealth/healthprotection/ghs/ihr/ihr-faq.html. Accessed 14 Jan 2021.

declares a PHEIC if at least two of the following four criteria are met: (1) the event has a serious public health impact; (2) the event is unusual or unexpected; (3) there is risk of international spread; and/or (4) there is risk of international trade or travel restrictions.[11] Some diseases always require reporting under the IHR, no matter when or where they occur, whereas others become notifiable when they represent an unusual risk or situation (Table 10.4).[10–13] From 2005 through 2016, WHO declared four PHEICs: H1N1 influenza (2009), polio (2014), Ebola (2014), and Zika virus (2016).[12]

In the field, one may encounter additional disease reporting requirements, such as those mandated by local, regional, or national public health authorities, and/or the military.[14,15]

Outbreak Investigation

PURSUING THE INVESTIGATION

An outbreak of disease is a number of cases in excess of an expected baseline. After detecting the presence of an outbreak, the decision must be made about whether to prioritize control measures or pursue further investigation. Generally, if the source or mode of transmission is known, then control measures that target the source or interrupt transmission can be implemented. If the source or mode of transmission is not known, then one cannot know what control measures to implement, so investigation takes priority.[7,16] Additionally, the severity of the illness, the potential for spread, political considerations, public relations, available resources, and other factors all influence the decision to launch a field investigation.[7]

INVESTIGATION COMPONENTS

Once the decision to conduct an outbreak investigation has been made, a systematic approach to proceeding is recommended (Box 10.1); depending on the outbreak, the investigation steps are adjusted.[7,17] It is important to note, even though the following components are presented in a stepwise fashion, it is often necessary to perform several components simultaneously.

By definition, an outbreak is a number of cases of disease in excess of anticipated baseline values. In determining whether the number of reported cases constitutes more than expected, one must attempt to contextualize the cases of reported disease. In outbreaks, the cases are usually presumed to have a common cause or to be related to one another in some way. Some disease clusters are true outbreaks with a common cause, some are sporadic and unrelated cases of the same disease, and some are unrelated cases of similar but unrelated diseases.[7] Incorrect diagnosis, faulty

> **BOX 10.1 ■ Components of an Outbreak Investigation**
>
> 1. Establish the existence of an outbreak
> 2. Prepare for fieldwork
> 3. Verify the diagnosis
> 4. Construct a working case definition
> 5. Find cases systematically and record information
> 6. Perform descriptive epidemiology
> 7. Develop hypotheses
> 8. Evaluate hypotheses epidemiologically. As necessary, reconsider, refine, and reevaluate hypotheses
> 9. Compare and reconcile with laboratory and/or environmental studies
> 10. Implement control and prevention measures
> 11. Initiate or maintain surveillance
> 12. Communicate findings

reporting, lack of baseline data, or sporadic surveillance occasionally result in the initial appearance of an outbreak where none actually exist—a phenomenon known as a pseudo-outbreak.

Preparing for a field investigation demands not only scientific and investigative preparation but also administrative and operational coordination. Understanding what is known about similar outbreaks and how to go about achieving the research objectives is important; however, understanding roles, communication strategy, logistics, and securing a plan for action are also critical for performing a successful investigation.[7]

Verifying the diagnosis is often done in tandem with establishing the existence of an outbreak. Investigators often review clinical findings and laboratory results; talk with one or more patients with the disease, elucidate clinical features, risk factors for illness, and the patient's understanding of possible cause(s); and summarize the clinical features using frequency distributions to help characterize the spectrum of illness, establish the credibility of the diagnosis (i.e., whether the clinical features are consistent with the purported diagnosis), and inform the refinement of case definitions.[7]

To construct a working case definition, one must identify a standard set of criteria for deciding whether an individual should be classified as having the health condition of interest.[7] Four typical elements of a case definition include: (1) clinical information about the disease (what signs and symptoms have been observed?); (2) characteristics about the persons who are affected (do any commonalities exist among those who have been ill?); (3) information about the location or place (where are the persons located?); and (4) specification of time during which the illness onset occurred (what place or time did the illness begin to occur, and how long did the symptoms last?). During an outbreak, case definitions often evolve, typically becoming more specific as additional information becomes available. Investigators sometimes create different categories of a case definition, such as confirmed, probable, and possible or suspect, to accommodate uncertainty. Usually, cases are confirmed if indicated by laboratory testing, probable if having typical clinical features of the disease without laboratory confirmation, and possible if all that is present are a few of the typical clinical features.[7]

Because only a small number of possible cases may be reported, it is important to find cases systematically, to ensure the complete burden and spectrum of disease is captured in the investigation. Usually, the first effort to identify cases is directed at healthcare practitioners and facilities where a diagnosis is likely to be made. Investigators may conduct what is sometimes called sentinel or enhanced passive surveillance by contacting these sources by mail and asking for reports of similar cases. Alternatively, they may conduct active surveillance by telephoning or visiting the facilities to collect information on any additional cases.[7] In the field, and especially in low-resource settings, determining when and where cases occurred will frequently require the ingenuity and assistance of local political, religious, cultural, and government authorities.[9] Essential to field surveillance efforts is striving to record information effectively, such as by abstracting selected critical items onto a form called a line listing.[7] Data collection is detailed elsewhere in this chapter.

After identifying and gathering basic information on the persons with the disease, investigators describe some of the key characteristics of those persons. This process, in which the outbreak is characterized by time, place, and person, is called descriptive epidemiology. It may be repeated or refined several times during the course of an investigation as additional cases are identified or as new information becomes available.[7] Visually depicting the time course of an epidemic is often helpful; an epidemic curve provides a sample visual display of the outbreak's magnitude and time trend. Additionally, epidemic curves (also called epi curves) can help classify outbreaks according to their manner of spread through a population. In a common-source outbreak (Fig. 10.3), a group of persons is exposed to an infectious agent or a toxin from the same source. Common-source outbreaks may further be classified according to whether persons have been exposed for a relatively short time within an incubation period (point-source outbreak); whether the case-patients have been exposed for a long duration (continuous common-source outbreak); or whether sporadic exposures over time have occurred (intermittent common-source outbreak). Other types of outbreak patterns discernible from epi curves include the propagated outbreak, where person-to-person transmission has resulted in increasing numbers of cases in each subsequent incubation period. In addition, mixed types of outbreaks can occur, containing features of both common-source and propagated outbreaks.[7]

Experienced investigators develop hypotheses and reconsider, refine, and reevaluate hypotheses throughout the outbreak investigation process. This process is informed by the data collection and analysis, and also serves as a discrete opportunity to compare and reconcile findings with laboratory and environmental studies when such resources are available.

The decision to implement control and prevention measures should be undertaken as early in the investigation process as possible. As mentioned earlier, once the source or mode of transmission is known, efforts to interrupt transmission can be implemented—sometimes even before an investigation is launched. For example, a child with measles in a community with other susceptible children may prompt a vaccination campaign before an investigation of how that child became infected.[7]

Initiating or maintaining surveillance is crucial to investigators who wish to monitor the situation and help determine whether control measures are working. Surveillance can identify whether the outbreak has spread, affording implementation of additional prevention and control efforts if required.[7] Surveillance also serves as the foundation for establishing the baseline rate of disease—a fundamental piece of information for determining the existence of future outbreaks.

To communicate findings in an effective way, one must develop an effective risk communication plan to relevant stakeholders. Additionally, briefings or reports should be provided to local authorities and other public health professionals to convey critical findings and lessons learned.[7] Principles of good risk communication are discussed later in this chapter.

General Epidemiologic Principles

"Epidemiology" is the study of the five "W"s (what, who, when, where, and why) as they relate to a population and disease:
- What: the disease (i.e., etiology)
- Who: demographics (e.g., sex, age)
- When: timing of exposure and disease onset
- Where: environment of exposure
- Why: risk factors and exposures

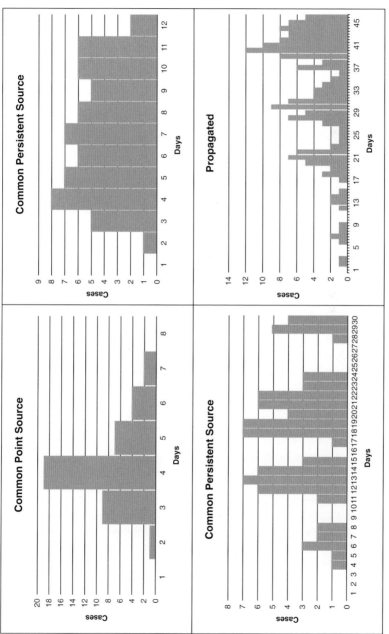

Fig. 10.3 Typical epi curves for different types of spread.

An epidemiologist studies the relationships between these five "W"s. The goal of most epidemiologic investigations is to better define one or more of the five "W"s, to most effectively allocate resources. The public health decisions based on epidemiologic investigations can have life or death implications; therefore, the data must be as accurate as possible. "Bias" is a systematic error that occurs during an epidemiologic investigation that can skew the results and occur at any stage of an epidemiologic investigation. Common types of bias include selection bias, recall bias, confounding, and random error.[18] It is nearly impossible to eliminate all sources of bias from an epidemiologic investigation. Instead, an epidemiologist aims to reduce bias as much as possible. This process starts with selecting a study design most appropriate to answer an investigator's key questions. The two most common epidemiologic study designs are a cohort study and a case-control study.[18]

COHORT STUDY

A cohort study is useful for identifying potential health outcomes that result from known exposures. In a cohort study, a group of individuals who share a set of common characteristics (i.e., a cohort) are followed for a given period of time to determine whether or not they acquire one or more health outcomes of interest. Follow-up can range from days to years. For example, a cohort might be defined as all refugees living in Turkey in September 2015; all children born to human immunodeficiency virus (HIV)-infected mothers during 2016 in Lusaka, Zambia; or all individuals who were displaced by 2015 Typhoon Koppu in the Philippines.

Cohort studies can be prospective or retrospective. Prospective cohort studies are typically resource intensive because they require first assembling a cohort, and then following the cohort population for months or years after a discrete exposure to identify potential outcomes. Retrospective cohorts use preexisting data and look back in time to determine who was exposed. A retrospective cohort study typically requires fewer resources, although it can be more prone to bias and exposure misclassification.

A cohort study usually requires more resources than a case-control study because it involves following individuals over time. Thus, they are usually more feasible for studying health outcomes that are common and/or that have a relatively short incubation period (i.e., the period of time from exposure to symptom manifestation).

CASE-CONTROL STUDY

In a case-control study, individuals who have acquired a particular health outcome (i.e., cases) are compared with individuals who have not acquired the health outcome (i.e., controls) to identify risk factors. A case-control study is usually employed when there is a single disease of interest and when multiple potential risk factors are being examined.

A case-control study usually takes fewer resources than a cohort study, and it can be used for studying rare diseases or diseases with a relatively long incubation period. However, it is more prone to bias than a cohort study. The largest source of bias in a case-control study comes from the selection of controls.

The ideal control group is selected in such a way that if the control had acquired the disease of interest, they would have been in the group of cases being studied. This means that the control group arises from the same population as the cases. For example, if you are studying risk factors for trachoma (i.e., a bacterial infection of the eyes that can cause scarring and blindness) in Nepal, and if your cases are individuals of any age who present to a particular Nepalese hospital with trachoma-induced corneal scarring, then you would want to identify controls who fall within that hospital's catchment area and who would have presented to that hospital if they had developed trachoma-induced corneal scarring. This means accounting not only for the geographic region/

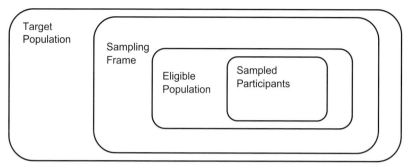

Fig. 10.4   The sequentially selective process of sampling.

catchment area but also for other factors such as socioeconomic status, insurance status, and access to transportation.

SAMPLING

Sampling is the scientific process of selecting participants for an epidemiologic investigation. To find participants, the investigator first identifies a target population for study. Within this population an investigator identifies a sampling frame; common sampling frames include a census, hospital records, and telephone directory. Ideal sampling frames capture as much of the target population as possible, while minimizing the capture of individuals outside the target population. Once a sampling frame has been determined, the investigators identify an eligible population, individuals from the sampling frame who meet certain eligibility criteria such as specific clinical or demographic characteristics. After applying inclusion and exclusion criteria, investigators arrive at the sampled participants, individuals from the eligible population who are selected, meet the eligibility criteria, can be contacted/reached, and agree to participate. Fig. 10.4 outlines the sequentially selective process of selecting a sample representative of a larger population.

SELECTION BIAS

Selection bias occurs when the sampled participants are not an accurate representation of the target population. Sampling bias can occur at any stage of the sampling process. For example, if a refugee who was sick upon entering the camp was more likely to go straight to the medical ward and skip the registration tent, then this means that the sampling frame might be less likely to include cholera patients compared with the target population. If a member of the eligible population is too weak to participate in the investigation, then the sampled participants would be less likely to have cholera compared with the target population.

SAMPLING METHODS

Three common sampling methods employed by epidemiologists are simple random sampling, cluster sampling, and stratified sampling.[19]

Simple random sampling means sampling participants completely at random from the sampling frame. For example, if the sampling frame (such as a list of names from a health clinic) is enumerated, a simple random sample could be performed by utilizing statistical software to generate random numbers that correspond to the enumerated individuals. Statistically, this sampling method will yield results that are more precise than cluster sampling or stratified sampling.

However, simple random sampling can be more resource intensive if the team needs to travel to a different location for each participant.

Cluster sampling involves breaking the target population into clusters. Ideally, clusters are formed such that individuals within a cluster are relatively homogenous but clusters are relatively heterogeneous from each other. For example, clusters might be neighborhood wards or hospital wings. Once clusters are formed, a predetermined number of clusters are randomly selected, and then a predetermined number of individuals within the chosen clusters are randomly selected. Results yielded from cluster sampling become more precise, as the within-cluster variation becomes smaller with respect to the between-cluster variation. Cluster sampling can be the least resource-intensive method, as it usually involves the least amount of travel.

Stratified sampling involves breaking the target population into strata and randomly selecting participants within each stratum. In contrast with cluster sampling, strata are formed to be different from each other. For example, strata could be income tertiles or disease severity. Participants are subsequently randomly selected from each stratum.

SAMPLE SIZE CALCULATION

Before beginning an epidemiologic investigation, investigators must decide how many individuals to include. As sample size increases, the results will become more precise, which will increase the likelihood of identifying statistically significant differences and answering objectives. However, as the number of participants increases, so does the amount of time, personnel, and resources required to conduct the investigation.

There are online resources available to assist in the calculation of the idea sample size.[20] These formulas take into account factors such as how big a difference is expected between cases and controls (or between exposed and unexposed participants).

EXISTING DATA

There are sometimes data available to responders to assist with an investigation. These include surveillance data, hospital/clinic records, and vital statistics. When planning to use existing data, such as data abstracted from hospital or clinical records, a data abstraction form can be developed to ensure data are collected systematically.

Data Collection

The key data collection tool employed during an epidemiologic investigation is the questionnaire. The questionnaire content should be driven by the investigation's objectives. The questionnaire should be as brief as possible while still collecting the necessary information.

Keep questions as specific as possible, and define all terms. For example, if a question asks about diarrheal illness, the questionnaire might need to include a definition of "diarrheal illness." For example, does it mean the passage of three or more loose or liquid stools per day, stools that are looser than usual for the participant, or something else? Time periods should also be specific. For example, "between the hours of 6 am to noon" is more precise than "morning."

Questions can be open-ended or closed-ended. An open-ended question allows the participant to answer freely: "Describe what you ate yesterday." A closed-ended question requires the participant to choose from a list of predefined answer options: "Did you eat chicken yesterday? (Yes/No/Don't remember)." Open-ended questions are typically used when investigators want to cast a broad net and collect as much data as possible, and they are sometimes more useful at the start of the investigation, when little is known.

Avoid double-barreled questions, which combine two questions. For example: "Did you take malaria prophylaxis and do you think it helped?" is a double-barreled question. If both of these questions are important to ask, then it should be restated as two questions: "Did you take malaria prophylaxis?" and "If you took malaria prophylaxis, do you think it helped?"

Once a draft questionnaire is developed, pilot test the questionnaire in the target population to make sure the questions are understood and correctly interpreted, and make sure the answer choices are comprehensive enough and appropriate.

Recall bias is a systematic bias in the way that cases answer a question compared with controls (or exposed participants vs. unexposed participants). For example, cases might be more likely to recall incidental exposures than controls, because they may have spent more time thinking about the days leading to their illness and analyzing where they went and what they did. Controls, however, would have had little reason for such self-reflection. Recall bias can be minimized by including cues in your questionnaire to facilitate recall of recent events. For example, if asking a control about what they ate three days previously, an investigator might ask the participant to describe their day and to remember where they went and who they spent time with.

DATA ENTRY

After administering questionnaires and collecting data, the data need to be entered into a database so that they can be analyzed. There are multiple software programs available that can be used for data entry. The simplest database is a two-dimensional spreadsheet, with each observation in a row and each variable in a column.

Data entry errors are easy to make and can cause erroneous results. All data entry should be double-checked. One method is to enter each observation twice. The two sets of observations can be compared with each other, and any discrepancies reviewed and corrected. Another method is to have one person enter the data, and then have a second person review a percentage of the observations for accuracy (typically around 10%).

Data Analysis
DESCRIPTIVE ANALYSES

Descriptive analyses describe the data. Common descriptive analyses include calculating ranges, medians, means, and standard deviations for continuous variables (i.e., variables that can have any value between two endpoints, such as age and height) and calculating frequencies for categorical variables (i.e., variables where the answer options are discrete categories, such as race and sex).

Common descriptive analyses include the following[21]:

- Attack rate: the proportion of exposed individuals who developed the outcome. It is commonly expressed as a percentage and is performed most commonly during an outbreak investigation to determine which exposures/risk factors are most strongly associated with the illness.

$$\text{Attack Rate} = \frac{\#\text{ exposed individuals developing health outcome}}{\#\text{ exposed individuals}}$$

- Incidence: The rate of new cases of an illness over a period of time. Incidence is always described with a time component.

$$\text{Incidence Rate} = \frac{\#\text{ new cases of disease}}{\#\text{ of people in population} * \text{length of time}}$$

- Prevalence: the proportion of individuals who have a particular disease at any one point in time. It is expressed as a percentage.

$$\text{Prevalence} = \frac{\text{\# cases of disease}}{\text{\# of people in population}}$$

ANALYTIC ANALYSES

Analytic analyses usually involve comparing exposures and risk factors between one or more groups. For example, if there is an outbreak of sudden severe, neurologic illness, investigators might want to compare exposures (drinking from well A) and risk factors (e.g., age, sex) between cases and controls, to identify the source of the exposure.

The type of comparisons that can be performed depends on the type of variable. For continuous variables, common analyses include the calculation of means and medians and use of t-tests. For categorical variables, common analyses include calculating chi-square values, odds ratios, and risk ratios. Risk ratios are used to analyze data collected during a cohort study; odds ratios are used to analyze data collected during a case-control study.[21]

	Case	Control	Total
Exposed	a	b	a + b
Not exposed	c	d	c + d
Total	a + c	b + d	a + b + c + d

$$\text{Risk Ratio} = \frac{\text{Risk among exposed}}{\text{Risk among unexposed}} = \frac{a/(a+b)}{c/(c+d)}$$

$$\text{Odds Ratio} = \frac{\text{Odds of exposure among cases}}{\text{Odds of exposure among controls}} = \frac{a/c}{b/d} = \frac{ad}{bc}$$

One common issue in epidemiologic analyses is confounding. Confounding occurs when a third variable is related to both the exposure and the outcome. For example, suppose you are investigating an outbreak of sudden severe, neurologic illness. Based on your descriptive analyses, drinking from well A seemed to be most strongly associated with exposure, with an odds ratio of 13.2.

	Case	Control	Total
Exposed	34	18	52
Not exposed	6	42	48
Total	40	60	100

$$\text{Odds Ratio} = \frac{\text{Odds of exposure among cases}}{\text{Odds of exposure among controls}} = \frac{34/6}{18/42} = \frac{34*42}{18*6} = 13.2$$

However, well A is near a school, and thus many of the participants who reported drinking from well A were children (i.e., age is related to the exposure). Children can be more susceptible to many illnesses (i.e., age might be related to the outcome). You would like to see if the relationship between case status and exposure is confounded by age. An analysis that controls for confounding is called an "adjusted analysis." In this scenario, we want to compare the age-adjusted odds ratio to the unadjusted odds ratio of 13.2.

In the simplest of scenarios, this can be performed by hand. However, in most cases, it is more feasible to conduct such analyses with statistical software. To perform the analysis by hand, we first look at the stratum-specific odds ratios. If the odds ratios are very different from one another, then interaction is present, and this must be dealt with. The topic of interaction is beyond this book, but more can be read in Rothman.[18]

CHILDREN

	Case	Control	Total
Exposed	25	5	35
Not exposed	5	15	15
Total	30	20	50

Odds ratio = 15.0

ADULTS

	Case	Control	Total
Exposed	8	9	17
Not exposed	2	31	33
Total	10	40	50

Odds ratio = 13.8

Here, the stratum-specific odds ratios of 15.0 and 13.8 are not too different, and thus one might decide that there is little interaction and proceed to calculate an adjusted odds ratio. One common adjusted odds ratio is the Mantel-Haenszel adjusted odds ratio.

$$\text{Adjusted Odds Ratio} = \frac{\dfrac{(25*15)}{50} + \dfrac{(8*31)}{50}}{\dfrac{(5*5)}{50} + \dfrac{(9*2)}{50}} = \frac{7.5 + 4.96}{0.5 + 0.36} = 14.5$$

In this scenario, the adjusted odds ratio of 14.5 would be reported.

Decision-Making

INTERPRETING RESULTS

Conducting a sound epidemiologic study will provide you with data upon which to make an informed decision. When trying to interpret the results of an epidemiologic investigation to make a decision about how to prevent future cases, there are three things that you will want to look at: (1) the strength of the association; (2) the results of the statistical hypothesis testing; and (3) biological plausibility. These three things taken together will help you to make a logical decision on what may have caused the outbreak.[22]

For example, let us look at an investigation of an epidemic of aflatoxicosis poisoning. Aflatoxin is a fungal toxin that can grow on maize and peanuts; when ingested in large amounts, it can cause liver failure, sometimes leading to death. You conducted an investigation, and you found that cases had a 3.5-times higher odds of eating maize flour from a particular producer, compared with controls. The first thing to look at is the strength of the association (in this case, the odds ratio). As the odds ratio increases, it becomes more suggestive that a particular exposure is truly associated with the illness. An odds ratio of 3.0 would be more compelling than an odds ratio of 1.2. In this example, an odds ratio of 3.5 would likely be considered fairly suggestive of a true association.

The second thing to look at is the result of the statistical hypothesis testing. Analytical data analyses will produce statistical estimates, such as p-values. A p-value is a number that ranges from 0 to 1, and it can be interpreted as the likelihood that the results seen in your investigation are a result of chance. A p-value that is closer to 0 indicates a stronger likelihood that there is a true association. Investigators will sometimes use a value of 0.05 as a cut-off, with p-values below 0.05 considered to be statistically significant. However, prudence is needed to not immediately discard a result with a p-value above 0.05. A p-value can be influenced by several factors, including sample size, and an investigation with a small sample size might not produce statistically significant results. If the p-value with the scenario above is 0.09, the investigators might still consider this suggestive of a true association.

Finally, investigators will want to look at biological plausibility. In other words, does it seem possible that the exposure caused the disease? In this example, because maize is a common source of aflatoxin exposure, it seems plausible. If the risk factor does not seem plausible, then the association might have been attributed to chance, or unmeasured confounding, or it could be a related factor. For example, in this example, if cases had a 4.0-times higher odds of attending school compared with controls, it might be that the exposure is occurring at school, or it might be that attending school is a proxy for the real association, such as being a child.

INTERVENTION

The end result of an epidemiologic investigation is to identify the cause or risk factors for illness to implement an intervention to reduce further risk. To do this, it is necessary to review the data interpretation with the key stakeholders and with those who most closely understand the population, to determine what type of intervention is feasible and appropriate. For example, in the above scenario, investigators might initially decide that the best course of action is to remove the implicated food product. However, it is possible that this might be the only food product available to the population, and removing the food product might cause more harm than good. In that case, they might work with local stakeholders to arrive at an alternative solution; in this case, perhaps they decide to mix the implicated food source with a safer food source, thereby reducing the dose of aflatoxin to below the toxic threshold, while still ensuring that enough food is available to eat.

Risk Communication

Communication during a public health crisis is different than routine communication. During a crisis, there can be emotional angst and outrage that may cause the public to perceive the risk as being much higher than the actual risk. Messages need to be simplified, and communication needs to be timely and frequent. Having a communication plan incorporated into the overall response plan is key.

There are six principles of crisis emergency risk communication[23]:

1. Be First. Crises are time sensitive, and the agency that gets the message out there first might be the most heard and accepted.

2. **Be Right.** The message should include three components: what is known, what is not known, and what is being done to address the situation and fill in the gaps.
3. **Be Credible.** Only provide facts in the communication. Do not speculate, and do not promise what cannot be delivered. If nothing is known, then state that nothing is known and explain what is being done.
4. **Express Empathy.** Empathy ("I understand there may be anger that this occurred and worry about what this means for your health") should not be confused with sympathy ("We feel sorry for you"). Empathy builds trust with the community. To be empathetic, it is important to choose the right spokesperson. The best spokesperson is not necessarily the person who is most knowledgeable or who is leading the response. Rather, the best spokesperson is the person who can best empathize with the community and those affected.
5. **Promote Action.** Providing an action can calm anxiety and restore a sense of control. People like to have something to do, and if an appropriate action is not suggested, then they might take an inappropriate action. Action steps should be provided as positives (e.g., "Drink only bottled water") rather than negatives (e.g., "Avoid drinking water from the faucet").
6. **Show Respect.** Respect is especially important when people feel vulnerable, and showing respect will promote cooperation within the community. Never use humor in the message.

Messages can be delivered to the public through a variety of channels, including a television interview, press releases, press conferences, websites, and social media. Regardless of the venue, a media interview or a press release should be practiced and prepared for in a similar fashion to a presentation. First, identify your audience. Then, determine what information can and cannot be shared. Messages delivered during a crisis must be short and to the point, and they will be most effective if they are repeated. The communication will be most effective if it is reduced to no more than four key messages (ideally two to three key messages). Finally, the spokesperson should practice and be prepared to answer common questions, such as the following: "Are my family and I safe?"; "What can I do to protect myself and my family?"; "Who is in charge?"; "Why did this happen?".

References

1. Sphere Project. *Sphere Handbook: Humanitarian Charter and Minimum Standards in Disaster Response.* 2011 Edition: Sphere Project; 2011. Available at: http://www.sphereproject.org.
2. Perrin P. *War and Public Health: Handbook on War and Public Health.* International Committee of the Red Cross; 1996. Available at: https://www.icrc.org/en/publication/0641-war-and-public-health-handbook-war-and-public-health.
3. Vaughan P, Morrow RH. *Manual of Epidemiology for District Health Management.* Geneva: World Health Organization; 1989.
4. German RR, Lee LM, Horan JM, et al. Updated guidelines for evaluating public health surveillance systems: recommendations from the Guidelines Working Group. *MMWR Recomm Rep.* 2001;50 (RR-13):1–35.
5. Lee LM, St. Louis ME, Teutsch SM, Thacker SB. *Principles and Practice of Public Health Surveillance.* 3rd ed. New York, NY: Oxford University Press; 2010.
6. Thacker SB, Qualters JR, Lee LM. Public health surveillance in the United States: evolution and challenges. *MMWR Surveill Summ.* 2012;61(suppl):3–9. https://www.cdc.gov/mmwr/preview/mmwrhtml/su6103a2.htm.
7. Centers for Disease Control and Prevention (U.S.) Office of Workforce and Career Development. *Principles of Epidemiology in Public Health Practice. An Introduction to Applied Epidemiology and Biostatistics;* 2012. Available at: http://www.cdc.gov/ophss/csels/dsepd/SS1978/SS1978.pdf.
8. St Louis M. Global health surveillance. *MMWR Suppl.* 2012;61:15–19.
9. Gregg MB. *Field Epidemiology.* 3rd ed. New York, NY: Oxford University Press; 2008.
10. World Health Organization. *Strengthening Health Security by Implementing the International Health Regulations;* 2005. Available at: http://www.who.int/ihr/about/en/. Accessed February 12, 2017.
11. Heymann DL. Association. *Control of Communicable Diseases Manual.* 20th ed. Washington, DC: American Public Health; 2015.

12. Centers for Disease Control and Prevention (U.S.) Center for Global Health. Global Health Security: International Health Regulations. (2012, August 19). Accessed January 17, 2016. Atlanta, Georgia, USA: U.S. Department of Health and Human Services. https://www.cdc.gov/globalhealth/healthprotection/ghs/ihr/index.html.

13. Centers for Disease Control and Prevention (U.S.) Center for Global Health (2015). What diseases are notifiable as a potential public health emergency of international concern (PHEIC) under the IHR? Frequently Asked Questions about the International Health Regulations (IHR). (2017, May 12). Accessed January 17, 2015. Atlanta, Georgia, USA: U.S. Department of Health and Human Services. https://www.cdc.gov/globalhealth/healthprotection/ghs/ihr/ihr-faq.html.

14. Centers for Disease Control and Prevention (U.S.), Office of Public Health Scientific Services Division of Health Informatics and Surveillance (2016). *2020 National Notifiable Conditions. (n.d.).* 2016. Accessed January 17, 2021. Atlanta, Georgia, USA: U.S. Department of Health and Human Services. https://wwwn.cdc.gov/nndss/conditions/notifiable/2020/.

15. Department of Defense (U.S.) AFHSC. Armed Forces Reportable Medical Event Guidelines & Case Definitions. Reports and Publications (n.d.). Accessed January 17, 2012. Silver Spring, Maryland, USA: U.S. Department of Defense. https://health.mil/Military-Health-Topics/Combat-Support/Armed-Forces-Health-Surveillance-Branch/Reports-and-Publications.

16. Goodman RA, Buehler JW, Koplan JP. The epidemiologic field investigation: science and judgment in public health practice. *Am J Epidemiol.* 1990;132:9–16.

17. Centers for Disease Control and Prevention (U.S.), Office of Public Health Scientific Services Division of Scientific Education and Professional Development. Public Health 101 Series, CDC. Introduction to Public Health Surveillance. Accessed January 17, 2021. Atlanta, Georgia, USA: U.S. Department of Health and Human Services. https://www.cdc.gov/training/publichealth101/index.html.

18. Rothman KJ. *Epidemiology: An Introduction.* New York: Oxford University Press; 2002.

19. Herold JM. Surveys and sampling. In: Gregg M, ed. *Field Epidemiology.* 3rd ed. New York: Oxford University Press; 2008:97–117.

20. Dean A, Sullivan K, Soe M. *OpenEpi: Open Source Epidemiologic Statistics for Public Health*; 2011. Available at: www.OpenEpi.com.

21. Centers for Disease Control and Prevention. *Principles of Epidemiology in Public Health Practice.* 3rd ed. Atlanta, GA: Centers for Disease Control and Prevention; 2012 https://www.cdc.gov/csels/dsepd/ss1978/ss1978.pdf.

22. Dicker R. Analyzing and interpreting data. In: Gregg M, ed. *Field Epidemiology.* 3rd ed. New York: Oxford University Press; 2008:199–236.

23. Centers for Disease Control and Prevention. *Crisis and Emergency Risk Communication.* CERC Manual. Atlanta, GA: Centers for Disease Control and Prevention; 2018. Accessed January 17, 2021. https://emergency.cdc.gov/cerc/manual/index.asp.

CHAPTER 11

Refugees and Internally-Displaced Persons

Rahma Aburas

Background

- Refugee (based on the 1951 Convention's Article One): an individual, who, because of actual and present fear of hostility and treatment, as a result of his/her ethnic group, religious belief, nationality, association with a specific social group, or views in politics, finds him/herself outside his/her country of origin or nationality, and, as such, fails to or is reluctant to avail of the said country's protection.[1]
- Internally displaced individual: a person with no other course but to flee the home or city they reside in to avert the impact of armed conflicts and generalized conditions of violence, human rights violations, or disasters that are either man-made or natural. By definition, internally displaced individuals have not stepped beyond internationally recognized borders of their state.[2]
- There are an unprecedented 65.6 million individuals all over the world today who have been forced out of their homes.
  - This includes almost 22.5 million refugees, of whom more than 50% are younger than 18 years[3]; they are especially vulnerable to exploitation.[4]
  - Adolescents are more likely to be victimized by armed conflict and without support than younger children, particularly with respect to child labor, sexual violence/exploitation, and forced combatant status. They are often denied basic education and experience sexual violence and exploitation.[2,5,6]
  - Many youth suffer posttraumatic stress disorder (PTSD), depression, and anxiety.[7]
- Case study: Syrian Civil War
  - Majority of citizens displaced.[8]
  - About 75% of Syrian refugees are women and children.[9]
  - According to the United Nations (UN), around 70,000 pregnant women run the risk of giving birth in unsafe conditions if further assistance is not extended to them.[10]
  - Some 80% (8.4 million) are Syrian child refugees or internally displaced persons (IDPs).

TABLE 11.1 ■ **Classification of the Principle Challenges Confronting Internally Displaced Persons/ Refugee Children**

Acute Emergency Situation	Subsequent Postemergency Phase
1. Physical and mental trauma	1. Restricted access to health care
2. Need for safe shelters	2. Outbreak of vaccine-preventable diseases such as poliomyelitis and measles
3. Need for food and clean water	3. Restricted access to education
4. Disrupted families, and loss of family members	4. Malnutrition
5. Need for health care including immunizations	5. Child labor
	6. Mental health issues
	7. Exposure to physical and sexual violence
	8. Other difficulties, for example, disrupted families and poor living conditions

- Majority refugees/IDPs are under 18 years old, 40% under 12 years old.[11]
- Some estimate that between 2011 and 2017, over 18,000 children were killed.[12]
- Refugee/IDP children are at higher risk than adults of physical and mental trauma, and lack of safe shelter, clean water, and food.
- Poor nutrition and health care present major threats.[13]
- Routine immunization unavailable to 33% of children under 5 years old; resulted in resurgence of measles and meningitis.[14]
- Polio had been eradicated from Syria in 1995, but returned; indeed, up to 80,000 children in Syria are thought to be carriers.[15]
- Access to education decreased; more than 4000 assaults on schools recorded.
- Half of school-age children not enrolled in school in the 2014–2015 school year.[16]

Table 11.1 shows acute emergency situations and the subsequent postemergency phase.

1. Restricted access to health care
   a. Up to 200,000 pediatric deaths have been attributed to lack of access to medical care in Syria.[17]
   b. Although many welcoming countries offer in principle some medical screening upon arrival, impact is often minimal because of poor quality or delay[18] (Table 11.2).
2. Outbreak of vaccine-preventable diseases and tuberculosis
   a. War and natural disasters increase risk for certain diseases and infection caused by degradation of infrastructure and immunization programs.
   b. In Syria, vaccination rates decreased from 91% to 45% between 2010 and 2013 in some places.
   c. Some 58% of 1.8 million children born in Syria are not vaccinated.[15]
   d. Immunization campaign efficacy is often impaired because of risks to volunteers in war zones.[18]
3. Restricted access to education
   a. Entire generations of refugee children from countries like Syria, Afghanistan, Palestine, and South Sudan have had to leave their homes and schools.[19]
   b. Recent UN High Commissioner for Refugees (UNHCR) data estimate that worldwide, 50% of primary school-age refugee children are out of school and 75% of adolescent refugees at the secondary education level are out of school. Refugee children and adolescents are five times more likely to be out of school than their nonrefugee peers.[19]

TABLE 11.2 ■ **Factors Related to Restricted Access to Effective Healthcare Acces**

	Internally Displaced Persons	Refugees
1.	Loss of healthcare personnel; in Syria, for example, about 160 doctors were killed and many more jailed, which resulted in about 80,000 doctors moving to other counties	Poor quality of screening programs
2.	Destruction of healthcare facilities	Legal restrictions impeding access
3.	Destruction of transportation routes	Host nation-imposed waiting periods before granting access to care
4.	Shortage of drugs and other pharmaceutics	Undocumented status of many refugees and uncertainties about entitlements for failed asylum seekers.
5.	Insecurity and lack of protective factors for healthcare personnel	Insufficient funds from the United Nations High Commissioner for Refugees and nongovernment organizations

    c. One and a half million school-aged Syrian refugee children live in Turkey, Jordan, and Lebanon, but approximately half of them do not have access to formal education.[20]

    d. In 2014–2015, half of Syrian children (about three-quarters in the worst-affected areas) did not go to school, one of the lowest school attendance rates globally.[21]

    e. Education in refugee and IDP camps is not given priority because of competing immediate demands, such as for food, clean water, safe shelter, control of communicable diseases, and security.[19]

4. Malnutrition and lack of clean water

    a. Food and nutrition insecurity accelerate in armed conflict areas.

    b. About 112 million malnourished children live in areas affected by armed conflict, accounting for two-thirds of all malnourished children in poor countries.[22]

    c. Poor nutrition is not only caused by lack of food; it is also related to poor hygiene, contaminated water, and lack of health education.

    d. Malnutrition is particularly injurious from birth to 2 years, contributing to irreversible mental and physical harm.[23]

    e. The World Food Program (WFP) reports that around 2000 of the displaced Syrian children in Lebanon are experiencing extreme intense poor health, which may lead to death without rapid interventions.

    f. Another 8000 Syrian children in Lebanon are experiencing less extreme hunger.

    g. The WFP likewise expresses that around 4% of exiled Syrian children in Jordan less than 5 years old need treatment for severe diseases.[24]

    h. Hunger is also an issue for internally displaced populations within Syria. Poor access to food and healthcare services and lack of potable water leads to diarrheal diseases, general poor health, and even death.[25]

5. Child labor

    a. Forcibly displaced and refugee children are particularly vulnerable to child labor.

    b. In conflicts and disasters, parents may lose their jobs, and schools may be damaged. In such situations, children often begin working.

    c. In other scenarios, children may end up separated from their parents in conflict areas and need to support themselves. However, working children may sacrifice their health, safety, and education to help their families or sustain their living expenses.[6]

d. In Syria's case, specific figures on the number of children in the Syrian labor market do not exist; a UN Children's Fund (UNICEF) report released in March 2017 estimates that around 1.7 million children are out of school. Large numbers of them are believed to have been forced to work in an expanding catastrophe that the UN says is only getting worse.[5]

e. Whether in Syria or in neighboring countries, children are forced to work in conditions that are mentally, physically, and socially dangerous.[17]

f. Save the Children and UNICEF outlined that inside Syria, children are contributing to the family income in more than 75% of reviewed families.

g. In Jordan, almost all displaced Syrian children are presently the joint or sole family providers in families studied.[23]

h. In Lebanon, children as young as 6 years of age are purportedly working.[23]

i. A spiraling number of children are regularly used in unsafe working conditions, being exposed to pesticides and poisonous chemicals, and working for extended periods of time with little pay, in dangerous and undesirable conditions.[5]

6. Mental health issues

a. Children are dependent on external sources for their protection and care and have their own individual developmental and psychological requirements.[4]

b. Refugee/IDP children are at substantial risk of experiencing emotional and psychological problems.

c. Starting from their native countries, many refugees/IDP children have been exposed to significant trauma.

d. Many children have been forced to flee their homes to escape war and have been confronted with violence, torture, and loss of close family and friends.[25]

e. The journey of refugees to a settlement place can be a source of further stress. It may take several weeks to months and expose the refugees to several life-threatening situations.[4]

f. Refugee children at these times may be exposed to separation from parents, either by accident or as a strategy to guarantee their safety.

g. Arriving at the final destination and starting a new life can be a source of additional difficulty, as many have to prove their asylum claims and also try to integrate in a new society.

h. Syrian displaced/refugee children are likewise in danger of a scope of issues related to their psychological well-being because of their horrendous experiences.

i. These children have experienced a high degree of trauma: 79% had encountered a demise in the family; 60% had seen somebody beaten, shot, or physically abused; and 30% had themselves been kicked, shot at, or physically hurt.[13]

j. Some 45% showed side effects of PTSD—10 times the usual rate in children—and 44% were suffering from depression as a side effect.[13]

k. Soykoek and his team studied a representative sample of 96 Syrian children (0–14 years) from a reception camp and detected PTSD in 11 (26%) of 42 children aged 0 to 6 years using the Posttraumatic Stress Disorder Semi-Structured Interview (PTSDSSI) and in 18 (33%) of 54 children aged 7 to 14 years using Kinder-DIPS.[26]

Approach to the Challenges Confronting Internally Displaced Persons/Refugee Children

- Approach to IDP/refugee children includes dealing with acute emergency situations and the subsequent postemergency phase. It is wise here to recall the 10 priorities set by Médecins Sans Frontières (MSF) for approaching refugee health in the emergency phase (Box 11.1).[27]

- Although the MSF priorities were established in 1997, after 20 years most of the parameters are still valid and need to be followed; if we need to change anything, it would probably be the second priority, which is related to measles immunization.

BOX 11.1 ■ The Médecins Sans Frontières 10 Priorities

1. Initial assessment
2. Measles immunization
3. Water and sanitation
4. Food and nutrition
5. Shelter and site planning
6. Health care in the emergency phase
7. Control of communicable diseases and epidemics
8. Public health surveillance
9. Human resources and training
10. Coordination

- Measles was noticed to affect many refugee camps and resulted in many preventable deaths in the 1990s and before; however, the situation nowadays is much worse, with a range of diseases preventable by immunization threatening the health and lives of refugee children, such as poliomyelitis, tuberculosis, and meningitis, in addition to measles.

In response to disasters, several national and international players will act:

- The Office for the Coordination of Humanitarian Affairs (OCHA) in collaboration with the Inter-Agency Standing Committee (IASC) is the arm of the UN responsible for bringing together national and international humanitarian providers to ensure a coherent response to emergencies.
- The other actors are the International Committee of the Red Cross (ICRC), leading international nongovernmental organizations (NGOs) working through volunteers, donors, and local committees.
- In the early phase of disasters, there will be a flood of refugees/displaced people seeking security and safety.
- There must be rapid action by the international community to make it possible to deal with these floods of refugees into regions that are sometimes difficult to reach, and where food, water, shelter, sanitary equipment, and so on must be urgently transported.[27]
- There are basic requirements that determine the well-being of refugees/displaced people in the early phase of disaster; these are safe shelter, clean water, food, and health care. All these requirements are covered by the UNHCR, which coordinates assistance to refugees, in close cooperation with other UN agencies, the local government, and different specialized NGOs.[27]

Postemergency Phase

After the initial assessment and coverage of emergency needs in terms of safe shelter; clean water and sanitation; provision of food and nutrition; and treatment of acute conditions, come long-term plans. These plans need to cover the principle challenges confronting IDP/refugee children (Box 11.2).

1. Restricted access to health care
   a. According to the 1951 Convention relating to the status of refugees, refugees should have access to medical care and schooling and have the right to work.[28]
   b. Host countries should recognize access to essential health services for refugees as a fundamental human right.[18]
   c. Donor countries should support efforts to ensure access for IDPs to secure essential healthcare services.

BOX 11.2 ■ **Postemergency Challenges Confronting Internally Displaced Persons/ Refugee Children**

1. Restricted access to health care
2. Outbreak of vaccine-preventable diseases such as poliomyelitis and measles
3. Restricted access to education
4. Malnutrition
5. Child labor
6. Mental health issues
7. Exposure to physical and sexual violence
8. Other difficulties, for example, disrupted families and poor living conditions

---

    d. As the global community moves toward the Sustainable Development Goals (SDGs), refugees' access to different aspects of health care has been pointed out in different targets including targets 1.4, 3.3, 3.7, and 3.8.[29]

    e. Greater efforts and serious consideration should be given to the right of IDPs/refugees to access timely, appropriate, and quality healthcare services.[18]

2. Outbreak of vaccine-preventable diseases (VPDs) such as poliomyelitis and measles

    a. The most affordable disease prevention strategy, which averts several childhood ailments and mortalities each year, remains vaccination.[30]

    b. Humanitarian crises may lead to the collapse of normal health services such as regular vaccination programs.[31]

    c. Among the VPDs reported in the literature during humanitarian crises were polio, measles, and, dependent on geographical setting, cholera, hepatitis A, yellow fever, and meningococcal meningitis.

    d. Campsite locations, particularly informal types, raise the vulnerability of a population to VPDs owing to poor nutritional status, shortage of safe water and hygiene, poor nutrition, suboptimal living conditions, and congestion.[31]

    e. Additional major challenges are communication problems and awareness in the host community, inadequate supplies and apparatus, inadequately trained personnel, and inadequate camp capacity following an enormous population influx.

    f. The World Health Organization (WHO) SAGE framework document, the UNICEF's code of conduct, the UNHCR handbook for emergencies, and the Sphere handbook all contain rules to guard people from VPDs in conflict situations, with globally accepted standards and universal minimum principles for action in humanitarian crises.[31]

        Table 11.3 lists some strategies that can improve vaccination coverage for IDP/ refugee children.

3. Security assessments

Security assessments assist immunization programs in knowledge of the threat profiles of regions where their operations are carried out, offering extra security management to health workers founded on the latest intelligence appraisals.

4. Negotiating secure physical access

However complicated, the negotiation of access to conflict areas is key to efficient delivery of vaccines and additional health necessities, and to conducting successful disease inspection in these locations. The identification and negotiation of secure access with every conflict participant, including state and nonstate actors, alongside their partners, may be significant to lessening field operational risks and facilitating the improvement of the odds of efficient vaccine delivery.

TABLE 11.3 ■ **Strategies to Improve Vaccination Coverage for Internally Displaced Persons/Refugee Children**

	Strategy	Description
1.	Security assessments	Security assessments help those running immunization programs to understand the risk profiles of areas where their work is performed, providing additional security guidance to health workers based on the most recent intelligence assessments.
2.	Negotiating secure physical access	Negotiating access to conflict areas, although complicated, may be key to effective delivery of vaccines and other health needs, and to conducting effective disease surveillance in these settings.
3.	Engaging local communities	Advocacy with local traditional and religious leaders, information sharing with communities, training of local residents as vaccinators, and building community mobilization networks with support from community "gatekeepers" may help in gaining trust and interest from and access to the community.
4.	Flexible age, schedule, and dosing options	Prioritizing flexibility about age and other eligibility criteria for receiving vaccines is a key strategy for preventing outbreaks among populations living in conflict and humanitarian-emergency settings.
5.	Permanent vaccination teams	These teams are usually drawn from local communities and tasked with vaccinating eligible local populations.
6.	Vaccination during days of settlement	This approach may also help improve population immunity in the communities living in inaccessible areas.
7.	Coordinating vaccine and other humanitarian aid delivery	Coordinating vaccine delivery efforts with other ongoing humanitarian response activities such as delivery of medicines, food, and clothing may be key to improving immunization coverage and efficient use of public health resources.
8.	Collaborating with military and other security personnel	Vaccination workers may embed with military contingents as they conduct routine security checks, providing an opportunity for vaccination during these missions. Members of medical corps can also be trained to administer vaccines and conduct disease surveillance.

5. Engaging local communities

Of significant value in vaccine delivery in conflict and humanitarian-emergency conditions, communication and community engagement are key components of successful vaccine delivery. Developing community mobilization systems with the aid of community gatekeepers, preparing the local residents to be vaccinators, propagating information within communities, and gaining support from local religious and traditional leaders assist in shedding light on the fundamental needs of the communities and developing trust between the program and the community. The key to gaining access to, and the interest and trust of, the community is to find solutions to a number of these necessities, such as working with other development ally agencies.

6. Flexible schedule, age, and dosing options

Access to essential healthcare services can be compromised by insecurity, often resulting in several infants missing age-appropriate vaccines. The main approaches to preventing outbreaks amongst populations residing in conflict and humanitarian-emergency situations are to prioritize flexibility in terms of age and to implement other appropriate measures for receiving the vaccines.

7. Permanent vaccination teams

Such teams are normally selected from local populations and given assignments to vaccinate eligible local people. These individuals live in limited security environments and, as local residents, have access to and the trust of local children that could not be reached by the agents of a formal vaccination plan. These enduring vaccination teams are often established as a distinct operation, are frequently supplied with vaccines, and may obtain direction as the security situation allows.

8. Vaccination on "days of tranquility"

This policy may entail establishing vaccination stations in areas unreachable by vaccinators. Because populations in these regions may continue to migrate in and out of communities, vaccination stations are put up at border crossings, security check positions, markets, commercial bus and taxi stations, and boundary settlement populations, to access communities passing through these areas.

9. Organizing vaccine and other humanitarian aid delivery

Because multifaceted humanitarian-emergency requirements regularly coexist in a number of conflict locations, the improvement of immunization coverage and effective use of public health resources can be achieved through the coordination of vaccine delivery endeavors with other progressive humanitarian response activities. In many situations, perfectly coordinated delivery of clothing, food, and medicines with the delivery of vaccine have facilitated the improvement of vaccine delivery to populations.

10. Working together with military and other security personnel

In conflict settings, military escorts have normally been employed in the delivery of humanitarian assistance and the escort of vaccination personnel throughout immunization activities. Vaccination workers in other places may be trained to be military agents as they perform their usual security checks, offering a chance for vaccination in these missions. Members of medical groups may also be taught to give out vaccines and perform medical examinations.[30]

11. Restricted access to education

To ensure that refugees and IDPs have access to quality education, there is a need for education providers and decision-makers to work on the various challenges that face these groups and establish ways to address them. It is evident that these challenges vary from one group to another depending on their needs and circumstances.[15] To formulate the right policy frameworks and an enabling environment for their implementation, strong collaboration between governments, development agencies, and humanitarian bodies is paramount. However, decision-making and responsibility for IDPs and refugees belong to states.[19] This is the reason why most nations take the initiative to include IDPs, refugees, asylum seekers, and stateless populations as part of their education plans at all costs. The state needs to respond in a flexible manner to ensure that they expand and strengthen formal education systems. As a result, more displaced children and youth from these affected populations will be absorbed into the education system.

Also, flexibility will ensure that certified education programs are offered to affected populations, and that other nonformal alternative pathways to the formal education system are designed.[19] The following points show the major policy directions for governments and their partners:

a. Enshrine the rights of forcibly displaced people to education in state laws and policies.

The extent to which refugees, stateless children, and IDPs enjoy protection is dependent on the national laws and policies in place and how effectively they are implemented. However, in various nations, these vulnerable groups encounter institutional barriers that may either directly or indirectly affect children's prospects of accessing quality education. Only 21 out of 50 nations with IDPs have incorporated IDP children in their policies and national laws.[19]

Columbia is one of the world's leading states with IDPs. The IDP population is estimated to be over 6 million. Columbia has clearly demonstrated that IDP opportunities can be extended by legal provisions.[19] For instance, in 2004, the constitutional court realized that the legal provisions of the government did not meet its obligations regarding IDPs. As a result, the court made a ruling that facilitated the development of an elaborate national plan for IDPs. Under the law, all children from internally displaced families are eligible to access free education within the state. Also, schools are required to accept them without necessarily asking for proof regarding their previous education.[32]

b. Incorporate children and youths IDPs into national education systems

Displaced children and youth should have access to accountable and certified education services (Box 11.3). This can be achieved by incorporating IDPs into national education systems. To ensure that IDPs access quality education, the inclusion calls for early and sustainable attention from both government and development partners to enhance national capacity and the required infrastructure. It also ensures that appropriate policy and legal frameworks are put in place, appropriate curriculum and instruction language are adopted, and that refugee children and displaced populations are prepared to transition to the education system of the host country. In cases where inclusion is not considered, the adoption of parallel education systems poses a number of challenges, as the curriculum of the host country and that of the country of origin are not the same. However, there is the challenge of lack of access to certification and examination that leaves IDP children unable to progress with their education.

c. Adoption of a double shift system

One of the common challenges that inclusion faces is inadequate infrastructure. To address the challenge of classroom shortages, the low-cost solution of a double shift system is adopted. For instance, in Lebanon during the academic year 2015–2016, Lebanese children attended 1278 public schools alongside Syrian children. Also, 259 schools offered special second-shift classes in the afternoon to accommodate the remaining Syrian children.[33]

d. Accelerated education programs

Such programs offer IDP and refugee children and adolescents viable alternatives for a certified education. Both IDPs and refugee populations have many learners who are over-age, as they have missed long periods of schooling. When these over-age children are offered a chance to study, they pose a number of risks, including overcrowding, the

---

BOX 11.3 ■ **Strategies to Improve Access to Education for Internally Displaced Persons/Refugee Children**

1. Enshrine forcibly displaced people's rights to education in national laws and policy
2. Include displaced children and youth in national education systems
3. Use a double shift system
4. Accelerated education programs
5. Flexible postprimary education
6. Assistance to enter higher education
7. Ensure an adequate supply of trained and motivated teachers

difficulties of teaching children of multiple ages, and the protection risks associated with mixing younger and older children in the same class.[19] Accelerated education programs are significant in allowing over-age children and adolescents access to condensed education services that are appropriate for their ages.

e. Flexible postprimary education

Refugees/IDPs face a number of challenges in accessing quality postprimary education. Some of these include a lack in their foundational skills, lack of capital to cover their education costs, or residence in areas where formal education systems are underserved. The Youth Education Pack of the Norwegian Refugee Council offers whole-year intensive full-time training to youths between the ages of 15 and 24 years in numeracy, literacy, and livelihood skills that are geared toward self-employment. Such programs have been implemented in about 13 countries, including Afghanistan and Timor-Leste. Upon completion of this course, graduates are given a start-up kit that assists them in establishing micro-businesses, enabling them to progress with their lives.[19]

f. Assistance to access higher education

One of the major ways of accessing higher education is through scholarships. The Albert Einstein German Academic Refugee Initiative program, DAFI, is a government-funded scholarship program that has supported over 2200 learners across 41 host nations. They provided children with scholarships to access higher education in 2014.[34] Increasingly, distance learning and e-learning are used, together with tutoring on site. This enables students to gain certifications from accredited institutions.

g. Ensure that there are enough motivated and trained teachers

Teachers who have been offering voluntary services for some time should be paid incentives to encourage them in their work. In 2015, over 4000 Syrian refugee teachers offering voluntary services in Turkey started receiving monthly incentive payments ranging between €130 and €190. These incentives were funded by various donors and enhanced the morale of the teachers. They also promoted the teachers' sense of professional value.[19]

12. Malnutrition

Refugees and internally displaced children living in camps are more vulnerable to malnutrition than children living in other hosting communities, yet none are immune.

Provision of food and nutrition inside camps is a shared responsibility. Nutrition partners to implement nutrition surveys, screenings, and nutrition programs may include the relevant ministry of health, NGOs (international or national), and UN agencies such as the WFP and UNICEF.[22]

The following are some recommendations set by the UNHCR in the fourth edition of the *Emergency Handbook for Nutrition in Camps* (Box 11.4)[35]:

a. Establish partnership agreements at field level early on so that interventions can be implemented rapidly.

BOX 11.4 ■ United Nations High Commissioner for Refugees Recommendations for Nutrition in Camps

1. Ensure coordination and collaboration between all those involved in a camp's nutrition activities.
2. Ensure that all refugees in a camp have access to food.
3. Establish programs to treat acute malnutrition and effective referral mechanisms (to services in the camp or in the host community where refugees have access to these services)
4. Establish infant and young-child feeding programs
5. Within the first 3 months conduct a Standardized Expanded Nutrition Survey and conduct regular mid-upper arm circumference-based nutrition programming screening

  b. A trained UNHCR public health officer, with knowledge of nutrition, to coordinate the response.
  c. Community outreach workers provide support in the camp (or surrounding community) and nutrition/health assistants at the nutrition centers, either from UNHCR or a partner organization.
  d. UNHCR must ensure that adequate food assistance, programs to treat acute malnutrition, and infant feeding support are provided to refugees residing in camps. These services are normally provided by NGO partners in collaboration with the WFP and UNICEF. Wherever required, UNHCR and WFP should provide appropriate food assistance, including fortified foods, to refugees in camps. UNHCR and partners must ensure that appropriate treatment programs are in place for acutely malnourished camp-based refugees by establishing new facilities or making facilities in the host community available to them.
  e. Public health and nutrition services and infrastructures in camps should also be accessible to the host community to ensure peaceful coexistence.
  f. Support services and facilities for infant and young-child feeding should always be available to IDPs/refugees living in camps (facilities based in the camp or by making facilities in the host community available to them). Skilled support and counseling should be on hand, along with safe, baby-friendly spaces in which mothers can feed and interact comfortably with their infants.
  g. UNHCR and partners must ensure that services and support are available for individuals who require help to breastfeed and for infants younger than 6 months who need alternatives to breast milk.
  h. There must be regular nutrition surveys and continuous screening for acute malnutrition in the community.
  i. Failure to provide adequate food or nutritional rehabilitation may generate longer-term risks. Refugees may take risks to acquire food or adopt unsafe coping strategies. These may adversely affect feeding and care (including breastfeeding) of infants and young children. Malnourished individuals may suffer long-term effects, such as impeded growth or development.
13. Child labor
  a. In 1989, the UN Convention on the Rights of the Child (CRC) was adopted, establishing a universally agreed set of nonnegotiable standards primarily specifying state obligations toward children under 18 years of age.
  b. Article 32 specifically addresses the protection of children from economic exploitation and from performing any work that interferes with his or her education or is harmful to his or her mental, spiritual, or social development (Box 11.5).[36]

BOX 11.5 ■ Strategies to Protect Children Away From Child Labor

1. Enable free access to education
2. Address the economic insecurity that compels refugee households to resort to child labor
3. Help to provide decent jobs to their parents
4. Legal regulations and effective inspections for keeping children away from the labor market
5. Overseeing and coordinating the implementation and monitoring of national programs to prevent and fight child labor
6. International nongovernment organizations provide cash vouchers to IDP/refugee families on the condition that they send their children to school

  c. Convention 138 concerns the Minimum Age (1973, No. 1384), and International Labor Organization (ILO) Convention 182 on the Worst Forms of Child Labour (1999, No. 1825). According to ILO Convention 138, the minimum age limit should not be below the age when compulsory schooling is completed—and, in any case, should not be below 15 years of age (Art. 3).

  d. Employment of persons aged 13 and upwards is allowed where this is not harmful to the health or development of a child and does not prejudice school attendance (Art. 5).[36]

  e. A high priority for labor market interventions is to address the economic insecurity that compels refugee households to resort to child labor.[37] Children should not have to sacrifice their health, safety, and education to bring in money.

  f. Governments should consider education for children affected by war and disasters a top priority and help to provide decent jobs to their parents.[19] In this way, giving adult refugees the right to work and granting them access to the labor market is both a vital protection tool for child refugees and a means of encouraging households to keep their children in school.[37]

  g. Establishing better conjuncture between rights, law, and economic interests and improving coordination between all stakeholders are key requirements for enhancing adult refugees' rights to work and access to labor markets.

  h. Governments should put legal regulations and effective inspections in place and raise awareness on the elimination of child labor. International NGOs provide cash vouchers to Syrian families on the condition that they send their children to school.[36]

Refugee/Internally Displaced Persons Women

- The total number of the world's refugees/IDPs at the end of 2016 reached 65.3 million; women and girls make up about 50% of that number.[38]
- However, women and girls were allocated only 4% of projects by UN inter-agencies in 2014. Also, only 0.4% funds were allocated for women's groups or women's ministries from 2012 to 2013.[38]
- It has been also noted that the numbers of women who have been affected by protracted displacement outnumber men.[38]
- Refugee and internally displaced women have very limited legal rights and are powerless and marginalized; their voices are hardly ever heard.[39]
- The UN reports that 60% of preventable maternal deaths happen in humanitarian settings, where at least one in five refugees or displaced women are approximated to have faced sexual violence.[38]
- Pregnant women are at a particular risk; many of them face lack of access to efficient antenatal care or a safe place with an expert attendant for delivery and a lack of access to postnatal care and birth control.
- Generally, refugees, in comparison to IDPs, are well protected by international laws.
- Women are highly vulnerable as they are easily violated. They are identified as losing livelihoods and the main documentation required for day-to-day activities.
- Women also have limited access to help, sufficient education, effective health care, livelihoods, and training. They are likely to experience hardship when fighting for their rights to land, housing, and property, and they are subjected to sexual and gender-based violence.[40]
- Additionally, women are seen to be excluded in times of decision-making. Conflict is the root of these experiences, where precrisis patterns of discrimination worsen.[41]
- The international community identified the need for integration of refugee matters from the end of World War One.

- Consequently, international and regional treaties have been established. National governments were forced to pass mechanisms and policies to incorporate refugee populations. However, refugees do not always benefit from these policies.
- There has been a need for focus on displaced women within the borders of their own countries in past years.
- This focus by states, international agencies, civil society organizations, and other relevant actors[41] started in the 1990s.
- The UN Guiding Principle on Internal Displacement 4.2 states that "Certain internally displaced persons, such as children, especially unaccompanied minors, expectant mothers, mothers with young children, female heads of household, persons with disabilities and elderly persons, shall be entitled to protection and assistance required by their condition and to treatment which takes into account their special needs."[41]

Refugee and internally displaced women and girls face all challenges faced by other refugees/IDPs, such as insecurity, poverty, mental health issues, and lack of access to health care and education. However, women and girls are subjected to other risks that affect women in particular. These are:

1. Reproductive health (RH), which includes pregnancy and delivery, family planning, sexual violence, prevention of sexual transmitted diseases
2. Poverty and lack of financial support, especially in female-headed families
3. Mental health issues

Reproductive Health

- Low priority has been given to RH in the humanitarian response's hierarchy. Establishment of the Inter-Agency Working Group (IAWG) for RH was as a result of RH needs awareness, which started in the mid-1990s.
- This was followed by the formation by the WHO of the IAWG for RH in refugee situations, who developed a central package of minimum RH interventions that should be put in place in emergency settings.[42]
- The Minimum Initial Service Package (MISP) was created, which is a set of guidelines for RH service delivery in crisis settings (Box 11.6). In addition to equipment kits and supplies, the MISP is a collection of activities requiring competent employees be used effectively.[42]
- The initiation of various activities ensures that RH is of high quality.
- Expanding and sustaining actions are needed through complete RH services.[42]
1. Ensure the health sector/cluster recognizes an organization to lead MISP implementation. The lead RH organization:
   a. Suggests an RH officer to offer technical and operational support to all healthcare agencies.
   b. Hosts constant stakeholder meetings to enable MISP implementation.

BOX 11.6 ■ Objectives of the Minimum Initial Service Package

1. Ensure an organization is identified to lead the implementation of the Minimum Initial Service Package
2. Prevent and manage the consequences of sexual violence
3. Reduce human immunodeficiency virus transmission
4. Prevent maternal and newborn death and illness
5. Plan for comprehensive sexual and reproductive health care, integrated into primary health care, as the situation permits

---

    c. Reports to the health sector/cluster meetings on any issues connected to MISP implementation.

    d. Shares information on accessibility of RH resources and supplies.[43]

2. Prevent and manage the consequences of sexual violence[43]

    a. Cautious site planning of camps

    b. Establish healthcare services for medical treatment of sexual violence survivors

    c. Offer training to all employees on the significance of early healthcare services referral of survivors

    d. Manage the response between health, community, security, and protection services.

3. Reduce transmission of human immunodeficiency virus (HIV)[43]

    a. Allow free access to condoms

    b. Impose universal precautions against HIV

    c. Ensure safe blood transfusion

4. Prevent extra neonatal and maternal morbidity and mortality

    a. Offer all pregnant women and birth attendants clean delivery kits

    b. Offer midwifery delivery kits to healthcare facilities and midwives

    c. Start the construction of a referral system to manage obstetrics emergencies

Important activities that enable prevention of excess maternal and newborn morbidity and mortality include:

- Ensuring accessibility of emergency obstetric care (EmOC) and newborn care services that include, at health facilities, competent birth attendants and supplies for normal births and management of obstetric and newborn complications, and at referral hospitals, competent medical staff and supplies for management of obstetric and newborn emergencies.

- Constructing a referral system to enable transport and communication from the community to the health center and between health center and the hospital.

- Offering clean delivery kits to visibly pregnant women and birth attendants to support clean home deliveries when access to a healthcare facility is impossible.

5. Plan for the provision of complete RH services, integrated into primary health care, when the situation allows

    a. Gather background data on RH mortality, sexually transmitted disease (STD)/HIV prevalence, and contraceptive prevalence

    b. Categorize applicable sites for the future delivery of complete RH services

    c. Examine the capability of staff and plan training/retraining

    d. Purchase equipment and supplies for complete RH services

RH intervention has been emphasized by the WHO, which tries to offer training to healthcare providers so that they can manage pregnant women appropriately.

- The provision of services in every humanitarian setting is monitored by the RH officer through use of the MISP checklist.

- This can sometimes be achieved through verbal reporting from RH managers and/or via observation visits. Monitoring is performed weekly at the start of the humanitarian response.

- This is followed by a monthly monitoring after complete establishment of services.

- Solutions are searched for and used through discussion of gaps and overlaps in service coverage in RH stakeholder meetings and through health sector/cluster coordination mechanisms.

Poverty and Lack of Financial Support

- Poverty and lack of financial support affects all refugees/IDPs; however, more women are becoming heads of households after losing male family members. Many of them lack the essential skills for employment, and they struggle to afford their families' needs. In Syria, for example, it is estimated that women now head three out of ten households.[44]
- Women refugees are vulnerable to gender-based violence (GBV) when attempting to access conventional refugee services and programs, including those provided by UNHCR and its partners.[45]
- Nearly 60% of refugees live in cities, a figure that will continue to increase, as camps become an option of last choice. Urban refugee women face multiple and complex challenges such as GBV; unmet social, medical, and economic needs; and cross-repression based on race, ethnicity, nationality, language, gender, and disability.[45]

This new situation calls for a massive shift in humanitarian response, necessitating policy makers, donors, and practitioners to create new programs that address the safety and security concerns of refugees in urban settings.[45]

Humanitarian representatives alone cannot achieve efficient urban protection and GBV prevention. The involvement of a broad network of other partners, such as police departments, school boards, hospital administrators, local shelters, medical facilities, social actors, and local community-based organization (CBOs),[45] is necessary.

Mental Health Issues

This subject will be discussed in Chapter 16.

Conclusion

Children and women are the most affected groups among refugees and IDPs. Children and adolescent refugees/IDPs are at risk of physical and mental trauma and frequently deprived of their essential needs such as nutrition, health care, education, and secure dwellings.

Women face their own challenges: they require well-being, health care, education, and economic opportunities. Pregnant women are at particular risk. Many women face lack of access to efficient antenatal care, a safe place with expert attendants for delivery, postnatal care, and access to birth control.

The international community needs to take full responsibility in a holistic manner to protect these vulnerable groups and join all efforts to meet their needs and alleviate their suffering.

References

1. Kleist JO. The history of refugee protection: conceptual and methodological challenges. *J Refugee Stud.* 2017;30:161–169.
2. Jorgensen E. *Refugee and Internally-Displaced Children.* Youth Advocate Program International; 2014. Available at: http://yapi.org/youth-wellbeing/refugee-and-internally-displaced-children/. Accessed September 8, 2017.
3. United Nations High Commissioner for Refugees. *Figures at a Glance.* UNHCR; 2017. Available at: http://www.unhcr.org/en-us/figures-at-a-glance.html.
4. Fazel M, Stein A. The mental health of refugee children. *Arch Disease Childhood.* 2002;87:366–370.
5. "There are many other kids here": Child tells of labor in Syria. *News Deeply.* July 24, 2017. Available at: https://www.newsdeeply.com/syria/articles/2017/07/24/there-are-many-other-kids-here-child-tells-of-labor-in-syria. Accessed November 15, 2017.
6. Raqib S. *How Wars and Disasters Fuel Child Labor.* Human Rights Watch; 2017. September 5, 2017.

7. Ehntholt KA Yule W. Practitioner review: assessment and treatment of refugee children and adolescents who have experienced war-related trauma. *J Child Psychol Psychiatry.* 2006;47:1197–1210.

8. World Vision. *Syrian Refugee Crisis: Facts, FAQs, and How to Help.* World Vision; 2017a. February 20, 2018.

9. United Nations High Commissioner for Refugees. UNHCR Syria Regional Refugee Response. Available at: http://data.unhcr.org/syrianrefugees/regio. Accessed May 14, 2017.

10. Akbarzada S, Mackey TK. The Syrian public health and humanitarian crisis: a "displacement" in global governance? *Glob Public Health.* 2018;13:914–930.

11. Berti B. The Syrian refugee crisis: regional and human security implications. *Strategic Assessment.* 2015; 17:41–53.

12. The Syrian Observatory for Human Rights; 2017. Available at: http://www.syriahr.com/en/?p=70012.

13. Ben Taleb Z, Bahelah R, Fouad FM, Coutts A, Wilcox M, Maziak W. Syria: health in a country undergoing tragic transition. *Int J Public Health.* 2015;60(suppl 1):S63–S72. World Health Organization. The Syrian Arab Republic. Fact sheet. Emergency Risk and Crisis Management. In.; 2014.

14. Roberton T, Weiss W, Jordan Health Access Study Team, Lebanon Health Access Study Team, Doocy S. Challenges in estimating vaccine coverage in refugee and displaced populations: results from household surveys in Jordan and Lebanon. *Vaccines.* 2017;5:22.

15. Sharara SL, Kanj SS. War and infectious diseases: challenges of the Syrian civil war. *PLoS Pathogens.* 2014;10:e1004438.

16. Black I. Report on Syria conflict finds 11.5% of population killed or injured. *The Guardian.* 2016:11.

17. Children of Syria. *Humanium—Together for Children's Rights;* October 15, 2016. Available at: http://www.humanium.org/en/middle-east-north-africa/syria/. Accessed May 23, 2017.

18. Langlois EV, Haines A, Tomson G, Ghaffar A. Refugees: towards better access to health-care services. *Lancet.* 2016;387:319.

19. United Nations Education, Scientific and Cultural Organization. *More Excuses: Provide Education to All Forcibly Displaced People.* UNESCO; 2016. Available at: http://unesdoc.unesco.org/images/0024/002448/244847E.pdf. Accessed February 19, 2018.

20. Human Rights Watch. *Following The Money, Lack of Transparency in Donor Funding for Syrian Refugee Education.* Human Rights Watch; September 2017. Available at: https://www.hrw.org/sites/default/files/report_pdf/crdsyrianrefugees0917_web.pdf. Accessed November 15, 2017.

21. Sirin SR, Rogers-Sirin L. *The Educational and Mental Health Needs of Syrian Refugee Children.* Migration Policy Institute; 2015.

22. Carroll GJ, Lama SD, Martinez-Brockman JL, Pérez-Escamilla R. Evaluation of nutrition interventions in children in conflict zones: A narrative review. *Adv Nutr.* 2017;8:770–779.

23. United Nations Childrens' Fund, Joint Nutrition Assessment Syrian Refugees in Lebanon. United Nations Human Rights Council: Report of the independent international commission of inquiry on the Syrian Arab Republic. In: United Nations; 2014 Sen K, Al-Faisal W, AlSaleh Y. Syria: effects of conflict and sanctions on public health. *J Public Health.* 2013;35:195–199.

24. World Food Program. *Annual Performance Report for 2014.* WFP; 2014. Available at: http://documents.wfp.org/stellent/groups/public/documents/eb/wfpdoc063825.pdf.

25. Hassan G, Ventevogal P, Jefee-Bahloul H, Barkil-Oteo A. Mental health and psychosocial wellbeing of Syrians affected by armed conflict. *Epidemiol Psychiatric Sci.* 2016;25:129–141.

26. Soykoek S, Mall V, Nehring I, Henningsen P, Aberl S. Post-traumatic stress disorder in Syrian children of a German refugee camp. *Lancet.* 2017;389:903–904.

27. Médecins Sans Frontières. *Refugee Health: An Approach to Emergency Situations.* Macmillan Education Ltd; 1997.

28. United Nations High Commissioner for Refugees. *Protecting Refugees: Questions and Answers.* UNHCR; 2002. Retrieved on February 24, 2018. Available at: http://www.unhcr.org/afr/publications/brochures/3b779dfe2/protecting-refugees-questions-answers.html. Accessed February 24, 2018.

29. Nijenhuis G, Leung M. Rethinking migration in the 2030 agenda: Towards a de-territorialized conceptualization of development. *Forum Develop Studies.* 2017;44:51–68.

30. Nnadi C, Etsano A, Uba B, et al. Approaches to vaccination among populations in areas of conflict. *J Infect Dis.* 2017;216(Suppl 1):S368–S372.

31. Lam E, McCarthy A, Brennan M. Vaccine-preventable diseases in humanitarian emergencies among refugee and internally-displaced populations. *Hum Vaccin Immunother.* 2015;11:2627–2636.

32. Cepeda MJ. *The Constitutional Protection of IDPs in Colombia. Judicial Protection of Internally Displaced Persons: The Colombian Experience*; 2009.

33. United Nations High Commissioner for Refugees. *200,000 Syrian Refugee Children to Get Free Schooling in Lebanon.* Geneva, Switzerland: UNHCR; 2015. Available at: http://www.unhcr.org/print/560e96b56. html.

34. United Nations High Commissioner for Refugees. DAFI scholarships. Available at: http://www.unhcr. org/pages/49e4a2dd6.html. Accessed March 10, 2016.

35. United Nations High Commissioner for Refugees. *Emergency Handbook. Nutrition in Camps.* UNHCR; 2015. Available at: https://emergency.unhcr.org/entry/85615/nutrition-in-camps.

36. Terre des Hommes. *Child Labour Report.* Terre des Hommes; 2016. Available at: data.unhcr.org/syrian-refugees/download.php?id=11674.

37. Zetter R, Ruaudel H. *Refugees' Right to Work and Access to Labor Markets—An Assessment. World Bank Global Program on Forced Displacement (GPFD) and the Global Knowledge Partnership on Migration and Development (KNOMAD) Thematic Working Group on Forced Migration.* KNOMAD Working Paper. Washington, DC: World Bank Group; 2016.

38. United Nations Women. *Women Refugees and Migrants.* United Nations Women; 2016. Available at: http://www.unwomen.org/en/news/in-focus/women-refugees-and-migrants.

39. Memela S, Maharaj B. Challenges facing refugee women. A critical review. In: Domínguez-Mujica J, ed. *Global Change and Human Mobility. Advances in Geographical and Environmental Sciences.* Singapore: Springer; 2016.

40. The Global Human Rights Education and Training Centre Rights of refugees and internally displaced persons; 2018. Available at: http://www.hrea.org/learn/elearning/refugees/. Accessed March 2, 2018.

41. Brookings Institution. *Improving the Protection of Internally Displaced Women: Assessment of Progress and Challenges.* Brookings Institution; 2014. Available at: https://www.brookings.edu/wp-content/uploads/2016/07/Improving-the-Protection-of-Internally-Displacement-Women-October-10-2014-FINAL.pdf.

42. United Nations Population Fund. *What Is the Minimum Initial Service Package?* UNPF; 2015. Available at: https://www.unfpa.org/resources/what-minimum-initial-service-package.

43. Inter-Agency Working Group on Reproductive Health in Crises. *Inter-agency field manual on reproductive health in humanitarian settings: 2010 revision for field review.* Inter-Agency Working Group on Reproductive Health in Crises; 2010.

44. Khalifeh R. Women refugees are not only vulnerable, they are resilient too! Does the resilience of women built the resilience of their families? Master Degree Thesis, Swedish Institute; 2017.

45. Women's Refugee Commission. Mean Streets: Identifying and Responding to Urban Refugees' Risks of Gender-Based Violence Women's Refugee Commission; 2016. Available at: http://www.refworld.org/docid/56d68f464.html. Accessed March 6, 2018.

CHAPTER 12

Austere Surgery and Anesthesia

John L. Tarpley ■ Donald E. Meier ■ Melinda S. New ■
George G. Johnston ■ Adam T. Soto

CHAPTER OUTLINE

Surgery
Pearls, Pitfalls, and Aphorisms

Anesthesia
Case Prioritization in Resource-Limited
    Environments
Medical Facilities/Drugs/Equipment
    Preparation

Patient Safety
Perioperative Care
Technology and Equipment
Techniques
Medications
Practical Pointers and Practice Pearls
Conclusion

Surgery

A significant number of Western physicians and other medical associates develop professional relationships with organizations involved with overseas medical care. The nature and extent of involvement ranges from brief educational or charitable exposures to longer periods of actual practice. This chapter seeks to start a brief preparation for both medical professionals and nonclinical medical planners with respect to the particular surgical management of issues often encountered in austere medical environments. Additionally, we want to highlight some common surgical conditions and pathologies while providing advice on how to triage, evaluate, temporize, stabilize, resuscitate, and refer patients.

From our perspective, austere surgery denotes surgical care in an environment that is infrastructure-, resource-, and/or technology-challenged. Whether or not one is a surgeon, nearly all healthcare professionals will be uncomfortable when faced with the issues encountered in rural or even urban areas in low-income countries (LICs) or low-middle income countries (LMICs). Those designations refer to a World Bank classification of countries with respect to per capita national income, per annum adjusted for purchasing power. The value for the United States in 2018 was about $63,000 and an LIC (many of which are in Africa) has a value of about $2400. Combining LICs and LMICs, that is, less than $10,600, generates a list of about 137 countries accounting for a large portion of the world's population.[1] Per capita governmental health expenditure of less than $24 per citizen exists in many areas of the world, including in sub-Saharan Africa.[2] The number of operative procedures annually also reflects the drastic differences in access, availability, and affordability between populations: Africa less than 200, United Kingdom 13,600, and United States 21,000 per 100,000 population, respectively. With socioeconomics and infrastructure being so critically important, "the pathology of poverty" derives from economic, political, social, and medical etiologies, with the medical being a function of the other three.

BOX 12.1 ■ Six Major Surgical Challenges

1. Safe anesthesia and airway management
2. Trauma: long bone; head and spine; thermal (burns)
3. Women's health issues: peripartum hemorrhage; obstructed labor
4. Cancer
5. Pediatric surgery
6. Analgesia: perioperative and palliative

Other than the trained medical workforce crisis per se, there are at least six major "surgical" challenges: (1) safe anesthesia and airway management; (2) trauma: particularly long bone, head and spine, and thermal (burns); (3) women's health issues: peripartum hemorrhage, obstructed labor; (4) cancer; (5) pediatric surgery; and (6) analgesia—perioperative and palliative (Box 12.1). These six challenges are the focus of joint initiatives by the World Health Organization (WHO), the Lancet Commission on Global Surgery (LCoGS),[3] the G4 Alliance (G4: surgery, trauma, anesthesia, obstetrics-gynecology), the Alliance for Surgical and Anesthesia Presence (ASAP), and similar organizations internationally. The growth of global cell-based and web-based capabilities facilitates access to up-to-date surgical atlases, texts, and information resources. *Primary Surgery Non-Trauma and Trauma* and *Primary Anesthesia* by M. King et al. (Oxford Press) and the revised *Primary Surgery* by Cotton[4-7] were/are key references for physicians and surgeons providing surgical care in austere environments from the 1980s forward. In 2015, the *Global Surgery and Anesthesia Handbook* edited by John Meara et al.[8] became available both in a portable paperback and an e-book edition that updates *Primary Surgery*. Links to free valuable resources, such as the International Committee of the Red Cross's (ICRC) *War Surgery, Volumes 1 and 2*,[9,10] the *Principles of Reconstructive Surgery in Africa, revised edition* edited by Louis Carter Jr. and Peter Nthumba,[11] and *Paediatric Surgery: A Comprehensive Text for Africa, Volume 1*,[12] address the spectrum of surgical challenges. The number of such resources continues to increase and helps provide needed instructions at the point of contact and in real time for those providing surgical management. Before traveling to an austere locale, one ought to load key texts and atlases onto a laptop or other device and/or carry one or more well-chosen texts, which can then be left behind for the hosts.

Prerequisites not always available but required to provide ongoing surgical care if one hopes to go beyond first aid include: water (potable is better); electricity (often inconsistent); a sterilizing capability (even if "homemade"); basic operating room (OR) equipment and supplies (sutures, instruments, lighting, head light, a suction capability); a pharmacy with intravenous (IV) fluids; basic imaging (usually limited to plain films); ultrasonography; and some level of laboratory capability (hopefully to include blood-typing, even if just an Eldon card). Any histopathology capability will likely experience a turnaround time in weeks or even months.

Evaluation of foreign medical facilities and dialogues/interactions with local/host medical providers are almost always more productive if conducted with consideration, circumspection, and respect. If you are visiting an overseas facility, you are likely the guest of someone affiliated with it. Preserving that relationship is critical to long-term success. Hosts are likely sensitive to the fact that their facility/practice is not equivalent to those in more affluent countries. The informed observer must look closely but quietly. Your hosts will likely appreciate any assistance provided but may be sensitive to criticism.

This chapter focuses on several common and a few less common conditions one may be called upon to manage that will likely be outside the usual practice for surgeons based in North America, Western Europe, and the Pacific high-income countries (HICs). By necessity, most comments must be terse.

PEARLS, PITFALLS, AND APHORISMS[13]

- Anesthesia: Safe anesthesia is the first requisite, with mandatory use of pulse oximeters.
- Typhoid perforations lead to secondary, bacterial, suppurative peritonitis in a patient immunologically and nutritionally compromised.
- Tetanus: Never presume a patient is immunized. No wounds are trivial.
- Trauma, burns, bites, and stings: Blunt and penetrating trauma, particularly from vehicular crashes, falls, farming, and industrial accidents, consume time, resources, and beds. Fracture and wound care are everyday procedures. Open fires, gasoline-tainted kerosene, and vehicular wrecks cause burns. Animal, human, and insect bites can lead to serious wounds.
- Osteomyelitis ensues from either open fractures or from hematogenous spread in patients with and without sickle cell disease.
- Gastrointestinal (GI) surgery and oncology: Sigmoid volvulus and incarcerated/strangulated hernias lead to colon resections. Common cancers include gastric, prostate, hepatocellular, breast, cervical, and lymphoma. Medical or radiation oncology, radiology, and pathology are rarely available.
- Critical care: An Ambu bag, a clock, and an OR technician may be the ventilator. Pressors and invasive monitoring, found mostly in teaching hospitals or capital cities, are uncommon. Creativity aids coping.
- Pediatric surgery, urology, and obstetrics: The surgeon must be a specialist in many areas. Neonatal and pediatric presentations include anorectal atresia, Hirschsprung's disease (HD), GI atresia, and intussusception. Urologic problems involve urinary retention, urethral strictures, torsion, and hypospadias. Obstetric issues include obstructed labor and ruptured ectopic pregnancies.
- Parasitic and mycobacterial diseases: Chagas disease, hydatid cysts, Buruli ulcer, schistosomiasis, lymphatic filariasis, and helminthoma vary by geographic locale.
- Surgical colleagues or referral specialists are likely unavailable, with professional isolation a norm, although the rapidly increasing use of wireless phone and Internet availability have improved this situation. Surgical practice is "the skin and its contents." Currently, telemedicine options are present and increasing in some countries. Listen to your hosts, whatever their specialty.
- "*Festina lente*"—make haste slowly.
- "If you argue for your limitations; they are yours" (Richard Bach); but likewise, "There is no condition that cannot be made worse with an operation" (Art Brooks).

Trauma

About 5 million die annually from injuries (accounting for 9% of all deaths globally), and deaths from trauma account for almost 1.7 times the total fatalities from malaria, tuberculosis, and human immunodeficiency virus (HIV)/acquired immunodeficiency syndrome (AIDS) combined.[14] Some 90% of injury-related deaths occur in LICs and LMICs. Prehospital emergency provider care is virtually nonexistent for managing trauma in resource-poor areas (RPAs). Emergency rooms are underequipped and understaffed, often without basics such as a suction capability. "Essentials" that surgeons in the developed world take for granted (e.g., timely imaging, a robust transfusion capability, and well-equipped/staffed ORs) are most often lacking.

    A. Blunt/Vehicular Trauma

        An "epidemic of trauma" afflicts much of the LICs and LMICs of the world, especially road traffic crashes. The proliferation of inexpensive, sturdy motorcycles, the use of motorcycle "taxis," and a lack of traffic control have led to a marked increase in motorcycle crashes over the past decade with consequent head and/or spine injuries and long bone fractures.

1. The fundamentals apply: that is, protect/immobilize the cervical spine; address the A, B, Cs of advanced trauma life support (ATLS); and complete the primary and secondary surveys. Mass casualty situations requiring triage are common. Establish and/or maintain the airway; ventilate the patient (even if not intubated); and address hypovolemia and optimize the circulation, usually relying on crystalloid rather than blood or blood products. Head, spine, abdominal, thoracic, and vascular injuries must be considered, ruled out, or addressed, often on the basis of clinical examination only. See the Meara and/or ICRC *War Injury* volumes.[8–10]

2. Extremity long bone fractures: stabilize, immobilize as you assess for pulses and neurologic status, motor and sensory. Options include traction, splinting, casting, external fixation, or open reduction with internal fixation, among others. Is there an open wound? Blood supply is "everything." The soft tissue envelope of skin and muscle is key to a successful outcome. What was the mechanism of injury? How much energy was applied to the tissues? Consider the "zone of injury" as with a crush injury. How long ago? "A fracture is a soft tissue injury complicated by a break in a bone" (CR Murray).

3. Abdominal trauma: Splenic injuries are frequent, perhaps in part because splenomegaly from malaria and other diseases is more prevalent. Management without computed tomography (CT), transfusion-readiness, or an interventional radiology presence dictates that early recognition and decision-making to proceed to the OR/theater are critical. The principles are similar to the practices stateside once the decision to proceed to laparotomy has been made. Various attempts at "galley pot" autotransfusions have been reported but are not clearly beneficial. A prompt decision to operate before irreversible physiologic exhaustion (the "golden hour" for adults or "platinum half hour" for children), judicious source control, packing, and perhaps "returning to fight again another day" are important. Avoid acidosis, hypothermia, and coagulopathy, known as the "lethal triad."

4. Vascular trauma: Patients with significant aortic or major venous injuries do not survive transport to casualty, triage, or the emergency room, not so different from what pertains in developed countries. Falls with fracture dislocations through the knee with popliteal arterial trauma with or without concomitant venous injury occur, notably if the patient was carrying a heavy load on their head. Vascular injuries associated with long bone fractures, notably about the elbow or the lower extremity, are encountered and present often hours postinjury.

5. Head and spine trauma: Both vehicular trauma and falls from heights during occupational pursuits are frequent and most unforgiving. Inspection burr holes without the benefit of a head CT can be performed based on the Glasgow Coma Scale and physical exam, but loss of life and function are the rule. Spinal cord patients can be treated with traction in hopes of some return of function, but outcomes are discouraging.

B. Penetrating Trauma

The incidence of penetrating trauma depends a great deal on the country and the political situation at any given time. Penetrating trauma from falls with impalement, encounters with wild animals, and machete, knife, and arrow injuries were formerly the rule. Historically, there were fewer gun-owning citizens with many of the guns used in hunting homemade and of low velocity. Yet in certain areas where extremists are active, sophisticated weapons such as high velocity automatic rifles, and bomb-laden suicide-terrorists, often produce mass casualty scenarios. The presence of improvised explosive devices (IEDs) and commercial land mines is now more common and can add "blast injuries" to the burden of penetrating trauma. The two Red Cross *War Surgery* texts[9,10] are useful guides for managing such patients.

C. Thermal Trauma (Burns)

Burns are an underappreciated crisis in much of sub-Saharan Africa, especially pediatric burns. Burns can occur from flame or scalding mechanisms and are associated with cooking, use of kerosene, kerosene adulterated with gasoline explosions, vehicular trauma, and even petrol tanker or pipeline disasters. Burn care entails incredible expenditures of time, effort, and supplies, and needs a physiotherapy/rehabilitation capability (often rudimentary or absent). In environments with open fires, without nonflammable garments for children, and with unsafe petrol storage, burn prevention is an inadequately addressed public health challenge.

Wound Care

The Pan-African Academy of Christian Surgeons (PAACS) e-book by Carter and Nthumba, the *Principles of Reconstructive Surgery in Africa*, and the Gionnou et al. *War Surgery* volume 2 have key principles on debridement, wound care, and coverage, in addition to management options.

- Wounds result from many causes: trauma, burn, postsurgical, decubitus, diabetic, pyomyositis/abscess, infections such as Buruli ulcer, vascular, and hemoglobinopathies, etc.
- Debridement refers to the resection of nonviable tissues back to bleeding, viable tissue and is one hallmark of the care for wounds and ulcers, where an ulcer is defined as "the loss of epithelial continuity." A thorough history and physical are mandatory. Questions to ask: What was the mechanism of injury? What type of wound? Clean and fresh versus dirty and old (>6 hours)? How did it happen? Is this a bite wound? How long ago did it happen? Does the patient have other medical issues? Ask about tetanus immunization status; "think" tetanus and suspect tetanus-prone wounds.
- Examine: hemorrhage, viability, foreign bodies, x-rays, motor/sensory function, proximity to vessels, nerves, ducts? Tetanus status? Consider antirabies treatment if an animal is involved.
- General principles: Most bleeding can be controlled by direct pressure. A tourniquet or blood pressure cuff can help to control bleeding, but be aware—and beware—of how long either has been in place. Consider pressure at adjacent pulse points: femoral artery at the groin, popliteal artery at the knee, or brachial artery in arm or elbow. "Blind" clamping into a wound is never a good idea!! The damage caused is often worse than the initial injury.
- If local anesthesia is to be used, the maximal dose for lidocaine is 4 mg/kg without epinephrine (epi) or 7 mg/kg with epi. Use diazepam or similar agent in addition. Note that a 50-cc vial of 1% lidocaine with epi has 500 mg of lidocaine, a safe amount for a 70 kg person who receives diazepam.

Obstetrics

An estimated 99% of world maternal deaths occur in Africa, Asia, Latin America, and the Caribbean. In LICs and LMICs, pregnancy-related complications are the leading cause of maternal death and disability for women 15 to 49 years of age. The lifetime risk of death in childbirth varies from 1 in 7 in Angola to 1 in 3500 in Europe to 1 in around 30,000 in Sweden. Annually, 45 million women deliver without a skilled birth attendant. A woman dies every 7 minutes from postpartum hemorrhage, the most common cause of maternal death. Infectious and hypertensive (preeclampsia/eclampsia) emergencies make up the remainder of the common causes of maternal mortality, which constitutes the single most disparate public health measure between rich and poor countries.

A. Peripartum Hemorrhage

Pre- and postpartum hemorrhage are ubiquitous obstetrical challenges, especially in areas with deficient antenatal care, instant-donor or nonexistent blood banks, and the absence of safe anesthesia, airway management, and knowledgeable personnel.

1. Antepartum

The three major concerns are placenta previa, placental abruption, and uterine rupture. An ultrasound (U/S) helps locate the placenta and gives some guidance on strategy.

If the placenta is not covering the cervix, a vaginal delivery can be attempted if both mother and baby are not in distress. If bleeding is heavy, continual, or with clots, or if either the mother or baby are in distress, then proceed straightaway to a cesarean section (C-section). If there is a history of prior C-section plus a low-lying placenta, consider placenta accreta. Abruptio placenta is separation of the placenta before delivery and can be accompanied by hypertension, preeclampsia, eclampsia with a hard, tender uterus and "pain out of proportion" to contractions. Fetal distress and death often occur. The goal is to save the mother which, if the cervix is not dilated, means resuscitation and an emergent C-section, often attended by coagulation disorders. Uterine rupture is seen primarily in women with prior C-sections or in grand multiparas (>5), those who present with long obstructive labors, or those with malpresentations. The bleeding may be intraabdominal rather than vaginal because the baby's head obstructs the birth canal. A midline laparotomy is indicated whenever a ruptured uterus is suspected, both for any chance to salvage the baby and to save the mother.

2. Postpartum

Uterine atony with prolonged labor or multiparity, genital tract trauma, retained placental tissue, inversion of the uterus, maternal bleeding disorders, and ruptured uterus produce postpartum bleeding.

a. Atony

Options include uterotonics (oxytocin, IV/intramuscular [IM]/intramyometrial and cytotec, methergine, carboprost), bimanual fundal "massage," removing all products of conception (swiping the uterine cavity with a lap sponge over one's hand), and uterine artery ligations ± ligation of the ovarian arteries, compressing sutures (B-Lynch suture), and ligation of the hypogastric (internal iliac) arteries. The last resort is hysterectomy.

b. Genital tract trauma

Lacerations to the cervix or lateral vaginal walls can occur with cephalopelvic disproportion (CPD)/larger infants, rapid labor, obstructed labor, or instrumented labor. Thorough vaginal examination with good lighting and the patient in the lithotomy position can abet detection of such lacerations. For retained products of conception, evacuate the uterus using a lap sponge over one's hand. Examine the maternal surface of every placenta to look for missing cotyledons. If uterine inversion is noted, use a closed fist to try and replace the uterus back into the pelvis; once replaced, perform immediate massage, and use oxytocin or other uterotonics. Note: reinversion can occur. If unsuccessful, proceed to laparotomy and "pull" the uterus back up and into the pelvis by pulling on the round ligaments from inside the abdomen. For maternal bleeding disorders, keep the patient warm and use blood products if available. When a ruptured uterus is diagnosed, try to repair it via laparotomy. Failing a successful repair, proceed to hysterectomy. Timely decision making to proceed to hysterectomy is key once you know such is required. The morbidity and mortality of the procedure climb with time and blood loss.

B. Cesarean Sections

C-sections are indicated for cephalopelvic disproportion, abnormal fetal presentations, placenta previa, fetal distress with a nondilated cervix, failure to progress (dystocia), abruption of the placenta, a prolapsed cord, etc. (See chapter 22, especially pages 237–238, by Groen and Kushner in Meara et al.[8]). Young age at conception and undernutrition with a small pelvis are a recipe for trouble, especially when coupled with late presentation, a bias against C-section, and the attendant fears of financial burden. This "perfect storm" combines to yield high fetal loss and obstetric fistula (vesicovaginal fistula [VVF] or vesicorectal fistula) in many RPAs. Timely C-section is the preferred treatment for obstructed labor.

In most centers, equipment and expertise for vacuum-assisted deliveries are not available. Symphysiotomy in obstructed labor entails dividing the symphysis pubis sharply to open up the pelvic ring and has a role in the second stage of labor if C-section is not available but with concerns about urethral injury and subsequent gait issues. Stateside symphysiotomy is generally reserved for a shoulder dystocia with the head already out. For the C-section, key areas to address follow.

1. Preparation
   Required are good anesthesia, illumination (a headlight helps), suction capability, a circulator, suture and equipment, and someone to focus on and resuscitate the baby once delivered, whether a nurse, midwife, colleague, or informed theater technician.

2. Positioning
   Place the mother in slight left lateral decubitus tilt to thwart inferior vena caval compression. Place a urinary catheter (Foley). Prep widely and include the perineum and the vagina.

3. Anesthesia
   Most agents cross the placenta and suppress the baby's subsequent breathing, etc. C-sections can be performed under general, spinal, or local anesthesia. The goals are a healthy mother and a healthy baby.

4. Abdominal incision
   For the nonobstetrician and in the emergent/urgent situation, use a lower midline incision, taking care not to enter the coelomic cavity. The uterus is extraperitoneal, below the peritoneal reflection. Try to avoid peritoneal cavity entry; but it is not a deal-breaker, more a style point. Incise the vesicouterine peritoneum and "push" the bladder down. Seek to avoid bladder entry. If you injure the bladder, repair it in two layers with absorbable sutures and keep the Foley in for a week or fortnight.

5. Uterine incision
   A horizontal lower uterine segment access is preferred over the "classical" vertical incision, given its lower uterine rupture potential with a subsequent pregnancy. Carefully enter the uterus via a 3 cm or so transverse incision above the bladder reflection, with care not to "stab" and injure the baby. Use digital retraction cephalad and caudally to enlarge the incision; use bandage scissors to extend the incision when needed. Take care: the myometrium may be only a few mm thick, that is, quite thin at this point.

6. Delivery
   Engage the presenting part with the palm of your hand, flex the neck of the fetus if possible, and cautiously deliver the baby. If the head is wedged in the pelvis, an assistant with gloved hands can push the fetus's head cephalad to abet delivery.

7. Postdelivery
   Place the baby, stably and securely, on the abdominal wall and clamp the cord. Note: the baby will be quite slippery. Once the cord has been divided, give the baby to the waiting assistant, and only then administer to the mother pharmacologic agents such as muscle relaxants, benzodiazepines, antibiotics, and, especially, oxytocin (5 units IV). Place atraumatic triangular, Babcock, or ring clamps on the lateral edges of the uterine incision to decrease blood loss.

8. Placental delivery
   Use slow, steady controlled cord traction to deliver the placenta followed by a spongestick or gauze removal of any remaining membranes.

9. Closure of the uterus
   Any heavy bleeding will usually abate with uterine closure if one takes care. Close with a careful running closure with 0 absorbable suture (catgut or polyglycolic) in one or two layers.

10. Abdominal wall closure
Use your preferred suture and technique. Absorbable polydioxanone suture (PDS) or nonabsorbable monofilament nylon all work if performed properly. Skin closure is your preference.

Abdomen and Abdominal Wall

A. Groin Hernias
Inguinal and femoral hernia, often incarcerated or strangulated. Hernias of the groin in children may present from birth, the first year of life, or childhood and represent a patent processus vaginalis. Hernias in infants are often bilateral and should be addressed with a high ligation of the sac.

Until recently, adults with inguinal or femoral hernias were treated via an open technique employing autogenous tissues utilizing a Bassini, McVay (Cooper's ligament), Shouldice, nylon darn, or other repair. Over the past 25 years, with the emergence of prosthetic repairs stateside and minimally invasive repairs, many surgeons have less experience with autogenous repairs. Mosquito net mesh with steam sterilization at 121°C × 15 minutes or 134°C to 137°C × 3.0 to 3.5 minutes has been found to be safe and economical with only 2 of more than 4000 patients requiring mesh excision during the past 6 years by Operation Hernia surgeons. If strangulation, perforation, or contamination are encountered, then an autogenous repair is indicated.

B. The Acute Abdomen
Acute abdomen does not equal "operative abdomen." Acute refers to a recent time since onset (a day or two, not weeks or longer) and not the characteristic of the pain, as with sharp versus dull. The "acute abdomen" bespeaks any of a myriad of disorders, excluding trauma, whose chief manifestation is in or abuts the abdomen and for which urgent operation may be necessary. If one visualizes the abdomen as a cylinder, then extraperitoneal processes such as pleurisy, pneumonia, pancreatitis, pelvic inflammatory disease, prostatitis, nephritis, and rectus muscle hematoma, among others, can cause pain and tenderness, which fall under the term "acute abdomen." Sir Zachery Cope enumerated a score of "medical conditions," including lues, diabetes, pancreatitis, sickle cell crisis, etc., that can present with an "acute abdomen" picture, for which operation is not indicated. The usual causes of the acute abdomen in Western practice relate to a perforated viscus, inflammation, obstruction, or ischemia. In the austere environment and in many LICs and LMICs, one must consider diseases such as typhoid with perforation, helminthoma, sigmoid volvulus, and more. For the surgeon, the history and physical examination are key because investigations (imaging and labs) are often unavailable or unaffordable. Whereas minimally invasive procedures (laparoscopy) are frequent in Western locales today, open procedures are the norm in underresourced areas. Open operations for perforated gastric and duodenal ulcers, appendicitis, cholecystitis, and diverticulitis of the colon (rare) will be similar to what pertains stateside and are not discussed here. Amoeba-related pathologies can confront the surgeon but are infrequent. Cholecystitis is quite rare in many parts of Africa, not so in other RPAs. Emergent abdominal operations include the aforementioned diagnoses plus perforated ileal ulcers from typhoid, sigmoid volvulus, bowel obstruction, especially from incarcerated or strangulated hernia, and rarer helminthic causes.

1. Perforated typhoid
The four classic pathological stages of intestinal typhoid, almost always ileal, are hyperplasia of lymphoid follicles, necrosis of mucosa, ulceration ± bleeding, and perforation. Perforated typhoid constitutes a threefold problem: generalized septicemia, generalized peritonitis, and dehydration and electrolyte imbalance. The key points of diagnosis and treatment include recognition, resuscitation, repair, and rehabilitation. Operative

options include local drainage, simple closure, ileostomy tube via perforation, wedge resection or segmental small bowel resection, closure and ileotransverse colostomy, and ileoright colectomy. A helpful aphorism at the time of the initial operation is to do "as much as necessary, as little as possible" in these compromised, critically ill patients requiring damage control. Close the fascia, but pack the skin and subcutaneous tissues. There is a role for healing by second intention or perhaps delayed primary closure. In these patients, intraabdominal deep space and interloop abscesses are frequent; second-look procedures and reoperation are common. "Preperforations" encountered at the initial operation should be over sewn and reinforced but may break down subsequently.

2. Sigmoid volvulus
   Per Denis Burkitt, sigmoid volvulus may be a downside of the "high fiber diet" and is often seen in many parts of Africa, notably the Horn. Although some advocate resection and primary anastomosis, with or without on-table lavage, most would resect the sigmoid, create an end colostomy and a mucus fistula, or close the rectosigmoid as in a Hartmann's procedure. At times, some small bowel can be caught up in the twist, the so-called "bowel in a knot" or "complex volvulus." Resect the compromised small bowel and perform a primary enteroenterostomy, and resect the twisted sigmoid as above. Volvulus of the cecum can occur but is infrequent. A right hemicolectomy is preferred to reduction and pexy procedures utilizing sutures or placement of a cecostomy tube.

Oncology

The WHO Cancer Today reported more than 18 million new cases with 9.5 million cancer-related deaths in 2018.[15] More than 60% of the world's cancer cases occur in Africa, Asia, and Central and South America, and these regions account for about 70% of the cancer deaths. Chemotherapeutic agents are not usually affordable, even if available. Few radiotherapy centers exist. Thus, for solid neoplasms, it is often the surgeon who is the provider of hope for a cure or, failing that, palliation. Patients often present late. Staging is usually based on a physical examination coupled with imaging via plain x-rays and abdominal U/S. In addition to lymphomas, the frequent solid cancers include breast, prostate, cervix uteri, hepatoma, Kaposi's, and stomach. Again there is much geographical variation: esophageal cancer in Kenya; oral cancer in Yemen (khat) and India (reverse smoking); and lung cancer anywhere tobacco use is prevalent. Childhood challenges include Wilms' tumor.

Urology

A. Acute urinary retention ensues from prostatic hypertrophy or cancer and urethral stricture. The history as always is vital. Ask about hesitancy in initiation of micturition, stream strength, interruption, frequency, terminal dribbling, etc. Percuss the bladder. Palpate the penile urethra and the perineum to assess for fibrosis. Watch the patient void and then attempt to pass a well-lubricated red rubber or urethral catheter. Is passage obstructed before the level of the prostate or at the prostate level? If the obstruction is prostatic, a 20 or 22 Fr catheter can more readily be passed than a smaller one. If the obstruction is from a stricture, use a filiform and follower technique to decompress the bladder. At times, neither a stout Foley nor a filiform can be passed, and a percutaneous (trocar-assisted) cystostomy can be performed to relieve the obstruction acutely before proceeding to further workup with either urethroscopy/cystoscopy or a retrograde urethrogram. Falls involving trauma to the perineum can injure or rupture the membranous urethra, and pelvic fractures with shear can disrupt the urethra at the mcmbranous/prostatic urethral junction. Gonococcal urethritis is on the decline but still a cause of urethral stricture.

B. Cancers of the prostate and bladder predominate, the latter associated with schistosomiasis in some regions. Most patients with cancer of the prostate present with advanced disease and treatment is hormonal or castration.

C. Congenital conditions. Hypospadias: do not perform circumcision on any male with abnormalities of the urethra/urethral orifice; preserve the valuable foreskin for later reconstruction via various urethroplasties. Undescended testis or testes: orchiopexy by 12 months of age maximizes the chances for spermatogenesis for boys with undescended testes. Posterior urethral valves in boys may not be diagnosed prenatally or shortly after birth. The child may present months later with chronic urinary difficulties with initiation of micturition and a weak stream. Consider a cystostomy to await expertise to permit valve destruction either endoscopically or via a perineal approach.

Osteomyelitis

Osteomyelitis may be either open (direct inoculation) or hematogenous, the latter at times often associated with hemoglobinopathies such as hemoglobin SS or SC. Presentations vary: acute, subacute, or chronic. View acute osteomyelitis as an abscess that requires incision and drainage (I&D), to not only drain the pus and allow speciation of the bacteria, but also to decompress the "hypertension" within the marrow cavity that causes further progression. Once the process has progressed to the chronic phase with involucrum (reactive cancellous bone formation) and sequestration (infarcted bone), the patient likely will have long-term drainage and intermittent flaring of infection until the sequestrum and any loculated pus are totally removed. Pathological fractures are a concern early on before significant involucrum formation occurs.

Common Neonatal/Pediatric Conditions

At least half of the population in RPAs are 15 years old or younger. African children have an estimated 85% cumulative risk of surgical disease by 15 years of age.

  A. Neonates: Up to 28 days

    1. Abdominal wall defects: omphalocele or gastroschisis. Membranes cover an omphalocele unless they have ruptured, whereas gastroschisis has no membrane. Children with omphalocele often have associated anomalies (cardiac, neurologic). If the membranes are intact, leave them alone, and do not perform any operation. Do not debride them. If left intact, the wound will eventually close by secondary intention. Omphaloceles with ruptured membranes or gastroschisis bowel must be covered somehow via either primary closure of the skin (make sure you have a ventilator available) or coverage with a silo (make one out of a sterilized IV bag).

    2. Anorectal malformations (ARMs)

      The most common male anomaly is a rectourethral fistula; the most common female defect is a fistula into the vestibule of the vagina just outside the hymen. Both of these are considered "high" defects and need a colostomy on the first or second day of life. Use a left lower quadrant incision to create a double-barrel, completely diverting colostomy with the distal descending or proximal sigmoid colon. The distal colon/rectum should be irrigated thoroughly at the time of colostomy creation to remove all meconium while it is soft. Definitive repair awaits someone with the expertise along with a safe anesthesia capability. If there is a perineal fistula, perhaps to the scrotal raphe, the fistula is considered "low" and can be repaired in the first day or two of life with a perineal anoplasty without colostomy. An anal cutback is easier for the nonpediatric surgeon and can be converted at a later time to a perineal anoplasty if needed.

    3. Small bowel atresia

      Atresias can occur anywhere in the intestine and are often multiple. Patients present with vomiting in the newborn period. Duodenal atresia can be treated with a duodeno-duodenostomy or duodenojejunostomy. Instill saline via the anastomotic opening of the intestine distal to the atresia to demonstrate and ensure transit to the cecum, because multiple atresias must be ruled out.

4. Malrotation with midgut volvulus

   Malrotation is a true emergency, because the torsed bowel, most often of the small bowel, can infarct. Suspect malrotation in any newborn or child with bilious vomiting. The upper gastrointestinal (UGI) series can help locate or identify the ligament of Treitz. When in doubt, explore. Reduce any malrotation found, lyse Ladd's bands in the right upper quadrant, make radial incisions in the peritoneal covering of the mesentery to widen the base of the mesentery to hopefully decrease repeat midgut volvulus, and then perform an appendectomy.

5. Esophageal atresia with or without a fistula

   Diagnosis can be made clinically, incorporating attempted passage of a red rubber catheter orally coupled with a chest/upper abdomen x-ray. Success will depend on surgical, anesthetic, and critical care/pediatric expertise and timeliness. If there is a fistula confirmed by air in the stomach but nonpassage of the catheter, then a thoracotomy is required to ligate the fistula and hopefully perform a definitive primary repair. If there is no fistula, as determined by nonpassage of the catheter without air in the stomach, then a cervical esophagostomy and gastrostomy are performed to await another day for definitive treatment with possibly a colon interposition. This differs from treatment in the United States, where there are intensive care nurseries where a gastrostomy can be performed but an esophagostomy avoided by using suction catheters in the esophageal pouch.

6. Congenital diaphragmatic hernia (CDH)

   The outcomes for children with CDH stateside are not outstanding even with critical care expertise and extracorporeal membrane oxygenation (ECMO). The neonate presents with "respiratory distress of the newborn" and has decreased or nil breath sounds on the left, with bowel in the left chest by x-ray and accompanying pulmonary hypoplasia. Pass an orogastric tube and treat expectantly, supportively for the first 5 days. If the child survives, then operation can be undertaken via a left subcostal incision or via the left chest to reduce the viscera and repair the diaphragm, either primarily or with prosthetic material if available.

7. Hypospadias—see Urology section previously.

8. Pyloric stenosis

   Suspect pyloric stenosis in any child in the first 2 months of life with progressive, projectile, nonbilious vomiting. One may palpate an "olive" in the epigastrium or right upper quadrant. If no "olive" is appreciated, use U/S if available, to confirm the diagnosis. Preoperative volume repletion until the child is voiding well is mandatory. When in doubt and no U/S is available, proceed to pyloroplasty based on clinical impression, via a transverse incision through the right rectus muscle midway between xiphoid and umbilicus. A longitudinal incision is made through the serosa and barely into the muscularis along the whole length of the hypertrophic pylorus. A pyloric spreader or hemostat is used to spread the halves of the pylorus. Great care is taken to avoid entering the mucosa; but if this occurs, carefully repair the defect and keep the child nil per os for 24 hours postoperatively.

9. Hirschsprung's disease

   A newborn with an anus who does not pass meconium in the first 48 hours should be suspected of having HD. Without contrast enemas and suction biopsy to confirm the diagnosis, one must operate based on clinical suspicion. Treatment is an initial colostomy in the distal portion of the grossly dilated colon (usually sigmoid) just above the transition zone funnel. A definitive pull-through procedure can be performed later electively, when expertise and safe anesthesia are available.

B. Infants

Intussusception is the leading cause of small bowel obstruction from 1 to 12 months. The child presents with intermittent colicky abdominal pain, perhaps with a "currant jelly stool," and at times with an empty right lower quadrant on physical exam. Diagnosis is often clinical. Reduction with air-contrast enemas is not the rule in RPAs. If suspected, explore. A key is to "push" the telescoped bowel from distal to proximal, not "pull" it. The bowel must be totally reduced to reveal the ileocecal valve area. The bowel is assessed for viability. If there is concern for infarction or ischemia that does not pinken up, then resection is indicated. A Meckel's diverticulum can serve as a "lead point," although usually the lead point is related to hyperplasia of Peyer's patches.

C. Children: 1 Year to Adolescence or Adulthood

  1. Groin hernia; umbilical hernia
     Inguinal hernias should be repaired when diagnosed unless in a neonate with immature lungs or other issues. The concerns are incarceration and strangulation. High ligation of the indirect sac usually without any floor repair is recommended. Consider exploring the contralateral groin in children under 10 years because there is a real possibility of bilaterality. Umbilical hernias are ubiquitous and spontaneous closure can occur until age 14 years. As a rule, there is no rush to repair them; incarceration episodes, with or without strangulation, are rare and the primary reason for repair.

  2. Appendicitis
     Open appendectomy via a right lower quadrant incision is the norm in RPAs. In advanced perforated appendicitis, conversion to a lower midline incision or a significantly extended right lower quadrant incision may be necessary to adequately perform peritoneal toileting.

Inflammatory/Infectious Conditions

A. Abscesses of the skin, subcutaneous tissue, muscles (pyomyositis), bones (osteomyelitis), joints (pyarthritis), thorax (empyema), and pericardial sac occur frequently and require drainage. *Staphylococcus aureus* is the most frequent pathogen. Multiple abscesses are common and may occur synchronously or metachronously. Early and wide drainage with antibiotic administration minimizes hematogenous spread of infection. Hand infections pose a special difficulty because most patients delay seeking medical care; even after drainage, antibiotics, elevation, and physiotherapy, residual hand deformity is frequently the outcome. Neonates may present with multiple metastatic abscesses, perhaps subsequent to the care of the umbilicus or male circumcision.

B. Inflammatory and mixed-synergistic infections include cancrum oris (noma, gangrenous stomatitis), Ludwig's angina, Fournier's gangrene, and necrotizing fasciitis. Cancrum oris, usually seen in malnourished children, is a destructive necrotic process that can produce oronasocutaneous fistulas and ankylosis of the temporomandibular joint. Treatment entails controlling the inflammation/infection, debriding and resecting the infarcted tissue, and restoring nutrition and immunocompetence, followed in time by a staged reconstruction with a vascularized flap. Ludwig's angina is a severe form of cellulitis of the submaxillary space and secondary involvement of the sublingual and segmental spaces subsequent to infection in the mandibular molar area or at times penetrating trauma to the floor of the mouth. For Ludwig's patients, maintaining and protecting the airway with adequate incision and drainage coupled with antibiotics are the initial treatments. These patients will need staged trips to the OR and vary in management from vascularized flap reconstruction for closure in the cancrum oris patients, to skin grafting versus healing by second intention via contraction and epithelialization for Fournier's gangrene patients. "Nec. fasc." patients warrant early and frequent (qd [daily] vs. qod [every other day] early on) debridement in the OR; some patients may require amputation or fecal diversion depending on location (extremity vs. perineum) and multiple trips to the OR theater. Necrotizing fasciitis can be like a fire and often lethal. Do not underestimate its virulence

Parasitic and Mycobacterial Diseases

A. Parasitic Diseases

It is claimed more people in the world have parasites than do not.

1. Ascariasis, historically, was ascribed as the leading cause of small bowel obstruction among patients where and when laparotomies were rare. Obstruction from worms seems rare at present, although in patients with a sizable biomass load, anthelmintics can create paralysis of the worms; obstruction can ensue after the initiation of treatment. Most patients can be successfully treated nonoperatively. Amoeba cause more medical problems than surgical as a rule, with either liver abscesses, usually treated with metronidazole rather than operations, or ameboma.

2. Other parasitic challenges for the surgeon often have a geographic track record such as the megasyndromes from Chaga' disease in South America and hydatid disease in the Middle East. A hookworm relative found in Ghana and Uganda, the nematode *Oesophagostomum*, evokes an intense inflammatory reaction and can present as appendicitis or even cancer. Most subside with medical therapy, but uncertainty as to diagnosis or complications such as abscesses, obstruction, or peritonitis can lead to exploration. Seek to learn and know the parasitic prevalences and patterns in whatever locale you find yourself. Listen to and learn from your hosts and their collective experience.

B. Mycobacterial Diseases

1. Tuberculosis (*Mycobacterium tuberculosis*) can fall into the domain of the surgeon because of pulmonary tuberculosis, empyema, Pott's disease with paraplegia potential, joint disease, and abdominal issues such as tuberculous peritonitis or ileal narrowing with bowel obstruction. In the present era, if a patient has tuberculosis, one must query if they have HIV infection and vice versa. Many patients are afflicted with the double burden of tuberculosis on top of HIV. A major concern, abetted by partial treatment, is the potential and emergence of multidrug resistant tuberculosis.

2. Hansen's disease (*M. leprae*, leprosy) patients present to the surgeon because of foot, finger, hand, and, at times, eye issues. The loss of protective sensation with subsequent neuropathic ulcers of the feet, mal perforans, and so on, are not dissimilar to what one encounters stateside in diabetic patients, albeit there is less associated vascular disease. Margaret Brand cautions us to *Mind the Eyes* of Hansen's patients who can proceed to blindness via about six mechanisms. The inability of the patient to completely blink (lagophthalmos) to cover and moisten the cornea can be treated by a lateral tarsorrhaphy.

3. Buruli ulcer (*M. ulcerans*) may be consequent to a trivial penetrating injury by a stick or twig, perhaps near a stream or river. The organism prefers a cooler environment and thrives in the subcutaneous tissue plane. Operative debridement and grafting may be required, but more recently, there is a role for antibiotic therapy with rifampicin combined with clarithromycin.[16] The infection may be increased in immunologically compromised patients. Treatment entails debridement of the margins of the ulcer, wound care, elevating the local temperature via a goose-neck lamp or other mechanism, nutritional replenishment if that is a cofactor, and often subsequent skin grafting.

Other Major Important Conditions—Not Addressed

A. Congenital Heart Disease

An estimated 40,000 infants per year are born in Nigeria with some form of congenital heart disease, yet perhaps only a few receive corrective operations.

B. Ophthalmologic Conditions; Blindness

About 80% of the blindness in RPAs is preventable. The major diagnoses are trachoma, cataract, xerophthalmia, onchocerciasis, and corneal scarring, whereas in the more resourced world the causes are macular degeneration, glaucoma, diabetes, cataracts, and congenital diseases. Most ophthalmologists reside in the resourced world; most folks who proceed to blindness in an RPA never see an ophthalmologist. Leprosy can produce blindness via a variety of mechanisms.

(Acknowledgment: Margaret Tarpley, MLS, Adjunct Lecturer, Department of Medical Education, University of Botswana and Adjunct Instructor, Surgery, Vanderbilt University, for editorial and technical support.)

Anesthesia

The global volume of surgery is estimated to be 313 million operations annually as of 2012. Approximately 29% of this total, 91 million operations, were performed in LICs.[3,17] Médecins Sans Frontières (Doctors Without Borders [MSF]) analyzed data over a 6-year period providing a sense of surgery patterns and anesthesia modalities most frequently used. Over the 6-year study, more than 75,000 anesthetics were provided to adult patients as follows: spinal anesthesia (46%); general anesthesia (GA) without intubation and often in conjunction with ketamine (34%); GA with intubation (10%); and regional anesthesia (RA) (7%). Given the inherent logistical challenges in austere and resource-limited environments, it is not surprising that spinal anesthesia was the most frequently used anesthetic in this large study. The most common types of procedures performed were C-sections (35%), followed by wound surgeries (25%), and herniorrhaphies (7%). Overall perioperative mortality was 0.25%, with the lowest rates associated with spinal anesthesia, RA, and GA without intubation.[18] Another retrospective study published by MSF showed that of over 79,000 procedures performed in a 7-year period, 45% were for trauma.[19]

Anesthesia and surgery will continue to play a pivotal role in managing the global burden of disease, especially because trauma remains a significant contributor to surgical volume. In addition, noncommunicable ailments potentially amenable to surgery, such as cardiovascular and pulmonary disease, are projected to surpass infectious diseases as the most important cause of mortality by 2020.[20] As the MSF analysis underscored, LICs and LMICs have underdeveloped and unreliable infrastructure, that is, inadequately maintained anesthesia equipment, unproven medical facilities, and constrained medical supply systems. Therefore, the austere anesthesia team should construct a standardized and streamlined anesthesia care model that can withstand challenging environments and uncertain logistics.

This chapter is intended to underscore the contextual framework for austere missions and identify high-yield considerations for austere anesthesia. This framework may be applied to short-term surgical missions that rely on the mission team's organic supplies and equipment, in addition to longer-term partner-support missions that may use host nation supplies and equipment. Less focus will be given to specific techniques of anesthesia or medication choices. Assumptions made with these recommendations are that anesthesia delivery will be overseen by a certified anesthesiologist (also recommended by the World Health Organization-World Federation of Societies of Anaesthesiologists [WHO-WFSA]), clinical anesthesia decisions made for individual circumstances will rest on the responsible anesthesia provider, and there may be multiple "right" answers to a given anesthesia scenario. Lastly, this document is not exhaustive and relies upon the anesthesia provider's appropriate application of anesthesia and creativity therein. Topics to be addressed are:

1. Case prioritization in resource-limited environments
2. Medical facilities, drugs, and equipment
3. Preparation
4. Patient safety
5. Technology and equipment
6. Techniques
7. Medications
8. Practical pointers and practice pearls

CASE PRIORITIZATION IN RESOURCE-LIMITED ENVIRONMENTS

Providing anesthesia services in the austere environment is highly demanding and can be stressful for the surgical/anesthesia team. Establishing common (team) goals and a common treatment philosophy before undertaking the medical mission is of utmost importance. Additionally, medical ethics, patient safety, and team capabilities and limitations should be considered. For example, should the team invest the most resources into the worst injuries/illnesses, or should the team strategize how to provide the most good for the most people, that is, a single long surgery versus many short surgeries? Should the team complete one complex surgery that requires complex postoperative care or one well-planned surgery that requires little to no postoperative care? These questions are simplified but serve to bring out the philosophical underpinnings of establishing surgical priorities and triage. Methods for selecting surgical candidates should therefore be established a priori, as it may be difficult to reconcile ethical issues in the heat of the moment and unexpected team conflict may result.

Safety standards must be established and agreed upon by the team. In LMICs anesthesia-related mortality can be as high as 1 in 300.[21] Many sources recommend that austere anesthesia providers adhere as closely as possible to HIC anesthesia standards of care. The team should decide beforehand if and how it will deviate from home country safety standards and which host nation safety standards are acceptable. The team should also determine beforehand when to stop providing medical care (e.g., when resources or safety capabilities are exhausted, and despite host nation pleas to continue). It is critical to understand that the team's capabilities in its home environment do not equal the same team's capabilities in the austere environment. Surgical team members will not likely be familiar with each other, further affecting patient care. Failure to acknowledge these limitations can be a significant source of team friction and can lead to increased patient harm.

In 2018, the WHO-WFSA jointly published an updated document detailing recommendations for international standards for safe anesthesia.[22] The WHO-WFSA document reconciled recommendations from other entities concerned with the same goal of safe surgery, such as the LCoGS, and illustrates the suggested degrees/capabilities of anesthesia care at three healthcare facility and infrastructure levels (see further in this section).[23] Also included are recommended standards for patient monitoring at each level. It is important to note that the recommended capabilities and standards will be unique to the specific environment and clinical situation. A complete review of this WHO-WFSA document is beyond the scope of this chapter; however, it is highly encouraged that the entire anesthesia team reviews it before undertaking an austere or resource-limited surgical mission.

Considering the WHO-WFSA safety standards document and the preponderance of anesthesia safety literature currently available, it is important to note that wherever and whenever possible anesthesia care should be provided or overseen by a certified anesthesiologist (Highly Recommended, see Patient Safety, Perioperative Care). As such, the ultimate provision of anesthesia, choice of medication and technique, risk assessment, and so on should be decided by the responsible anesthesia provider and even more importantly by a provider who has experience providing anesthesia care in the austere setting. Many recently trained anesthesiologists, for example, may have never used older anesthetics with significant hemodynamic implications such as halothane, which are still in use in other countries. The exact prevalence of worldwide use of halothane for GA is unknown, however, the WHO Model List of Essential Medicines (August 2017) lists halothane as an essential medicine along with isoflurane, nitrous oxide, and oxygen (available at http://www.who.int/medicines/publications/essentialmedicines/en/).

MEDICAL FACILITIES/DRUGS/EQUIPMENT

The WHO and the WHO-WFSA safe anesthesia standards documents describe three levels of medical facilities and associated services, capabilities, equipment, and drugs. Tables 12.1 and 12.2

TABLE 12.1 ▉ World Health Organization Healthcare Facility Levels: Infrastructure/Capability/
Procedures/Personnel

	Level 1 Small Hospital/ Health Center	Level 2 District/ Provincial Hospital	Level 3 Referral Hospital
Infrastructure	• Rural with small number of beds, sparsely equipped OR/procedure room	• 100–300 beds, adequately equipped major and minor ORs	• 300–1000 or more beds, intensive care facilities
Capability	• Emergency treatment of 90%–95% of trauma and obstetric cases (excluding cesarean section) • Referral of other patients (e.g., obstructed labor, bowel obstruction) to a higher level	Same as Level 1, with addition of: • Short-term treatment of 95%–99% of major life-threatening conditions	Same as Level 2, with addition of: • Intensive care treatment • Limited care for: hemodialysis, complex neurosurgical/cardiac surgery, prolonged respiratory failure
Procedures	• Normal vaginal delivery • Uterine evacuation • Circumcision • Hydrocele reduction, incision and drainage • Wound suturing • Control of hemorrhage with pressure dressings • Debridement and dressing of wounds • Temporary reduction of fractures • Cleaning/stabilization of open/closed fractures • Chest drainage (limited)	Same as Level 1 with addition of: • Cesarean delivery • Laparotomy (usually not for bowel obstruction) • Amputation • Hernia repair • Tubal ligation • Closed fracture treatment/application of cast • Eye operations, including cataract extraction • Removal of foreign bodies (e.g., in the airway) • Emergency ventilation and airway management for referred patients such as those with thoracic and head injuries	Same as Level 2 with addition of: • Facial and intracranial surgery • Bowel surgery • Pediatric and neonatal surgery • Thoracic surgery • Major eye surgery • Major gynecologic surgery (e.g., vesicovaginal repair)
Personnel	• Paramedical staff without formal anesthesia training • Nurse-midwife	• 1–2 trained anesthetists • District medical officers, senior clinical officers, nurses, midwives • Visiting specialists/ resident surgeon/ obstetrician-gynecologist	• Clinical officers and specialists in anesthesia and surgery

Modified from World Health Organization. *Guide to Infrastructure and Supplies at Various Levels of Health Care Facilities. Emergency and Essential Surgical Care.* Available at: http://www.who.int/surgery/publications/ s15983e.pdf?ua=1. Accessed August 2018.

TABLE 12.2 ■ World Health Organization Healthcare Facility Levels: Drugs

	Level 1 Small Hospital/ Health Center	Level 2 District/ Provincial Hospital	Level 3 Referral Hospital
Drugs	• Ketamine • Lidocaine 1% or 2% • Diazepam injection • Epinephrine 1 mg/mL (limited) • Atropine 0.6 mg/mL (limited)	Same as Level 1, with addition of: • Thiopental 500 mg/1 g powder • Suxamethonium bromide 500 mg powder • Atropine 0.5 mg injection • Epinephrine 1 mg injection • Diazepam 10 mg injection • Halothane, 250 mL inhalation • Bupivacaine 0.5% heavy or plain, 4 mL • Hydralazine 20 mg injection • Furosemide 20 mg injection • Dextrose 50%, 20 mL injection • Aminophylline 250 mg injection • Ephedrine 30/50 mg ampoules	Same as Level 2, with addition of: • Vecuronium 10 mg powder • Pancuronium 4 mg injection • Neostigmine 2.5 mg injection • Trichloroethylene, 500 mL inhalation • Calcium chloride 10%, 10 mL injection • Potassium chloride 20%, 10 mL injection (for infusion)

Modified from World Health Organization. *Guide to Infrastructure and Supplies at Various Levels of Health Care Facilities. Emergency and Essential Surgical Care.* Available from: http://www.who.int/surgery/publications/s15983e.pdf?ua=1. Accessed August 2018.

summarize this information. The LCoGS article mentioned previously notes that all Level 2 hospitals should aim to provide Bellwether procedures defined as laparotomy, cesarean delivery, and treatment of an open fracture. These procedures are acute and high value, and the consistent performance of these procedures is suggestive of a capable surgical system with broad service delivery.

The WHO-WFSA also defines recommendations for safety standards and minimum equipment requirements based on three levels: Highly Recommended (minimum standard, essentially mandatory), Recommended, and Suggested (standards practiced when resources allow and if appropriate for the care being provided). Tables 12.3 and 12.4 summarize these recommendations.

Briefly summarizing Table 12.1 through Table 12.4, a Level 1 facility represents a small rural hospital or clinic with very limited surgical equipment that provides emergency services for trauma, minor surgery, and obstetric cases (excluding Caesarean delivery). A Level 1 facility refers more complex surgical care (e.g., obstructed labor, bowel obstruction) to a higher level. Level 1 drugs include ketamine, lidocaine 1% or 2%, diazepam/midazolam, morphine, epinephrine, atropine, dextrose, normal saline or Ringer's lactate, oxygen, and appropriate inhalation anesthetic if a vaporizer is available and the machine is functional.[22,23]

A Level 2 facility represents a district or provincial hospital with 100 to 300 beds and adequate surgical capabilities to handle major life-threatening conditions such as laparotomy and cesarean delivery. Level 2 drugs include Level 1 drugs plus thiopental/propofol, succinylcholine/suxamethonium bromide, pancuronium/atracurium, neostigmine, inhalation anesthetic (e.g., halothane, isoflurane, or other agent), lidocaine 5% heavy spinal solution, bupivacaine 0.5% heavy or plain, hydralazine, furosemide, dextrose 50%, aminophylline, ephedrine, norepinephrine, phenylephrine, hydrocortisone, ± nitrous oxide.[22,23]

A Level 3 facility represents a referral hospital with 300 to 1000 beds capable of handling complex subspecialty surgical cases and managing prolonged intensive care cases. Level 3 drugs include Level 2 drugs plus propofol, nitrous oxide, sevoflurane, rocuronium/cisatracurium,

TABLE 12.3 ■ **World Health Organization-World Federation of Societies of Anaesthesiologists: Standards for Drugs by Recommendation Level**

Drugs: WHO-WFSA (recommendation level)	HIGHLY RECOMMENDED	RECOMMENDED Same as HIGHLY RECOMMENDED with addition of:	SUGGESTED Same as RECOMMENDED with addition of:
	• Ketamine • Diazepam or midazolam • Morphine • Local anesthetic (e.g., lidocaine/bupivacaine) • Dextrose • Normal saline (injection) • Normal saline or Ringer's lactate (infusion) • Oxygen • Epinephrine • Atropine • Dextrose • Morphine • Acetaminophen • Nonsteroidal antiinflammatory • Magnesium	• Thiopental or propofol • Inhalational anesthetic gas (e.g., isoflurane) • Succinylcholine • Nondepolarizing neuromuscular blocker (e.g., pancuronium or atracurium) • Neostigmine • Mannitol, Plasma-lyte • Amiodarone • Ephedrine, metaraminol, norepinephrine, or phenylephrine • Hydrocortisone • Salbutamol • Calcium gluconate (or chloride) • Hydralazine • Furosemide	• Propofol • Alternative inhalational anesthetic gas (e.g., sevoflurane) • Alternative nondepolarizing neuromuscular blocker (e.g., rocuronium or cisatracurium) • Tramadol • Gabapentin • Oxycodone • Nitroglycerin • Heparin

Modified from World Health Organization. Model list of essential medications. 2017. Available at: http://apps.who.int/iris/bitstrea/handle/10665/273826/EML-20-eng.pdf?ua+1. Accessed August 2018.

inotropic agents, intravenous antiarrhythmic agents, IV nitroglycerine, tramadol, gabapentin, oxycodone, calcium chloride 10%, potassium chloride 20%, and heparin. Recommended durable and disposable equipment for each level is similarly detailed in Tables 12.4 and 12.5.[22]

PREPARATION

Preparation for austere conditions will challenge the clinical decision-making of any medical team. The unpredictability of circumstances and conditions simply cannot be underestimated (e.g., hurricane Katrina in 2005 crippled the southeast United States infrastructure and medical systems). Creative solutions will be necessary for some situations in austere or resource-limited environments and many factors must be taken into consideration:

1. Physical safety of the clinical area (armed conflict vs. natural disaster)
2. Surgical facility (fixed or mobile)
3. Logistical supply chain (use of organic mission team equipment with sterilization of reusable items, and so on vs. host nation supplies [compatibility issues] vs. austere with few durable or disposable supplies and low probability of timely resupply).
4. Power source ("clean" established reliable power vs. variable duration of rationed power vs. unpredictable power from outdated unreliable grid vs. local generator power vs. no electrical power).

TABLE 12.4 ■ **World Health Organization-World Federation of Societies of Anaesthesiologists: Standard for Equipment by Recommendation Level**

Equipment: WHO-WFSA (Recommendation level)	HIGHLY RECOMMENDED	RECOMMENDED Same as HIGHLY RECOMMENDED with addition of:	SUGGESTED Same as RECOMMENDED with addition of:

	• Adequate lighting
	• Tilting operating table
	• Supply of oxygen (concentrator, cylinders, or pipeline)
	• Oropharyngeal airways
	• Face masks
	• Laryngoscope + blades (adult and pediatric)
	• Endotracheal tubes (adult and pediatric)
	• Intubation aids (e.g., Magill forceps, bougie, stylet)
	• Suction device + catheters
	• Self-inflating bags (adult and pediatric)
	• IV infusion equipment (adult and pediatric)
	• Regional and neuraxial block equipment
	• Sterile gloves
	• Access to defibrillator
	• Stethoscope
	• Pulse oximeter
	• Carbon dioxide detector (Single use)
	• Noninvasive blood pressure monitor with cuffs (adults and pediatric)
	• Electrocardiography
		• Work surface and storage for equipment and medications
		• System for delivering inhalation anesthesia (draw-over or plenum)
		• For plenum systems
		  ○ Inspired oxygen concentration monitor
		  ○ Antihypoxia device (prevent delivery of a hypoxic gas mixture)
		  ○ System to prevent improper connection of gas sources
		• Automated ventilator with disconnect alarm
		• IV pressure infusor bag
		• IV fluid warner
		• Nonsterile examination gloves
		• Waveform capnography
		• ECG
		• Temperature monitor (intermittent)
		• Nerve stimulator (twitch monitor)
		• Dedicated space for recovering patients
			• Dedicated space for preoperative assessment
			• System for delivering inhalation anesthesia (plenum)
			• Inhalational gas concentration monitor
			• Adult and pediatric supraglottic airways
			• IV infusion pumps
			• Warming blanket
			• Overhead heater (neonates)
			• Incubator (neonates)
			• ICU ventilator
			• Invasive (intraarterial) blood pressure monitor
			• Temperature monitor (continuous)

ECG, electrocardiogram; *ICU,* intensive care unit, *IV,* intravenous.
Modified from World Health Organization. *Guide to Infrastructure and Supplies at Various Levels of Health Care Facilities. Emergency and Essential Surgical Care.* Available at: http://www.who.int/surgery/publications/s15983e.pfd?ua=1. Accessed August 2018; Gelb AW, Morriss WW, Johnson W, et al. World Health Organization-World Federation of Societies of Anaesthesiologists (WHO-WFSA) International Standards for a Safe Practice of Anesthesia. *Anesth Analg.* 2018;126:2047–2055. Accessed August 2018.

To oversimplify, one should consider the environment as either a safe environment where no physical threat to the medical team exists or a critical unsafe environment where the safety of the medical team is threatened. Provision of anesthesia and surgical care in the latter is not recommended unless the proper resources (e.g., host nation security elements), are in place to ensure the physical safety of the surgical team and patients. Once physical security is established, the

TABLE 12.5 ■ World Health Organization Healthcare Facility Levels: Equipment

	Level 1 Small Hospital/Health Center	Level 2 District/Provincial	Level 3 Referral Hospital
Equipment (reusable)	• Adult and pediatric resuscitators • Manual suction • Oxygen concentrator	Complete anesthesia, resuscitation and airway management system: • Oxygen source • Vaporizer • Hoses/valves/bellows or bag to inflate lungs • Face masks (sizes 00–5) • Work surface and storage • Pediatric anesthesia system • Adult and pediatric resuscitator sets • Pulse oximeter • Laryngoscope blades (Mac 1–3, ± 4) • Oxygen concentrator (storage cylinder) • Suction (electric) • IV pressure infusor bag • Magill forceps (adult and child) • Intubation stylet and/or bougie	Same as Level 2, and addition: • Pulse oximeter and spare probes (adult and pediatric) • ECG monitor • Anesthesia ventilator (electric with manual override) • Infusion pumps (two per OR/ICU bed) • Defibrillator (one per OR/ICU bed) • Automatic noninvasive blood pressure machine • Capnograph • Oxygen analyzer • Temperature probe • Warming blanket • Warming heater • Infant incubator • Laryngeal mask airways sizes 2, 3, 4 (three sets per OR) • Intubating bougie, adult and pediatric (1 set per OR)
Equipment (disposable)	• IV equipment • Suction catheters, size 16 Fr • Examination gloves	Same as Level 1, with addition of: • Normal saline, Ringer's lactate dextrose 5% • Nasogastric tubes, sizes 10–16 Fr • Oral airways, sizes 000–4 • Endotracheal tubes, sizes 3–8.5 • Spinal needles, sizes 22 G and 25 G • Batteries, sizes AA and C	Same as Level 2, with addition of: • ECG electrodes • Ventilator circuits • Yankhauer sucker • Filter tubing for transfusion • Disposables for suction machine • Disposables for capnography/oxygen analyzer (sample lines, water traps, connectors, filters–fuel cells)

ECG, Electrocardiogram; ICU, intensive care unit; IV, intravenous; Mac, minimum alveolar concentration; OR, operating room.
Modified from World Health Organization. Guide to Infrastructure and Supplies at Various Levels of Health Care Facilities. Emergency and Essential Surgical Care. Available at: http://www.who.int/surgery/publications/s15983.pdf?ua=1. Accessed August 2018.

above-mentioned factors can be evaluated to determine the most appropriate anesthetic for the given clinical and environmental setting.

Although there are many resources to augment planning and preparation, three recent texts published in 2015 and 2017 are highlighted here and worthy of review: (1) *Essential Surgery: Disease Control Priorities*; (2) *Combat Anesthesia: The First 24 Hours*; (3) *Pediatric Surgery and Medicine for Hostile Environments*.[20,24,25]

PATIENT SAFETY

The WHO *Surgical Safety Checklist* provides recommendations to optimize safety during three critical perioperative phases: before induction, before incision, and before leaving the OR. "Before induction" focuses on ensuring correct patient, procedure, laterality, allergies, critical equipment functionality (anesthesia machine and medication check, pulse oximeter function), and anticipated airway or hemorrhage risks. "Before incision" covers OR team roles and dynamics, focusing on critical stages of surgery and critical events for nursing and anesthesia. "Before leaving" the OR covers instrument counts, confirmation of procedure performed, equipment issues, and anesthesia/nursing concerns for recovery and management of the patient (available at http://www.who.int/patientsafety/topics/safe-surgery/checklist/en/). This checklist in combination with the WHO-WFSA document can be used to facilitate a standardized approach to safety.[22]

PERIOPERATIVE CARE

The American Society of Anesthesiologists (ASA) Task Force on Preanesthesia Evaluation published a practice advisory supported by extensive literature correlating risks and benefits of various screening tests.[26] Many of the references are published using data from HICs that may not be generalizable to the austere LMIC demographic or environment. The austere anesthesia provider must make a determination of which, if any, screening tests to obtain before surgery to enhance appropriate patient selection and ensure needed equipment is available. A simple test, such as a pregnancy test, may be offered to female patients of childbearing age and for whom the result would alter the patient's management.[26] At a minimum, a history with a review of systems should be obtained and a physical examination performed. Often the patient's self-reported history will provide the most relevant clues to the underlying pathology, allowing specific preparation to mitigate morbidity or mortality.

In the *WHO-WFSA International Standards for a Safe Practice of Anesthesia* document, standards for safety and monitoring are ranked by priority: Highly Recommended (minimum standard, essentially mandatory), Recommended, and Suggested (standards practiced when resources allow and if appropriate for the care being provided). See Table 12.6 for details. Note that the anesthesia provider should be adhering to the Recommended and Suggested standards when providing elective surgery in any environment, austere or otherwise. In some austere or resource-limited settings, the Highly Recommended standard may not be met, and the provision of anesthesia should be restricted to those emergency procedures critical to preserving life, limb, or eyesight. The authors further suggest that in cases of elective procedures, if Highly Recommended standards cannot be met "provision of anesthesia for elective surgical procedures is unsafe and unacceptable."[22]

TECHNOLOGY AND EQUIPMENT

Modern anesthesia in HICs relies heavily on sophisticated equipment and technology that is frequently ill-suited for austere environments because of deficiencies in the power grid, extremes of environmental temperatures, lack of technical training/expertise, and unreliable access to maintenance and replacement parts.[27,28] One comprehensive clinical engineering source cites upwards

TABLE 12.6 ▓ **World Health Organization-World Federation of Societies of Anaesthesiologists: Standards for Monitoring by Recommendation Level**

Monitoring (recommendation level)	HIGHLY RECOM-MENDED	RECOMMENDED Same as HIGHLY RECOM-MENDED with addition of:	SUGGESTED Same as RECOMMENDED with addition of:
	• Clinical oversight by a certified anesthetist	• Inspired oxygen concentration monitor	• Continuous measurement of:
	• Pulse rate and quality	• Device to prevent hypoxic gas delivery	• Inspired and expired gas volumes
	• Tissue oxygenation and perfusion	• Disconnect alarm (mechanical ventilation)	• Inspired and expired inhalation anesthetic concentrations
	• Respiratory rate and quality	• Continuous ECG	• Continuous arterial blood pressure monitoring (when appropriate)
	• Breathing system bag movement	• Nerve stimulator (Twitch monitor, when muscle relaxants used)	• Continuous temperature monitoring
	• Breath sounds	• Continuous waveform capnography (during general anesthesia or deep sedation)	• Urine output monitoring
	• Heart sounds (e.g., precordial stethoscope)	• Intermittent tempera-ture monitoring	• EEG monitoring (when appropriate)
	• Audible signals and alarms at all times		
	• Continuous pulse oximetry		
	• Intermittent noninva-sive blood pressure monitoring		
	• Carbon dioxide (for intubation)		
	• Assessment of pain store (age appropriate)		

ECG, Electrocardiogram; *EEG,* electroencephalogram.
Modified from Gelb AW, Morriss WW, Johnson W, et al. World Health Organization-World Federation of Societies of Anaesthesiologists (WHO-WFSA) International Standards for Safe Practice of Anesthesia. *Anesth Analg.* 2018;126:2047–2055.

of 80% of medical devices fail in the austere environment.[29] Furthermore, austere environments frequently lack access to consumable and disposable resources, which may further affect the functioning of medical equipment. For these reasons and because anesthesia machines, medical-grade gases, and other adjunct monitors may not be consistently available or reliable, it is important to consider and plan for alternative techniques and modalities not reliant upon these technologies. The WHO-WFSA document may be used as a starting point when considering which equipment or machines may be available or should be used in the austere setting. Keep in mind that the Highly Recommended safety standards and standards for monitoring are essentially mandatory and apply to any modality of anesthesia, be it monitored anesthesia care, RA, neuraxial anesthesia, or GA. Also keep in mind that equipment considered to be ubiquitous in HICs, such as portable U/S machines and anesthesia infusion pumps, may not be commonly accessible in the resource-limited environment; if equipment is available, it may be reserved only for the high-risk locations such as the cardiac rooms.

Depending on the type of surgical mission, the anesthesia team will need to prioritize what resources to bring. For example, a short-term mission with all the equipment, supplies, and medications supplied by the mission team versus a long-term partner-assist mission utilizing primarily host nation resources. This decision on what to bring can be informed by a predeployment site survey or a comprehensive visit to the host nation, paying particular attention to the anticipated patient load, facilities' operational status, local support, medical contingencies using host nation services, clean water availability, electricity availability and type, piped gases availability to include oxygen concentrators versus cylinders of compressed medical-grade oxygen, etc. It is conceivable that the mission team will need to bring all equipment, supplies, and medications to last the duration of the surgical mission.

TECHNIQUES

1. Inhalational anesthesia, sometimes referred to as volatile gas anesthesia (VGA), is performed with five agents that are in use today: nitrous oxide (nonvolatile), halothane, isoflurane, desflurane, and sevoflurane. Nitrous oxide is commonly used as an inhalational adjunct for induction or maintenance of GA or for moderate sedation to assist with procedures. Consider not using nitrous oxide where inhaled oxygen concentrations cannot be measured, otherwise a potentially hypoxic mixture may be delivered. Although halothane is no longer in use in North America, it is still in use in LMICs, although the prevalence of its use worldwide is uncertain. Halothane and sevoflurane are less pungent, lending to their effectiveness with inhalational inductions, especially in children. Of particular importance with halothane is its dose-dependent myocardial depression. Isoflurane is pungent, and therefore should not be used for inhalational induction, but it is well suited for cases where cardiac stability is important because of minimal cardiac depression. Desflurane exhibits a high vapor pressure requiring a special heated vaporizer for safe use and has an ultrashort duration of action with moderate potency. Sevoflurane is nonpungent and is the most commonly used agent for inhalational inductions. Sevoflurane exhibits mild cardiac depression and may prolong the QT interval.

2. Total intravenous anesthesia (TIVA) is particularly amenable to austere settings and is a practical alternative to VGA. Although target-controlled infusion (TCI) devices are not yet US Food and Drug Administration (FDA) approved in the United States, these devices are in use in Europe and elsewhere and therefore may be available in austere environments. A TCI device is a computer-controlled system that is intended to deliver a target plasma concentration of a drug. Exact knowledge of an individual patient's pharmacokinetics is difficult to ascertain or measure, making use of the TCI device an imperfect science.

   TIVA has both logistical and physiologic advantages over VGA in the austere setting. In essence, all that is needed for TIVA is an appropriate IV anesthetic such as propofol and/or ketamine, which may be combined with other IV adjuncts such as midazolam and/or opioids to achieve surgical anesthesia. A programmable syringe driver (TCI device), a standard syringe or IV fluid pump, or drop counting using given sets of IV tubing with known drops/mL combined with close monitoring of vital signs could be used to maintain anesthesia. There are numerous drop counter apps for tablets or smart phones to make drop counting more precise. The alternative, VGA, requires machines, vaporizers, volatile gases, monitors, and reliable supplies of oxygen and power. Should a patient require transport to another location while sedated, TIVA facilitates this movement with the least interruptions of anesthesia.[30]

   Compared with even the newer VGA agents, postsurgery nausea, vomiting, antiemetic use, and headache were found to be lowest following propofol-based TIVA.[30,31] This outcome is especially appreciated in the Level 1 facility. Postanesthesia recovery complications strain existing personnel requirements, diverting valuable resources away from the OR. Because it is not predictable that the austere surgical theater will have a robust recovery capability, any element that diverts resources away from surgery should be avoided or mitigated.

Another reason to consider TIVA in the austere setting is a physiologic benefit. The metabolic consequences of severe illness or trauma can significantly affect both the perioperative course of anesthesia and the postoperative surgical outcome. Elevated inflammatory markers and stress hormones are found in victims of disaster, trauma, or severe illness and create a protein imbalance that can impair wound healing following surgery. When TIVA is used, versus VGA, these inflammatory markers and stress hormones are measurably less.[32,33] Although not singularly conclusive, this does suggest a tangible and potentially long-lasting benefit to using this modality. Unrelated to the metabolic derangements of malnutrition and trauma is the hypermetabolic state of malignant hyperthermia (MH), which may occur after exposure to VGA and/or succinylcholine. Although rare, with an estimated incidence of 1 in 15,000 in general anesthetics, MH is potentially fatal, requiring tremendous personnel and logistical resources to treat and manage.[34] TIVA (without the use of succinylcholine) eliminates this grave albeit rare complication. Another rare complication associated with TIVA is unrecognized awareness with explicit recall (AWR) during surgery. This is mainly because, despite the use of TCIs, a verifiable monitor value for depth of anesthesia, such as the minimum alveolar concentration (MAC) used with VGA, does not exist. Available literature suggests that AWR may be more likely with TIVA and consideration of brain monitoring during surgery may be reasonable; however, this is a field requiring greater study. That said, the reported incidence of AWR is approximately 1 to 2 cases in 1000 (0.1%–0.2%).[35] Assuming that anesthesia machines, compressed medical-grade gases, and modern volatile agents are not available, and recognizing the limitations in monitoring depth of anesthesia, TIVA is still a practical option for GA in settings where GA is required and the supply chain is constrained.

3. RA boasts many advantages in the austere environment and can supplement GA or serve as the primary means to achieve surgical anesthesia.[36] As discussed earlier, GA requires a relatively large logistical footprint to include personnel (postoperative monitoring and management of complications), equipment, and supplies. RA, however, reduces the total general anesthetic dose including opioids and maximizes the patient's participation in postoperative recovery. This minimizes the clinical "overhead" required to manage patients in the postoperative recovery environment. RA delivers excellent operating conditions including profound perioperative analgesia, stable hemodynamics, limb-specific anesthesia, reduced need for additional anesthetics, improved postoperative alertness and participation, minimal side effects, and rapid recovery from anesthesia, and uses easily transported equipment.[37] In conventional settings, RA has been used in the OR following surgery for postoperative pain control. RA in the acute trauma setting and during the initial transport of patients to definitive care is promising and has been associated with a reduced stress response to injury.[38]

U/S machines are more portable and readily available, further enhancing the safety margin for RA, especially for the placement of continuous peripheral nerve blocks (CPNBs) using indwelling catheters.[39,40] Some providers may still prefer the nerve stimulator technique and although the overall outcome is heavily influenced by provider experience, data suggest that adverse outcomes, including nerve damage and local anesthetic systemic toxicity (LAST), are similarly low between both nerve stimulator and U/S-guided techniques.[41] RA via CPNB can provide days of improved pain control, allowing for serial surgical procedures and transport.[40,42] In addition to improved pain control, modalities such as epidural (neuraxial) RA reduce morbidity and mortality in the setting of major thoracic surgery or thoracic trauma, such as multiple rib fractures. Thoracic epidurals, although not feasible in all Level 1 hospitals, have been associated with greater restoration of pulmonary function and reduced incidence of nosocomial pneumonia in settings of thoracic surgery or trauma.[40,43] The portable programmable pumps used with CPNBs and epidural catheters are straightforward and run off common batteries, simplifying use in both the OR and postoperative settings where electrical power can be unreliable. The portable nature of these pumps also provides for uninterrupted analgesia from the intraoperative phase through recovery ± transport to another facility. A creative application for the CPNBs, for example, is the continuous transversus abdominus plane (TAP) block, which has been used successfully in thoracoabdominal trauma.[44] The single injection TAP block or the continuous TAP block is reasonable when an epidural is not appropriate or feasible. The quadratus lumborum (QL) block may be similarly used. Neuraxial RAs, such as spinal and continuous epidural, are excellent modalities for surgery from the thorax to the lower extremities and have been used in modern combat to transport wounded casualties to higher levels of care. Recall that the MSF study found that of the 75,000 anesthetics used, 46% were spinal anesthetics.[18]

The WHO-WFSA Table 12.4 classifies equipment for spinal anesthesia and regional blocks as a Highly Recommended (mandatory) standard.[22] Please note that the WHO-WFSA document does not identify specific RA/neuraxial equipment to have available; however, the *Military Advanced Regional Anesthesia and Analgesia Handbook* is an excellent resource covering topics from recommended RA equipment and local anesthetics to advanced RA techniques complete with images (available at https://www.dvcipm.org/clinical-resources/dvcipm-maraa-book-project/). Given the utility of spinal anesthesia, the austere anesthesia team should consider having generous quantities of spinal anesthetic drugs and equipment (spinal needles) on hand, in addition to RA supplies.

According to the available literature, the disadvantages of RA seem to center primarily on provider proficiency. Because RA is an invasive procedure, standard risks such as bleeding, infection, nerve injury, perforation of a hollow viscus, and LAST apply. These risks are amplified in the traumatized or severely ill patient who may be suffering from coagulopathy or other metabolic derangements not favorable to optimal coagulation. The theoretical concern for RA masking a compartment syndrome has been discussed in various sources; however, literature has not demonstrated cases of unidentified compartment syndrome with a functioning peripheral nerve block (PNB).[40,45]

The ASRA and the ASA recommended minimum monitors for RA are: (1) pulse oximetry (WHO-WFSA Highly Recommended); (2) blood pressure monitoring (WHO-WFSA Highly Recommended); (3) and electrocardiography tracing (WHO-WFSA Recommended). Additionally, ASRA and ASA recommend having appropriate resuscitation equipment and medication on hand and readily available to treat sedation complications or LAST. RA and neuraxial anesthesia require significantly less equipment and logistical support when compared with GA; therefore it is reasonable that whenever and wherever possible, the austere anesthesia team should maximize RA and neuraxial anesthesia. Pertinent to the surgical and/or traumatized patient is the issue of prophylactic or therapeutic anticoagulation. The WHO-WFSA lists heparin as a Suggested standard, meaning that it should be available when resources allow. Not all trauma patients will be appropriately started on prophylactic anticoagulation. Placement of a PNB or CPNB catheter in the setting of anticoagulation should follow guidelines published by ASRA but is ultimately up to the judgment of the responsible anesthesia provider after weighing the risks and benefits and after discussion with the patient. A recent publication in April 2018, *Regional Anesthesia in the Patient Receiving Antithrombotic or Thrombolytic Therapy*, covers this topic in detail and, given the different anticoagulant medications from heparin and warfarin to the novel anticoagulants, each having a different recommended safety window for invasive procedures, a detailed review is beyond the scope of this chapter.[46]

MEDICATIONS

It is expected that the qualified anesthesia provider will determine appropriate drugs and doses for bolus or infusion appropriate for the clinical scenario and in accordance with the WHO-WFSA guideline. This section is a cursory orientation to commonly used drugs and is only a guide. Efforts have been made to ensure accuracy consistent with recent publications, but note that the author is not responsible for specific doses of drugs, uses in any particular patient, adverse effects, or errors. Anesthesia providers must exercise individual clinical judgment. Inhalational anesthetic agents are not covered in depth in this section. (See Techniques: 1. Inhalational anesthesia.)

Agents commonly used for GA and TIVA are propofol and ketamine. Propofol has an excellent and predictable physiologic profile including a low incidence of allergy, high familiarity, and reduction in postoperative nausea and vomiting.[30,47] Propofol has a rapid onset and a short duration of action, making it desirable when rapid awakening is needed, such as during emergence following surgery or during a sedation "holiday," where interval assessment of neurologic function is important, in the intensive care unit (ICU) setting, for example. One rare but potentially fatal complication of propofol infusion is referred to as propofol infusion syndrome (PRIS), which is more common in children and at high infusion doses/rates for prolonged periods of time, such as during sedation in the ICU. Propofol is known to result in vasodilation, which could be problematic in cases of trauma, shock, or other volume-depleted or cardiovascular-impaired states, leading to significant hypotension. A noteworthy logistical limitation for propofol (and all anesthetic drugs for that matter) is that it should be stored between 4°C and 25°C (available at https://www.accessdata.fda.gov/drugs atfda_docs/label/2014/019627s062lbl.pdf). There are theoretical potency and sterility concerns with medications stored in austere environments because climate control is not reliable and extreme temperature ranges may far exceed maximum recommended storage temperatures for long periods of time. Propofol may be used for induction of GA in adults and children, for maintenance of anesthesia as in TIVA, and for procedural sedation when combined with an appropriate analgesic.

Ketamine has many properties that make its use ideal in austere environments and trauma. Among these properties are hemodynamic stability with preserved cardiac output; maintenance of protective airway reflexes and respiratory drive; bronchodilation; analgesia; and synergy with opioids.[30,48] Despite historic concerns with increased intracranial pressure, ketamine has been gaining acceptance as being safe for use in traumatic brain injury.[49] A more present concern with ketamine is the dissociative and psychotropic effect, which could require greater postoperative observation. This effect is mitigated by the concomitant use of benzodiazepines. Ketamine is also associated with increased salivation and secretions, which can be mitigated by the concomitant use of an anticholinergic such as glycopyrrolate or atropine, favoring atropine for its lower volume for IM use and faster onset of action. Ketamine may also exhibit direct cardiac depression unmasked by catecholamine depletion as in chronic disease, prolonged stress, or trauma. Ketamine may be used in adults and children via IV or IM route for induction of GA (add glycopyrrolate for children to mitigate aspiration risk and laryngospasm from secretions), for maintenance of anesthesia as either a single agent or for balanced anesthesia, and for procedural sedation.

Midazolam has the main actions of sedation, anxiolysis, and anterograde amnesia. When combined with ketamine, midazolam can attenuate adverse dissociative and psychotropic effects. When used as a bolus, such as for preoperative sedation, it has a short duration of action. A minor drawback is that higher doses result in moderate cardiorespiratory depression. Fortunately, a supratherapeutic dose of midazolam may be reversed by flumazenil; however, the availability of this reversal agent in austere settings could be variable. Midazolam is commonly used for preoperative or procedural sedation; however, it may also be used for induction of GA in adults.

Opioids are commonly used in the perioperative area for procedural, surgical, and postoperative analgesia. Opioids are also used as infusions as part of a TIVA protocol and when combined with propofol result in synergy, that is, a reduced Cp50 of propofol (the plasma equivalent to MAC).[30,50] This synergistic effect allows for less propofol to achieve surgical anesthesia, which in turn allows for greater hemodynamic stability. Use of ultrashort-acting opioids such as remifentanil further reduces cardiovascular fluctuations; however, use may be limited by cost and availability. Fentanyl is commonly used for induction of anesthesia in adults and children and may also be used as an infusion in balanced anesthesia. Morphine has the added benefit of a longer duration of action, allowing for a single bolus dose to be used for both induction of anesthesia and intraoperative analgesia during a short case, with analgesia possibly lasting into the postoperative period. A drawback to morphine is its propensity to result in histamine release and the associated side effects.

Dexmedetomidine has a useful therapeutic range from sedation to analgesia and can be used without significant respiratory depression.[51,52] Significant adverse reactions associated with dexmedetomidine in one review were hypotension (30%), hypertension (12%), and bradycardia (9%).[53] Of note, the bradycardia and hypotension most often occurred with a loading dose and may be exaggerated in patients with preexisting hypovolemia. Dexmedetomidine may be used in adults and children for induction of GA (in children beware of bradycardia), for procedural sedation, and to smooth emergence approximately 30 minutes before wakeup (adults/children). Care should be taken to avoid rapid IV boluses, as the incidence of significant bradycardia may be higher.

Neuromuscular blocking drugs are commonly grouped as depolarizing and nondepolarizing. Succinylcholine is the only depolarizing neuromuscular blocker in use today. Succinylcholine is commonly used for rapid sequence induction (RSI), has a very short duration of action, and does not require a reversal agent. Succinylcholine may cause severe hyperkalemia in burn patients or following massive trauma. In children, succinylcholine is relatively contraindicated because of the risk of hyperkalemia, rhabdomyolysis, and cardiac arrest from undiagnosed myopathies. Succinylcholine is also a known trigger for MH.

Rocuronium is a steroidal nondepolarizing neuromuscular blocker that can be used for routine surgical paralysis and RSI in higher doses. Rocuronium is eliminated primarily by the liver and may be reversed with sugammadex or neostigmine coupled with glycopyrrolate.

Pancuronium is a steroidal nondepolarizing neuromuscular blocker with primarily renal excretion. Pancuronium is vagolytic with atropine-like effects such as tachycardia, sympathetic stimulation, and hypertension.

Atracurium and cisatracurium are benzylisoquinolone neuromuscular blockers that undergo organ-independent ester hydrolysis and Hofmann elimination (spontaneous breakdown), making these drugs ideal in clinical scenarios involving organ failure where paralysis is required. Atracurium is known to exhibit histamine release.

PRACTICAL POINTERS AND PRACTICE PEARLS

The following section represents lessons learned and best practices, compiled from anesthesiologists experienced in austere medical missions.

Preparation

1. Review the WHO-WFSA International Standards for a Safe Practice of Anesthesia; pay special attention to the recommended drugs and equipment one may expect at each of the three medical infrastructure levels.[22] The anesthesia provider can extrapolate what equipment, supplies, or medications to bring if the austere team is tasked with bringing its own supplies. Keep in mind that any elective surgery should abide by the Highly Recommended and Recommended WHO-WFSA international standards.
2. Obtain the proper safety monitors (pulse oximeter, continuous capnography, continuous electrocardiogram, etc.) before beginning the austere mission; consider contacting one of

the many humanitarian agencies or medical device manufacturers to inquire if they will donate the needed safety monitors for the mission.

3. Any new mission should be preceded by a site visit 6 to 12 months in advance to assess and plan for anticipated patient load, facilities operational status, medical logistics, local support, medical contingencies using host nation services (lab, x-ray, blood bank, escalation of care, medical transport between facilities, etc.), and to develop relationships with host nation medical staff.

4. Comprehensively assess and mitigate physical security risks in the region before departing home country and again before commencing anesthesia.

5. Anticipate deficiencies in host nation anesthesia equipment and logistics.

6. Anticipate technical challenges with HIC equipment and associated technology operating in austere environments; develop alternative modalities and backup options before you need them.

7. Thoroughly function-check all equipment provided by the host nation before use; some devices may have limited operability or be inoperable, particularly the sensitive electronic anesthesia devices.

8. Have a plan for obtaining oxygen or working without it.

9. Have backup breathing systems (self-inflating bag, Jackson-Rees, etc.) available.

10. Reuse what can be reused and be prepared to sanitize/disinfect equipment.

11. Bring or obtain appropriate chemicals to sanitize/disinfect reusable equipment.

12. Have adequate quantities of batteries (laryngoscope handles, CPNB pumps, portable pulse oximeters, etc.).

13. Establish a method to chart/document care given; will a chart be created for each patient and secured to them? How will drugs administered be tracked? Will office supplies be provided in-country? And so on.

Triage

1. Establish a reasonable operative schedule commensurate with the team's established priorities and austere capabilities; start thinking about this during the site visit 6 to 12 months before the mission.

2. Establish what cases the team will not attempt. Abide by the maxim "to do no harm."

3. Intentionally start the mission with simple surgical cases on either older children or relatively healthy adults. This allows the team to identify and resolve system/team/equipment issues and challenges before attempting more complex surgical cases.

4. Ethics: should the team perform a single 6-hour surgery or six life-transforming 1-hour surgeries?

5. Establish exclusion criteria for surgery based on post-anesthesia care unit (PACU)/recovery capabilities (e.g., severe anemia, malnourishment, "new" heart murmur, obstructive sleep apnea [OSA]).

6. Know which consultants/specialists are available in the local region and obtain contact information ahead of time. Use these resources to aid in risk stratification and operative triage decisions.

7. Be aware of regional infectious disease incidence rates that may complicate recovery (e.g., parasitic infections such as ascariasis and associated invasive pulmonary disease).

Anesthesia Techniques

1. Expect the unexpected and do not experiment. Stick to standard procedures that are adaptable to the host nation's infrastructure.

2. Prepare for limited/no blood products or colloid being available, for example, understand the benefits and limitations of employing a strategy of permissive hypotension.

3. Standardize as best as possible the organization and storage of anesthesia drugs, equipment, supplies. Organization is essential to anesthesia and surgical safety. Devices used in HICs (anesthesia cart, code cart, etc.) will likely be absent. Furthermore, emergency supplies will be limited and should be in a central location accessible to all team members (nurses, surgeons, anesthetists, etc.).
4. Be aware of microshock. Most austere ORs are not grounded and/or grounded electrical outlets do not exist. Know the power system, 110 V versus 220 V, and bring appropriate converters.

Conclusion

In summary, the austere environment will frustrate and challenge even the most seasoned anesthesia providers. Prior experience in resource-limited environments will serve the team well. Proper planning for contingencies is essential. A realistic and honest evaluation of the surgical team's austere capabilities will assist with surgery allocation, planning, scheduling, and resource stewardship. Forming a cohesive team requires intentionality, a willingness to address team friction, and a focus on team dynamics. While maximizing patient safety throughout the duration of the mission should be a top priority, special attention should also be focused on the health and well-being of the mission team members. Ultimately, the austere mission will refine the team's clinical skills and creativity, bringing healing and hope to patients in need.

Acknowledgments

For such a vast academic topic, special thanks and recognition go to Cynthia Shields, MD, Quentin Fisher, MD, and Honorato Nicodemus, MD for gracious assistance reviewing this chapter and helping to distill the most practical and useful pearls for the austere mission and austere anesthesia in particular.

Disclaimer

The views expressed in this chapter are those of the author and do not reflect the official policy of the Department of the Army/Navy/Air Force, Department of Defense, or US government.

References

1. World Bank Data. GDP per capita, PPP (current international $). Available at: https://data.worldbank.org/indicator/NY.GDP.PCAP.PP.CD?view=chart. Accessed June 13, 2020.
2. World Bank Data. Domestic general government health expenditure per capita, PPP (current international $). Available at: https://data.worldbank.org/indicator/SH.XPD.GHED.PP.CD?locations=XM. Accessed June 13, 2020.
3. Meara JG, Leather AJM, Hagander L, et al. Global surgery 2030: evidence and solutions for achieving health, welfare, and economic development. *Lancet*. 2015;386:569–624.
4. King M. *Primary Anesthesia*. Oxford: Oxford University Press; 1986.
5. King M, Bewes P, Cairns J, et al. *Primary Surgery Volume One: Non-Trauma*. Oxford: Oxford University Press; 1990.
6. King M, Bewes P, Cairns J, et al. *Primary Surgery Volume Two: Trauma*. Oxford: Oxford University Press; 1987.
7. Cotton M. *Primary Surgery Volume One: Non-Trauma*. 2nd ed. Seattle: Global Help; 2016. Available at: http://www.primary-surgery.org/assets/help_primarysurgery.pdf. Accessed June 13, 2020.
8. Meara J, McClain CD, Rogers SO Jr, Mooney DP, eds. *Global Surgery and Anesthesia Handbook: Providing Care in Resource-Limited Settings*. Boca Raton: CRC Press; 2015. Available at: http://ecx.images-amazon.com/images/I/51aOtObFtsL._SX384_BO1,204,203,200_.jpg. Accessed June 13, 2020.

9. Gionnou M, Baldan M. *War Surgery: Working With Limited Resources in Armed Conflict and Other Simulations of Violence, Volume 1*. Geneva: International Committee Red Cross; 2010. Available at: https://www.icrc.org/eng/assets/files/other/icrc_002_0973.pdf. Accessed June 13, 2020.

10. Gionnou M, Baldan M, Molde A. *War Surgery: Working With Limited Resources in Armed Conflict and Other Simulations of Violence, Volume 2*. Geneva: International Committee Red Cross; 2013. Available at: https://www.icrc.org/eng/resources/documents/publication/p4105.htm. Accessed June 13, 2020.

11. Carter L, Nthumba P. *Principles of Reconstructive Surgery*. Revised ed. PAACS; 2016. Available at: https://www.paacs.net/wp-content/uploads/2012/09/PAACS-Reconstructive-Surgery-Text-v.-2-072516.pdf. Accessed June 13, 2020.

12. Ameh EA, Bickler SW, Lakhoo K, Nwomeh BC, Poenaru D. *Paediatric Surgery: A Comprehensive Text for Africa*. Vol. 1. Seattle: Global HELP Organization; 2010. Available at: http://www.global-help.org/publications/books/help_pedsurgeryafricavolume01.pdf. Accessed June 13, 2020.

13. Tarpley JL, Meier DE. Tropical medicine for the general surgeon. In: Bland KI, Büchler MW, Csendes A, Garden OJ, Sarr MG, Wong J, eds. *General Surgery: Volume 2: Principles and International Practice*. 2nd ed. New York: Springer; 2008:1971–1982.

14. World Health Organization. Violence and injury prevention. Available at: https://www.who.int/violence_injury_prevention/media/news/2015/Injury_violence_facts_2014/en/. Accessed June 13, 2020.

15. World Health Organization, International Agency for Research on Cancer. *Cancer Today*; 2018. Available at: https://gco.iarc.fr/today/home. Accessed June 13, 2020.

16. Johnson PDR. Buruli ulcer: cured by 8 weeks of oral antibiotics? *Lancet*. 2020;395:1231–1232.

17. Weiser TG, Regenbogen SE, Thompson KD, et al. An estimation of the global volume of surgery: a modelling strategy based on available data. *Lancet*. 2008;372:139–144.

18. Ariyo P, Trellis M, Helmand R, et al. Providing anesthesia care in resource-limited settings: a 6-year analysis of anesthesia services provided at Médecins Sans Frontières facilities. *Anesthesiology*. 2016;124:561–569.

19. Wong EG, Dominguez L, Trelles M, et al. Operative trauma in low-resource settings: the experience of Médecins Sans Frontières in environments of conflict, postconflict, and disaster. *Surgery*. 2015;157:850–856.

20. Debas HT, Donkor P, Gawande A, Jamison DT, Kruk ME, Mock CN. *Essential Surgery. Disease Control Priorities. Vol. 1*, 3rd ed. Washington, DC: World Bank; 2015.

21. Braz LG, Braz DG, da Cruz DS, et al. Mortality in anesthesia: a systematic review. *Clinics (Sao Paulo)*. 2009;64:999–1006.

22. Gelb AW, Morriss WW, Johnson W, et al. World Health Organization-World Federation of Societies of Anaesthesiologists (WHO-WFSA) International Standards for a Safe Practice of Anesthesia. *Anesth Analg*. 2018;126:2047–2055.

23. Merry AF, Cooper JB, Soyannwo O, Wilson IH, Eichhorn JH. International standards for a safe practice of anesthesia 2010. *Can J Anaesth*. 2010;57:1027–1034.

24. Buckenmaier CC 3rd, Mahoney PF. *Combat Anesthesia: The First 24 Hours*. US Army Medical Department Center and School, Fort Sam Houston, Texas Borden Institute; 2015:571.

25. Creamer KM, Fuenfer MM. *Pediatric Surgery and Medicine for Hostile Environments*. 2nd ed. US Army Medical Department Center and School, Fort Sam Houston, Texas Borden Institute; 2017:825.

26. Apfelbaum JL, Connis RT, Nickinovich DG, et al. Practice Advisory for Preanesthesia Evaluation: An Updated Report by the American Society of Anesthesiologists Task Force on Preanesthesia Evaluation. *Anesthesiology*. 2012;116:522–538.

27. Rosen MA, Lee BH, Sampson JB, et al. Failure mode and effects analysis applied to the maintenance and repair of anesthetic equipment in an austere medical environment. *Int J Qual Health Care*. 2014;26:404–410.

28. McCormick BA, Eltringham RJ. Anaesthesia equipment for resource-poor environments. *Anaesthesia*. 2007;62(suppl 1):54–60.

29. Dyro JF. Donation of medical device technologies. In: *Clinical Engineering Handbook*. Burlington, VT: Elsevier Academic Press; 2004:696.

30. Lewis S, Jagdish S. Total intravenous anaesthesia for war surgery. *J R Army Med Corps*. 2010;156(4 suppl 1):301–307.

31. Gupta A, Stierer T, Zuckerman R, et al. Comparison of recovery profile after ambulatory anesthesia with propofol, isoflurane, sevoflurane and desflurane: a systematic review. *Anesth Analg*. 2004;98:632–641.

32. Crozier TA, Muller JE, Quittkat D, Sydow M, Wuttke W, Kettler D. Effect of anaesthesia on the cytokine responses to abdominal surgery. *Br J Anaesth*. 1994;72:280–285.

33. Ledowski T, Bein B, Hanss R, et al. Neuroendocrine stress response and heart rate variability: a comparison of total intravenous versus balanced anesthesia. *Anesth Analg*. 2005;101:1700–1705.

34. Strazis KP, Fox AW. Malignant hyperthermia: a review of published cases. *Anesth Analg*. 1993;77:297–304.

35. Avidan MS, Mashour GA. Prevention of intraoperative awareness with explicit recall: making sense of the evidence. *Anesthesiology*. 2013;118:449–456.

36. Greengrass RA. Regional anesthesia for ambulatory surgery. *Anesthesiol Clin North Am*. 2000;18:341–353 vi.

37. Buckenmaier CC 3rd, Lee EH, Shields CH, Sampson JB, Chiles JH. Regional anesthesia in austere environments. *Reg Anesth Pain Med*. 2003;28:321–327.

38. Malchow RJ, Black IH. The evolution of pain management in the critically ill trauma patient: emerging concepts from the global war on terrorism. *Crit Care Med*. 2008;36(7 suppl):S346–S357.

39. Plunkett AR, Brown DS, Rogers JM, Buckenmaier CC III. Supraclavicular continuous peripheral nerve block in a wounded soldier: when ultrasound is the only option. *Br J Anaesth*. 2006;97:715–717.

40. Wu JJ, Lollo L, Grabinsky A. Regional anesthesia in trauma medicine. *Anesthesiol Res Pract*. 2011;2011: 13281.

41. Orebaugh SL, Kentor ML, Williams BA. Adverse outcomes associated with nerve stimulator-guided and ultrasound-guided peripheral nerve blocks by supervised trainees: update of a single-site database. *Reg Anesth Pain Med*. 2012;37:577–582.

42. Buckenmaier CC III, McKnight GM, Winkley JV, et al. Continuous peripheral nerve block for battlefield anesthesia and evacuation. *Reg Anesth Pain Med*. 2005;30:202–205.

43. Simon BJ, Cushman J, Barraco R, et al. Pain management guidelines for blunt thoracic trauma. *J Trauma*. 2005;59:1256–1267.

44. Allcock E, Spencer E, Frazer R, Applegate G, Buckenmaier CC III. Continuous transversus abdominis plane (TAP) block catheters in a combat surgical environment. *Pain Med*. 2010;11:1426–1429.

45. Mar GJ, Barrington MJ, McGuirk BR. Acute compartment syndrome of the lower limb and the effect of postoperative analgesia on diagnosis. *Br J Anaesth*. 2009;102:3–11.

46. Horlocker TT, Vandermeuelen E, Kopp SL, Gogarten W, Leffert LR, Benzon HT. Regional anesthesia in the patient receiving antithrombotic or thrombolytic therapy: American Society of Regional Anesthesia and Pain Medicine Evidence-Based Guidelines (Fourth Edition). *Reg Anesth Pain Med*. 2018;43:263–309.

47. Gan TJ, Diemunsch P, Habib AS, et al. Consensus guidelines for managing postoperative nausea and vomiting. *Anesth Analg*. 2003;97:62–71, table of contents.

48. Smith CE. *Trauma Anesthesia*. 1st ed. New York: Cambridge University Press; 2008:606.

49. Chang LC, Raty SR, Ortiz J, Bailard NS, Mathew SJ. The emerging use of ketamine for anesthesia and sedation in traumatic brain injuries. *CNS Neurosci Ther*. 2013;19:390–395.

50. Smith C, McEwan AI, Jhaveri R, et al. The interaction of fentanyl on the Cp50 of propofol for loss of consciousness and skin incision. *Anesthesiology*. 1994;81:820–828; discussion 26A.

51. Gerlach AT, Dasta JF. Dexmedetomidine: an updated review. *Ann Pharmacother*. 2007;41:245–252.

52. Gerlach AT, Murphy CV, Dasta JF. An updated focused review of dexmedetomidine in adults. *Ann Pharmacother*. 2009;43:2064–2074.

53. Bhana N, Goa KL, McClellan KJ. Dexmedetomidine. *Drugs*. 2000;59:263–268; discussion 269–270.

CHAPTER 13

Mental Health in Crisis Regions

Jan Ilhan Kizilhan

Introduction

Armed conflicts and natural disasters cause significant challenges to the long-term mental health and psychosocial well-being of the affected population. Millions of people in many countries of the world experience war and conflict, and flight and displacement, over long periods of time and are severely affected by these experiences. This state of crisis also leads to intergenerational changes in traditional family and social structures. This often leads to severe emotional instability and a rapid increase in mental disorders such as trauma, anxiety, and depression. State professional mental healthcare services are rarely available in crisis countries. Even if they do exist, people who need psychological care are often not recognized as being in the need of help. Consequently, they are not referred to these services. There is an urgent need for high-quality mental health services and psychosocial support in crisis areas.

In 2019, the United Nations refugee agency (UNHCR) registered 70.8 million people who had been forcefully displaced. Of these, 25.9 million people were classified as refugees who had been forced to leave their homeland on account of persecution, war, or violence.[1]

In 2014, people in Iraq and Syria, in particular, were subjected to considerable stressors owing to "Islamic State" terror, when the Islamic State of Syria and Iraq (ISIS) overran vast areas of Syria and Iraq.[2] They used severe brutality, especially against long-established peoples and religious minorities in the countries, particularly the Yazidis. Huge numbers of men were executed, and thousands upon thousands of women and children were kidnapped and deliberately subjected to sexual violence.[3] This situation led to massive movement of refugees. The Duhok region in Iraq was one of the areas most affected by this movement. It borders Turkey in the north and Syria in the southwest and had a population of approximately 1.5 million in 2015.[4] This area took in the vast majority of the internally displaced persons (IDPs). In the Duhok region alone, there are currently (2019) 350,231 IDPs and 21 refugee camps. Throughout Iraq there are 2,045,718 IDPs in such camps.[5]

Above all, it has been shown that the experience of violence and torture can increase the risk of developing a mental disorder, especially an affective disorder or posttraumatic stress disorder (PTSD).[6,7] The life of many refugees is characterized by competition when looking for work, a difficult living situation in the camps, rejection in the homeland, the experience of sexual and physical violence, and cultural uprooting. This, in turn, leads to conflicts in the social environment and feelings of helplessness, worry, insecurity, and hopelessness.[3,8,9]

Prevalence

Several studies have examined the prevalence rates of psychological disorders among refugees and IDPs in 21 countries.[9] These studies have found different prevalence rates of mental disorders. However, a systematic review points out that PTSD (3%–88%), depression (5%–80%), and various forms of anxiety disorders (1%–81%) are the most prevalent disorders. These and other studies have drawn attention to a process in which trauma caused by human action (torture and predominantly sexual violence) precede the emergence of PTSD[10,11] and comorbid depression.[12]

The World Health Organization's (WHO) review of 129 studies in 39 countries showed that among people who have experienced war or other conflicts in the previous 10 years, one in five people (22%) will have depression, anxiety, PTSD, bipolar disorder, or schizophrenia.[10]

According to the WHO's review, the estimated prevalence of mental disorders among conflict-affected populations at any specific point in time (point prevalence) is 13% for mild forms of depression, anxiety, and PTSD and 4% for moderate forms of these disorders. The estimated point prevalence for severe disorders (i.e., schizophrenia, bipolar disorder, severe depression, severe anxiety, and severe PTSD) is 5%. It is estimated that 1 in 11 people (9%) living in a setting that has been exposed to conflict in the previous 10 years will have a moderate or severe mental disorder. In conflict-affected settings, depression and anxiety increase with age. Depression is more common in women than in men.[10]

These studies and the systematic review suggest that demographic and socioeconomic factors shaping the environment of displaced groups, for example, internal displacement, potentially influence psychological health significantly. For instance, the coincidence of living in a refugee camp, unresolved conflict issues, unpromising prospects, and financial and material insecurity is frequently associated with reduced psychological health.[11,12]

People with severe mental disorders can be especially vulnerable during and after emergencies, and they need access to basic needs and clinical care. A review from 2014 analyzed health information systems from 90 refugee camps across 15 low- and middle-income countries. It found that 41% of healthcare visits for mental, neurologic, and substance use disorders were for epilepsy/seizures, 23% for psychotic disorders, and 13% for moderate and severe forms of depression, anxiety, or PTSD.[13]

Mental Health and Psychosocial Care

In Northern Iraq, for example, there are currently 28 psychiatrists and 26 licensed psychotherapists who work in three psychiatric institutions or for local nongovernmental organizations (NGOs), for 6 million people. Financial problems frequently represent an obstacle to psychiatric support. For instance, health insurance companies do not cover psychiatric outpatient support. Moreover, organizational difficulties hamper psychiatric support. For example, difficult and precarious conditions in refugee camps and a poor infrastructure in towns and rural areas cause difficulties in providing psychiatric care. Finally, up to now, the work of local psychotherapists and psychotherapists in general is not recognized professionally.[14]

According to the WHO figures (2018), there are 22 international and 8 national NGOs focusing on healthcare work in Iraq at the moment, in addition to the meagre care structures mentioned above. Only nine of these are working in the Dohuk region. NGOs frequently work according to the Mental Health and Psychosocial Support (MHPSS) approach. MHPSS describes all types of support, local or otherwise, geared to protecting or strengthening psychosocial welfare.[15] This includes consultations with trained laypersons and with specialized psychotherapists. In 2018, relief agencies were able to take care of approximately 1.3 million people in need. In this context, merely 10,294 people out of 360,000 IDPs were provided with MHPSS up to now. Insufficient healthcare structure, a low number of professional staff, limited financial resources, and other causes[16] make an adequate professional and nationwide psychotherapeutic treatment system impossible.[14]

Implementation of Programs in the Aftermath of War and Terror

Several programs have been designed and implemented, such as the Inter-Agency Standing Committee (IASC) by the heads of a broad range of United Nations (UN) and non-UN humanitarian organizations.[15] The programs have highlighted that mental health with a psychosocial care program is highly relevant.[17]

For example, the IASC incorporates the following into crisis prevention: (1) preexisting social problems (e.g., poverty, discrimination, ethnic and religious conflicts, domestic violence), (2) preexisting distress (e.g., grief, nonpathological distress and distress, substance abuse, psychological disorders), and (3) humanitarian aid (e.g., undermining of community structures or traditional support mechanisms, and lack of information about food distribution or poor management of the information that is provided).

Some studies show that it is not of primary importance to apply psychosocial interventions immediately after disasters. This approach is based on the principles of psychological first aid.[18,19]

It is crucial primarily that people feel safe and that their anxiety decreases immediately after a disaster. This necessitates agents providing information, psychosocial support, and sufficient food, housing, and access to medical care if necessary or wanted, or accompanying those who are affected to a safe place (Table 13.1). The philosophy of psychosocial and mental health interventions can be formulated as follows: based on their proximity, services should provide immediacy of response, expectancy of recovery, and simplicity.[20]

People should be provided the ability to reduce stress and feel psychologically and physically comfortable. Those suffering from pain or from injuries should be given medication if necessary, to stop or reduce the pain.

It should be stressed that psychosocial help on the ground and immediately after the disaster will not prevent mental disease; it is strictly to help people overcome their anxiety and reduce the stress that has arisen. A possible mental disease that would require psychiatric or psychotherapeutic treatment cannot automatically be prevented. In addition to first psychological aid, an expert will subsequently diagnose mental disorder and provide appropriate treatment.

In many war and crisis regions, there are not always enough physicians, therapists, or psychiatric hospitals. For this reason, it is recommended that survivors are integrated into communities and societies they are more likely to trust and where they know the culture and local conditions. General practitioners are more likely to be consulted here. Consequently, a training program for general practitioners in mental health diagnostics, psychopharmacology,[21] and basic knowledge of psychotherapeutic treatment is necessary, as they are the most common contact persons for people who need long-term treatment.[22] A training program enables general practitioners to learn quickly and effectively to determine whether survivors need psychosocial care or specialized psychiatric and psychotherapeutic treatment.[23]

At this stage, some people may develop an acute stress reaction. This can be described as an acute stress disorder (ASD) if the experiences are severe and cause a functional disorder (panic, anxiety, shortness of breath, feelings of insecurity, tension, nervousness, etc.).[24] At first glance, these symptoms seem similar to those of PTSD. However, PTSD should only be diagnosed after a month or longer if symptoms such as anxiety, nightmares, sleep disorders, flashbacks, and

TABLE 13.1 ■ **Interventions in the Aftermath of Disasters**

Intervention	Target Population	Examples of Interventions	Intervention Conducted by
Finding people and protecting them from further threats	Most of the people who are affected	Professionals and any person who can help to protect them	Military Policy Community
Take to a safe place if possible	Most of the people who are affected	Put in a safe place (house, building, tent, etc.)	Police Health staff
First medical emergency aid	Most of the people who are affected	Physical examination, first treatment of injuries	Physician Aid workers
Medical examination	Most of the people who are affected	Physical examination, outpatient or inpatient treatment	Physician
Psychological first aid	Most of the people who are affected	Restoring immediate safety Restoring contact with loved ones	All responders and aid workers
Psychological examination and diagnostics	People with first psychological symptoms, such as acute stress disorder (ASD)	Anxiety, seizures, state of shock, first depressive symptoms, sleep disorder, nightmares, social isolation	Psychiatrist Psychotherapist Clinical psychologist
Psychological examination and diagnostics after one month	People who meet the criteria for posttraumatic stress disorder (PTSD)	Psychological screening and assessment	Long-term psychotherapy
Skills for psychosocial recovery	People whose distress is sustained by bereavement or secondary stressors	Brief assessment of needs, problem-solving, social support	Healthcare practitioners and workers with expertise in the required skills and in conveying these skills effectively
Psychosocial interventions for medium- and long-term problems Outpatient and/or inpatient psychiatric treatment	People whose distress is sustained and associated with functional impairment	Culture-sensitive adapted psychotrauma therapy	Staff of mental healthcare facilities Psychiatrist, Psychotherapists, Clinical Psychologist, Social workers specialized in trauma

intrusions, and so on continue to exist. The symptoms of acute trauma (ASD) can persist for up to 1 month.[25]

Not all people who experience such disasters develop a mental disorder such as PTSD. This depends on their resilience and coping mechanisms.[26] Studies show that people with ASD recover more slowly. These findings have led the National Institute for Health and Clinical Excellence in the United Kingdom[27] to recommend watchful waiting for about 4 weeks after the onset of events before starting treatment for PTSD. During this period, survivors should be offered support, based on the principles of psychological first aid,[20] and further assessment.

For this reason, one of the main objectives at this stage is to screen affected people and to provide some assessment of those who are at particular risk in the future. However, in the case of unusual or particularly intense suffering, earlier treatment should be provided.

In the rescue and early recovery phases, it is best to use local health providers, if possible, because they are established in the affected communities, trusted, and know the culture and local circumstances. During this phase, it is also critical to develop a training program for general practitioners who are likely to be the contact points for people who require long-term services. Even if they are not particularly skilled in the mental health domain at this point, they are the people who tend to be consulted by survivors in the aftermath of the disaster. They are well placed to distinguish people who require psychosocial care from those who need specialist mental health care.[28]

The general objective of intervention programs is to reduce the risk of posttraumatic stress events, primarily PTSD, at the early stages of obvious psychological reaction.[25] To meet this goal, different types of emergency response units need to be established in health centers, hospitals (if they exist), and the community. Such a system of mental health care will also enable the prevention of secondary traumatization. This can occur when helping staff or agents see severely injured and traumatized victims, and hear stories of capture, rape, observation of people being killed, torture, hunger, and other deprivations.[29]

To maximize effectiveness, programs should be culturally sensitive and attempt to avoid cultural biases, that is, to meet the mental health needs and beliefs of people with different cultural backgrounds (ethnic, religious, etc.). For example, it is a typically Western approach to ascribe importance to emotional expression in the treatment of trauma. In this point of view, emotional expression is a crucial means of sharing feelings of grief and distress with those around. In this perspective, sharing feelings and talking about the event experienced or observed may cause an individual to become overwhelmed by a trauma and fall ill. In contrast, some cultural groups believe that emotional expression is detrimental to health. In our experience, the strengthening of problem-oriented strategies is a more effective way to cope with posttrauma distress than emotion-oriented coping.[26,30,31]

Conclusions

Mental health is crucial to the overall social and economic recovery of individuals, societies, and countries after emergencies. Global progress in mental health reform will happen more quickly if, during every crisis, efforts are initiated to convert the short-term increase in attention to mental health issues combined with a surge of aid into momentum for long-term service development. However, mental health services should always be a part of national healthcare policy, despite possible difficulties.

Additionally, it should be noted that many mental health and psychosocial care professionals find it difficult to cope with the many burdens and emergencies experienced by their patients. This implies the significance of secondary trauma. In connection to secondary trauma, there is evidence that people working in crisis and postconflict areas are more likely to have a traumatic experience than the general population.[32] Consequently, prevention programs are just as important for professionals in crisis regions. They enable them to help effectively and to maintain their health with a long-term perspective.

In crisis areas, there will not always be sufficient aid available, such as infrastructure and staff in the mental health sector. For this reason, alternative resources in the community should always be explored.

Community self-help and social support can be strengthened in such difficult times, for example, by creating or restoring community groups in which members solve problems together and participate in activities such as emergency relief or learning new skills, while ensuring the inclusion of people who are vulnerable and marginalized, including people with mental disorders.

References

1. United Nations Refugee Agency. *Figures at a Glance*; 2019. Available at: https://www.ncbi.nlm.nih.gov/pmc/articles/PMC6160546/pdf/fpsyt-09-00433.pdf. Accessed January 24, 2020.
2. Kizilhan JI, Noll-Hussong M. Individual, collective and transgenerational traumatization in the Yazidi. *BMC Med*. 2017;15(198).
3. Gerdau I, Kizilhan JI, Noll-Hussong M. Posttraumatic stress disorder and related disorders among female Yazidi refugees following Islamic State of Iraq and Syria attacks—a case series and mini-review. *Front Psychiat*. 2017;8:282.
4. Kurdish Regional Statistics Office. *The Total Number Population of Duhok Governorate*. Erbil: KRSO; 2015.
5. World Health Organization. *Iraq: Health Cluster Emergency Response May 2018*. Geneva: WHO; 2018.
6. Steel Z, Chey T, Silove D, et al. Association of torture and other potentially traumatic events with mental health outcomes among populations exposed to mass conflict and displacement: a systematic review and meta-analysis. *JAMA*. 2009;302:537–549.
7. Ibrahim H, Hassan CQ. Post-traumatic stress disorder symptoms resulting from torture and other traumatic events among Syrian Kurdish refugees in Kurdistan region, Iraq. *Front Psychology*. 2017;8:241.
8. Cetorelli V, Burnham G, Shabila N. Health needs and care seeking behaviours of Yazidis and other minority groups displaced by ISIS into the Kurdistan Region of Iraq. *PLoS One*. 2017;12:e0181028.
9. Independent International Commission of Inquiry on the Syrian Arab Republic. *They Came to Destroy: ISIS Crimes Against the Yazidis*; 2016.
10. Morina N, Akhtar A, Barth J, Schnyder U. Psychiatric disorders in refugees and internally displaced persons after forced displacement: a systematic review. *Front Psychiatry*. 2018;9:433.
11. United Nations High Commissioner for Refugees. *Global Trends*. UNHCR; 2016. Available at: http://www.unhcr.org/5943e8a34.pdf. Accessed December 20, 2016.
12. Nickerson A, Schick M, Schnyder U, Bryant RA, Morina N. Comorbidity of posttraumatic stress disorder and depression in tortured, treatment-seeking refugees. *J Trauma Stress*. 30:409–415.
13. Bogic M, Njoku A, Priebe S. Long-term mental health of war-refugee: a systematic literature review. *BMC Int Health Human Rights*. 2015;15:29.
14. Wolf S, Seiffer B, Hautzinger M, Othman MF, Kizilhan JI. Aufbau psychotherapeutischer Versorgung in der Region Dohuk, Nordirak. Gründung des Instituts für Psychotraumatologie und Psychotherapie sowie Durchführung eines Masterstudiengangs für Psychotherapie und Psychotraumatologie. *Psychotherapeut*. 2019;64:328.
15. Inter-Agency Standing Committee. *IASC Guidelines on Mental Health and Psychosocial Support in Emergency Settings*. Geneva: IASC; 2007.
16. Porter M, Haslam N. Predisplacement and postdisplacement factors associated with mental health of refugees and internally displaced persons: a meta-analysis. *JAMA*. 2005;294:602–612.
17. Tol WA, Ommeren MV. Evidence-based mental health and psychosocial support in humanitarian settings: gaps and opportunities. *Evid Based Ment Health*. 2012;15:25–26.
18. Meewisse ML, Olff M, Kleber R, Kitchiner NJ, Gersons BR. The course of mental health disorders after a disaster: predictors and comorbidity. *J Trauma Stress*. 2011;24:405–413.
19. World Health Organization. *War Trauma Foundation, and World Vision International, Psychological First Aid: Guide for Field Workers*. Geneva, Switzerland: WHO; 2011.
20. Forbes D, Lewis V, Varker T. Psychological first aid following trauma: implementation and evaluation framework for high-risk organizations. *Psychiatry*. 2011;74:224–239.
21. Choe HM, Farris KB, Stevenson JG. Patient-centered medical home: developing, expanding, and sustaining a role for pharmacists. *Am J Health Syst Pharm*. 2012;69:1063–1071.
22. Luoma JB, Martin CE, Pearson JL. Contact with mental health and primary care providers before suicide: a review of the evidence. *Am J Psychiatry*. 2002;159:909–916.

23. Loeb DF, Bayliss EA, Binswanger IA. Primary care physician perceptions on caring for complex patients with medical and mental illness. *J Gen Intern Med.* 2012;27:945–952.

24. Morina N, Ajdukovic D, Bogic M, et al. Co-occurrence of major depressive episode and posttraumatic stress disorder among survivors of war: how is it different from either condition alone? *J Clin Psychiatry.* 2013;74:212–218.

25. Kizilhan JI. Impact of sexual violation of ISIS terror against Yazidi women after five years. *JSM Sexual Med.* 2020;4:1025.

26. Wright AM, Talia YR, Aldhalimi A, et al. Kidnapping and mental health in Iraqi refugees: the role of resilience. *J Immigr Minor Health.* 2017;19:98–107.

27. National Institute for Health and Care Excellence. Post-traumatic stress disorder (PTSD): the management of PTSD in adults and children in primary and secondary care. Available at: www.nice.org.uk/nicemedia/pdf/CG026NICEguideline.pdf. Accessed March 12, 2020.

28. Perlman SE, Friedman S, Galea S. Short-term and medium-term health effects of 9/11. *Lancet.* 2011; 378:925–934.

29. Lusk M, Terrazas S. Secondary trauma among caregivers who work with Mexican and Central American refugees. *His J Behav Sci.* 2015;37:257–273.

30. Kindermann D, Schmid C, Derreza-Greeven C, et al. Prevalence of and risk factors for secondary traumatization in interpreters for refugees: a cross-sectional study. *Psychopathology.* 2017;50:262–272.

31. Lahav Y, Kanat-Maymon Y, Solomon Z. Secondary traumatization and attachment among wives of former POWs: a longitudinal study. *Attach Hum Dev.* 2016;18:141–153.

32. Püttker K, Thomsen T, Bockmann AK. Sekundäre Traumatisierung bei Traumatherapeutinnen. *Zeitschrift für Klinische Psychologie und Psychotherapie.* 2015;44:254–265.

CHAPTER 14

Radiological, Biological, and Chemical Agents

Frédéric Dorandeu ▦ Richard Pilch

Further Reading

Although this material is provided as a convenient initial reference, readers are strongly recommended to refer to the resources listed at the end of this chapter for more detailed information, particularly the website for radiation-associated injury, which is updated periodically.

Biological Warfare Agents

1. Bacteria
   a. Anthrax: *Bacillus anthracis* is a gram-positive, spore-forming bacteria that can cause cutaneous, gastrointestinal (GI), or pulmonary symptoms, depending on route of infection. Weaponized anthrax is delivered via aerosol for inhalation of the spores; the following information is for pulmonary anthrax.
      i. Signs and symptoms: incubation period is 1 to 6 days, followed by an initial phase (1–5 days) of nonspecific symptoms such as low-grade fever, malaise, fatigue, nonproductive cough, and mild chest discomfort. This may be followed by 1 to 3 days of apparent improvement before an abrupt onset of high fever and severe respiratory distress with dyspnea, diaphoresis, stridor, and cyanosis. Shock and death ensue within 24 to 36 hours after onset of severe symptoms.
      ii. Diagnosis: physical findings are nonspecific. A widened mediastinum may be seen on chest x-ray (CXR) (or chest computed tomography [CT] if CXR is negative and exposure is strongly suspected). Detectable by gram stain (gram-positive rods) and blood culture. Nasal swab, sputum, and induced sputum will reveal pathogen. Blood and cerebrospinal fluid (CSF) will be used for culture, polymerase chain reaction (PCR), and antibody studies.
      iii. Treatment: although effectiveness may be limited after symptoms have developed, high-dose antibiotic treatment with penicillin, ciprofloxacin, or doxycycline should be undertaken. Supportive therapy may be necessary. Anthrax Vaccine Adsorbed is available under investigational new drug (IND) for postexposure use in conjunction with above drug therapy.
      iv. Prophylaxis: doxycycline, ciprofloxacin levofloxacin, and penicillin G may be considered for preexposure prophylaxis. For postexposure prophylaxis, consider 60 days of ciprofloxacin or doxycycline plus a three-dose series of anthrax vaccine.

     v. Isolation/decontamination: standard precautions for healthcare workers. After an invasive procedure or autopsy, instruments and affected area should be disinfected with sporicidal agent such as 5% sodium hypochlorite. Autoclaving, steam sterilizing, or burning is required for complete eradication of spores. Decontamination of patients using water and soap is sufficient (collecting the effluent to prevent spreading of the displaced spores).

b. Cholera (*Vibrio cholera*)

     i. Signs and symptoms: incubation period is 4 hours to 5 days (usually 2–3 days). Asymptomatic to severe with sudden onset. Vomiting, headache, intestinal cramping with little or no fever, followed rapidly by painless, voluminous diarrhea. Fluid losses may exceed 5 to 10 L/d. Without treatment, death may result from severe dehydration, hypovolemia, and shock.

     ii. Diagnosis: clinical. "Rice water" diarrhea and dehydration. Microscopic examination of stool reveals few/no red or white cells. Organisms can be visualized with darkfield or phase contrast microscopy, or by observation of darting motile vibrio under direct microscopy.

     iii. Treatment: fluid and electrolyte replacement. Antibiotics (tetracycline, ciprofloxacin, or erythromycin) may shorten the duration of diarrhea and reduce the shedding of the organism.

     iv. Prophylaxis: a licensed, killed vaccine is available but provides only about 50% protection which lasts no longer than 6 months. Vaccine is given at 0 and 4 weeks, with boosters every 6 months.

     v. Isolation/decontamination: standard precautions for healthcare workers. Bactericidal solutions such as hypochlorite may be used to decontaminate areas.

c. Pneumonic plague (*Yersinia pestis*)

     i. Signs and symptoms: pneumonic plague usually requires 1 to 6 days of incubation before acutely presenting with high fever, chills, headache, malaise, myalgias, cough, and tachypnea within 24 hours, eventually producing bloody sputum (hemoptysis). The pneumonia progresses rapidly to dyspnea, stridor, and cyanosis. Death from respiratory failure, circulatory collapse, and a bleeding diathesis. Bubonic plague incubates for 2 to 10 days and may present with malaise, high fever, and tender lymph nodes (buboes); may progress spontaneously to the septicemic form, with spread to the central nervous system (CNS), lungs, and so on.

     ii. Diagnosis: presumptive diagnosis can be made by gram, Wright, Wright-Giemsa or Wayson stain of lymph node aspirates, sputum, or CSF. Plague bacilli may also be cultured on standard media.

     iii. Treatment: early administration of antibiotics is necessary. Supportive therapy is required.

     iv. Postexposure prophylaxis: doxycycline or ciprofloxacin for 7 days.

     v. Isolation/decontamination: standard precaution for healthcare workers for those exposed to bubonic plague, and droplet precautions are mandatory for pneumonic plague (for at least 48 hours of therapy antibiotics). Heat, disinfectants (2%–5% hypochlorite) and exposure to sunlight inactivates the bacteria.

d. Tularemia (*Francisella tularensis*)

     i. Signs and symptoms: after an incubation period of 3 to 6 days (up to 21 days), ulceroglandular tularemia presents with a local ulcer and regional lymphadenopathy and a sudden fever, chills, headache, and malaise. Typhoidal tularemia presents with a nonspecific febrile syndrome consisting of abrupt onset of fever, headache, malaise, myalgias, substernal discomfort, prostration, weight loss, and a nonproductive cough.

ii. Diagnosis: clinical. Physical findings are usually nonspecific. CXR may reveal a pneumonic process, mediastinal lymphadenopathy, or pleural effusion. Routine culture is possible but difficult. The diagnosis can be established retrospectively via serology.

iii. Treatment: administration of antibiotics (streptomycin or gentamicin) with early treatment is effective.

iv. Postexposure prophylaxis: a 2-week course of tetracycline, ciprofloxacin, or doxycycline is effective when given after exposure.

v. Isolation/decontamination: standard precautions for healthcare workers. Organisms can be inactivated by exposure to 55°C for 10 minutes or with standard disinfectants. Control of ticks, mosquitoes, deer flies, and lice is important in disrupting transmission.

e. Q fever (*Coxiella burnetii*)

i. Signs and symptoms: after an incubation period (7–21 days, or up to 41 days), abrupt onset of high fever, fatigue, severe headache, chills, myalgias, dry cough, nausea, and pleuritic chest pain. Patients are usually not critically ill, and the illness lasts from 2 days to 2 weeks.

ii. Diagnosis: Q fever is not a clinically distinct illness and may resemble a viral illness or other types of atypical pneumonia. The diagnosis is confirmed serologically.

iii. Treatment: Q fever is generally a self-limited illness without treatment. Tetracycline or doxycycline are the treatments of choice and are given orally for 14 to 21 days. Q fever endocarditis is much more difficult to treat but is fortunately quite rare.

iv. Postexposure prophylaxis: treatment with doxycycline or tetracycline for 7 days during the incubation period (start 8–12 days postexposure) may delay but not prevent the onset of symptoms.

v. Isolation/decontamination: standard precautions for healthcare workers. Patient decontamination may be accomplished with soap and water or after a 30-minute contact time with 5% microchem plus (quaternary ammonium compound) or 70% ethyl alcohol.

f. Brucellosis (*Brucella* spp.)

i. Signs and symptoms: incubation period 5 to 60 days (usually 1–2 months). Nonspecific findings include irregular fever, headache, profound weakness and fatigue, chills, diaphoresis, arthralgias, myalgias, depression, and mental status changes. May see osteoarticular changes (i.e., sacroiliitis, vertebral osteomyelitis). Rarely fatal.

ii. Diagnosis: blood cultures require a prolonged time for growth, and bone marrow cultures may be of higher yield. Confirmation requires phage-typing, oxidative metabolism, or genotyping procedures. Enzyme-linked immunosorbent assays (ELISAs), followed by Western blotting are used.

iii. Treatment: doxycycline and rifampin (or streptomycin or gentamycin) for at least 6 weeks. For complicated disease (i.e., endocarditis, meningoencephalitis), treat with rifampin, a tetracycline, and an aminoglycoside.

iv. Prophylaxis: no approved vaccine. Avoid consumption of unpasteurized milk and cheese.

v. Isolation/decontamination: standard precautions for healthcare workers. Environmental decontamination can be accomplished with a 0.5% hypochlorite solution.

g. Inhalational glanders (*Burkholderia mallei*)

i. Signs and symptoms: incubation ranges from 10 to 14 days after inhalation of causative organism. Fever, rigors, diaphoresis, sweats, myalgia, headache, pleuritic chest pain, cervical adenopathy, splenomegaly, and generalized papular/pustular eruptions may occur. Almost uniformly fatal without treatment.

    ii. Diagnosis: methylene blue stain of exudates may reveal scant small bacilli. CXR may show miliary lesions, small multiple lung abscesses, or bronchopneumonia. *B. mallei* can be cultured from infected secretions using meat nutrients.

    iii. Treatment: ciprofloxacin, doxycycline, and rifampin have in vitro efficacy. Extrapolating from guidelines for melioidosis, a combination of trimethoprim-sulfamethoxazole (TMP-SMX) + ceftazidime ± gentamicin might be appropriate. The intravenous (IV) therapy will be continued for a minimum of 10 to 14 days before maintenance oral therapy is initiated for weeks to months.

    iv. Prophylaxis: no approved vaccine. Postexposure prophylaxis may be tried with TMP-SMX.

    v. Isolation/decontamination: standard precautions for healthcare workers. Environmental decontamination may be achieved with 0.5% hypochlorite solution.

2. Viruses

  a. Smallpox

    i. Signs and symptoms: after an incubation period of 7 to 19 days (average 12 days): begins acutely with malaise, fever, rigors, vomiting, headache, and backache. Two to three days later lesions appear in the oropharynx, followed by (or concomitantly with) a rash on the face, then forearms and legs, then trunk, and subsequently hands and feet. The lesions will quickly progress from macules to papules, and eventually to pustular vesicles. They are more abundant on the extremities and face and develop synchronously.

    ii. Diagnosis: electron and light microscopy are not capable of discriminating variola from vaccinia, monkeypox, or cowpox. PCR may be more useful. Samples should be sent to international reference laboratories such as Centers for Disease Control and Prevention (CDC), the World Health Organization (WHO), or other reference laboratories such as the French Armed Forces Biomedical Research Institute (IRBA) in France.

    iii. Treatment: no effective specific chemotherapy. Supportive care should be given.

    iv. Prophylaxis: immediate vaccination or revaccination should be undertaken for all exposed personnel. Vaccinia immune globulin (VIG) is of value in postexposure prophylaxis of smallpox when given within the first week following exposure.

    v. Isolation/decontamination: droplet and airborne precautions for a minimum of 16 to 17 days following exposure for all contacts (3–6 feet of person). Patients should be considered infectious until all scabs separate.

  b. Venezuelan equine encephalitis (VEE)

    i. Signs and symptoms: following a 1 to 6 -day incubation period, sudden onset of illness with generalized malaise, spiking fevers, rigors, severe headache, photophobia, and myalgias (prominent in the thighs and lower back). Nausea, vomiting, cough, sore throat, and diarrhea may follow. Full recovery takes 1 to 2 weeks.

    ii. Diagnosis: clinical—physical findings are nonspecific. Complete blood count (CBC) often demonstrates a striking leukopenia and lymphopenia. Virus isolation may be achieved from serum and in some cases from throat swab specimens. Both neutralizing or immunoglobulin (Ig)G antibody in paired sera or VEE-specific IgM present in a single serum sample indicate recent infection.

    iii. Treatment: supportive only.

    iv. Isolation/decontamination: standard precautions for healthcare workers. Control mosquito vectors and vaccinate horses in the vicinity.

  c. Viral hemorrhagic fevers (VHFs)

    i. Signs and symptoms: febrile illnesses often complicated by easy bleeding, petechiae, hypotension/shock, flushing of the face and chest, and edema. Malaise, myalgias, headache, vomiting, and diarrhea may occur as well.

    ii. Diagnosis: specific virologic techniques or PCR are required.

    iii. Treatment: intensive supportive care may be required. Antiviral therapy with ribavirin may be useful in several of these infections. Convalescent plasma may be effective for Argentine hemorrhagic fever.

    iv. Prophylaxis: the only licensed VHF vaccine is for yellow fever. Prophylactic ribavirin may be effective for Lassa fever, Rift Valley fever, Crimean-Congo hemorrhagic fever (CCHF); not recommended for pulmonary virus hantavirus hemorrhagic fever with renal syndrome (HFRS).

    v. Isolation/decontamination: contact preparations for healthcare workers. Decontamination is accomplished with hypochlorite or phenolic disinfectants. Isolation measures and barrier nursing procedures are indicated.

3. Biological toxins

  a. Botulinum

    i. Signs and symptoms: after 12 to 36 hours (range 2 hours to 8 days after inhalation): ptosis, generalized weakness, dizziness, dry mouth and throat, blurred vision and diplopia, dysarthria, and dysphagia, followed by symmetrical descending flaccid paralysis and development of respiratory failure.

    ii. Diagnosis: clinical. No routine laboratory findings.

    iii. Treatment: intubation and ventilatory assistance for respiratory failure—anticipate possible need for tracheostomy. Administration of heptavalent botulinum antitoxin (IND product) may prevent or decrease progression to respiratory failure and hasten recovery.

    iv. Isolation/decontamination: standard precautions for healthcare workers. Toxin is not dermally active, and secondary aerosols are not a hazard from patients. Soap and water suffice for patient decontamination.

  b. Staphylococcal enterotoxin B

    i. Signs and symptoms: from 2 to 12 hours (range 1.5–24 hours) after aerosol exposure, sudden onset of nonspecific flu-like symptoms: fever, chills, headache, myalgia, and nonproductive cough. Later symptoms depend on the route of exposure. Inhalation: some patients may develop shortness of breath and retrosternal chest pain, dyspnea (may progress to pulmonary edema). Upper respiratory tract infection (URTI) symptoms (rhinorrhea, sinus congestion, pharyngitis) are observed in approximately one-third of the cases. Fever may last 2 to 5 days, and cough may persist for up to 4 weeks. Ingestion: patients may also present with nausea, vomiting, and diarrhea if they swallow toxin. Presumably, higher exposure can lead to septic shock and death.

    ii. Diagnosis: clinical. Patients present with a febrile respiratory syndrome without CXR abnormalities. If performed with 24 hours postinhalation, nasal swabs and induced respiratory secretions will be used for different toxin assays (PCR, Ag ELISA, electrochemiluminiscent tests). Leukocytosis is common.

    iii. Treatment: limited to supportive care, including ventilatory support with meticulous fluid management.

    iv. Prophylaxis: use of protective mask. No vaccine available.

    v. Isolation/decontamination: standard precautions for healthcare workers. Soap and water should suffice to remove potential contamination. Destroy any food that may have been contaminated.

  c. Ricin

    i. Signs and symptoms: 4 to 8 hours after exposure weakness, fever, chest tightness, cough, dyspnea, nausea, and/or diaphoresis with sublethal doses in humans. Higher inhaled doses would lead to labored breathing within 18 to 24 hours, and then to pulmonary edema, followed by severe respiratory distress and death from hypoxemia in 36 to 48 hours. After 1 to 2 hours following ingestion, the clinical presentation is different: severe nausea, vomiting, abdominal cramps, followed by diarrhea, vascular collapse shock, and possibly death at higher doses. Organ necrosis starting with the GI tract is observed.

ii. Diagnosis: aside from clinical suspicion, serum ELISA is available for acute and convalescent sera. Nasal swabs and induced respiratory secretions would be used for toxin assays (PCR, Ag ELISA) within 24 hours of aerosol exposure.

iii. Treatment: management is supportive, directed primarily toward pulmonary edema. Gastric decontamination measures should be used if ingested (vigorous gastric lavage, cathartics such as magnesium citrate).

iv. Prophylaxis: no vaccine or prophylactic antitoxin available. Use of protective mask is currently the best protection against inhalation.

v. Isolation/decontamination: standard precautions for healthcare workers. Secondary aerosols should generally not be a danger to healthcare providers. Weak hypochlorite solutions (0.1% sodium hypochlorite) and/or soap and water can decontaminate skin surfaces.

  d. T-2 mycotoxins

i. Signs and symptoms: exposure causes skin pain, pruritis, redness, vesicles, necrosis and sloughing of epidermis. Nose and throat pain, nasal discharge, itching and sneezing, cough, dyspnea, wheezing, chest pain, and hemoptysis may follow inhalation. Ingestion or eye contact leads to local symptoms as well. Severe poisoning results in prostration, weakness, dizziness, ataxia and loss of coordination, collapse, shock, and death.

ii. Diagnosis: should be suspected if an aerosol attack occurs in the form of "yellow rain" with droplets of yellow fluid contaminating clothes and the environment. Confirmation requires testing of blood, tissue, and environmental samples.

iii. Treatment: no specific antidote. Superactivated charcoal should be given orally if the toxin is swallowed.

iv. Prophylaxis: protective mask and clothing during an attack.

v. Isolation/decontamination: standard precautions for healthcare workers. Outer clothing should be removed and exposed skin should be decontaminated with soap and water (even 4–6 hours after exposure), although a quicker decontamination (<1 hour) may prevent toxicity entirely. Eye exposure should be treated with copious saline irrigation. Once decontamination is complete, isolation is not required. Environmental decontamination requires use of hypochlorite solution under alkaline conditions such as 1% sodium hypochlorite and 0.1 M NaOH with 1-hour contact time. Secondary aerosols are not a hazard.

Chemical Warfare Agents

1. Nerve agents (GA, GB, GD, GF, VX)

  a. Mechanism of action: inhibiting acetylcholinesterase, leading to excess acetylcholine in synapses and other parts of the body.

  b. Symptoms and signs

i. Vapor: small exposure leads to miosis, rhinorrhea, mild difficulty breathing. Large exposure leads to sudden loss of consciousness, convulsions, apnea, flaccid paralysis, copious secretions, and miosis.

ii. Liquid on skin: small to moderate exposure leads to localized sweating, nausea, vomiting, feeling of weakness with a delay of minutes-hours. Large exposure, as with vapor exposure, results in sudden loss of consciousness, apnea, flaccid paralysis, copious secretions.

    c. Decontamination: Fuller's earth (decontamination mitt), followed by soapy water used with a sponge/towel (0.5% hypochlorite solution does not have a clear benefit) or Reactive Skin Decontamination Lotion (RSDL) sponge, large amounts of water if nothing else (efficacy of the latter depends on the agent considered: sarin is fully soluble in water, whereas VX has limited solubility).

    d. Immediate management: atropine sulfate and pralidoxime chloride (or other salts). Add diazepam (or other benzodiazepine) if severe poisoning with signs of CNS involvement (e.g., seizures); intubation and ventilation with aggressive pulmonary toilet for respiratory distress.

  2. Vesicants

    a. Mustard (HD, H)

       i. Signs and symptoms: asymptomatic latent period up to several hours, followed by skin erythema and blisters, eye irritation with conjunctivitis and corneal opacity, respiratory embarrassment, GI effects, and bone marrow suppression.

      ii. Decontamination: Fuller's earth (decontamination mitt), followed by soapy water used with a sponge/towel (0.5% hypochlorite solution does not have a clear benefit) or RSDL sponge, large amounts of water if nothing else.

     iii. Immediate management: decontaminate, symptomatic treatment.

    b. Lewisite (L)

       i. Signs and symptoms: immediate pain or irritation of skin and mucous membranes. Skin and eye lesions, and airway damage similar to that seen with mustard gas exposure develop later.

      ii. Decontamination: hypochlorite, large amounts of water.

     iii. Management: immediate decontamination, symptomatic management of lesions as with mustard agents—giving bronchoalveolar lavage (BAL) will decrease systemic effects but beware of the adverse effects (including for person allergic to peanuts).

    c. Phosgene oxime (CX)

       i. Signs and symptoms: immediate burning and irritation followed by wheal-like skin lesions and eye and airway damage.

      ii. Decontamination: large amounts of water.

     iii. Management: immediate decontamination, symptomatic treatment.

    d. Cyanide (AC, CK)

       i. Signs and symptoms: few—if very high exposure, may see seizures, respiratory and cardiac arrest.

      ii. Decontamination: skin decontamination usually not necessary because highly volatile, but wet, contaminated clothing should be removed and underlying skin decontaminated with water or other standard decontaminants.

     iii. Management: antidote = IV sodium nitrite and sodium thiosulfate or IV hydroxocobalamine; supportive oxygen and acidosis correction helpful.

  3. Pulmonary agents (CG)

    a. Signs and symptoms: eye, airway irritation, dyspnea, chest tightness, and delayed pulmonary edema.

    b. Decontamination: vapor → fresh air; liquid (rare situation)→ copious water irrigation.

    c. Management: termination of exposure, ABC's, rest and observation, oxygen ± positive pressure ventilation, other supportive care.

  4. Riot control agents (CS, CN, pepper spray)

    a. Signs and symptoms: burning and pain on exposed mucous membranes and skin, eye pain and tearing, burning in the nostrils, respiratory discomfort, paresthesia in exposed skin.

   b. Decontamination: flush eyes thoroughly with water or isotonic solution such as normal saline. Flush skin with copious amounts of water, alkaline soap and water, or a mildly alkaline solution (sodium bicarbonate or sodium carbonate). Generally, decontamination is not needed if the wind is brisk. Hypochlorite may exacerbate the skin lesions induced by CS and should not be used.
   c. Management: usually none is necessary as effects are self-limiting.

Nuclear Weapons

1. Nomenclature and introduction to ionizing radiation
   a. Charged particles: alpha-particles (essentially ionized helium nuclei with a charge of 2+), beta-particles (essentially liberated electrons), and positrons (positively charged electrons).
   b. Uncharged, indirectly ionizing x-rays (electromagnetic radiation), gamma-rays (electromagnetic radiation), and neutrons.
   c. Units of radiation measurement
      i. Measures of activity: Curie (1 Ci = 1 g of Ra-226), Becquerel (1 Bq = 1 disintegration/s).
      ii. Measures of exposure: Roentgen (number of ion-pairs produced in a volume of air, defined only for x-rays, gamma-rays).
      iii. Measures of absorbed: rad—radiation absorbed dose (energy deposited by any ionizing radiation per unit mass of any absorber: 1 rad = 100 erg/g ~100 mosquito push-ups); gray is the SI unit (1 Gy = 1 J/kg = 100 cGy = 100 rad). $LD_{50/60} = 3.5$–4 Gy for average person.
2. Determinants of biological effects
   a. Density of tissue: high-density tissue (muscle) is affected more severely than low-density tissue (lung). Also, for particulate radiation, damage is proportionate to charge and size; for both photon and particulate radiation, damage is inversely proportionate to energy (higher energy means less time spent passing through tissue).
   b. Type of radiation
      Must "weigh" relative effects of different types of radiation. For example, one Gy of alpha absorbed is much more damaging than one Gy of gamma-radiation absorbed.
      i. W_R x-rays, gamma-rays, beta-particles.
      ii. Neutrons: continuous function of neutron energy #peak at 20 at about 1 MeV, for low and high energy under 5.
      iii. Alpha 20.
   c. Measurements of dose equivalents
      i. Rad equivalent mean (rem): measure of relative effectiveness of radiation in causing biological damage: DE(rem) = Dose (rad) × W_R.
      ii. The sievert (Sv): SI unit of dose equivalent: 1 Sv = 1 J/kg (if W_R = 1), 1 Sv = 100 rem.
      iii. Sources of energy.
         ▪ If weight is 2 neutrons and 2 protons, their mass is greater than the weight of a helium nucleus; this discrepancy is termed the "mass defect" and is converted into the binding energy of a nucleus.
         ▪ In a typical U^{235} fission, the neutrons perpetuate a chain reaction which liberates additional neutrons as well as gamma- and beta-radiation.
         ▪ In both fission and fusion, the end mass is less. Fusion liberates three times as much energy as fission.
         ▪ Bremsstrahlung ("braking radiation"): in a nuclear explosion, x-ray photons ionize the surrounding air, forming the surface or "radiation front" of the fireball.

3. Physical effects of nuclear weapons

   a. Of the energy released from a standard fission weapon: 50% is dissipated as mechanical blast, 35% as thermal energy, 5% as initial radiation, and 10% as residual radiation with several hundred different nuclides/isotopes formed along with x-rays.

   b. The blast results in an initial compression, followed by a suction phase. At blast strengths of 1 psi, windows are shattered; at 5 psi, brick houses are destroyed and tympanic membranes burst; 15 psi causes lung damage; and 50 psi is lethal to the average person 50% of the time. Additionally, wind effects can lead to deceleration injuries (injury threshold 5 mph, LD_{50} = 55 mph) and missile injuries.

   c. Thermal injuries can cause conventional body burns and ophthalmic trauma in the form of retinal burns and flash blindness.

   d. If have some degree of warning, effects can be reduced with some postural changes. Once a blast occurs, lie head toward ground zero if wearing helmet, feet toward ground zero if not wearing helmet. Any clothing or protective barriers can be beneficial.

   e. Nuclear fallout: early fallout arrives within the first day and is concerning for whole-body exposure from gamma-radiation, external burns from beta-radiation, and internal exposure from ingested/inhaled alpha-particles (0.01–1-cm diameter particles). During the first weeks, I^{131} is a great concern. Delayed fallout arrives after the first day, with smaller particles, and can be a global concern. Primary risk is from ingestion of long-lived fission products such as $Sr^{90/89}$ and Cs^{137}, with half-lives of 30 years or more. Generally, rate of decay falls logarithmically; after every 7 hours, there is one-tenth of the activity as before.

4. Biological effects of radiation

   a. Ionizing radiation damages through ionization and excitation, which either directly ionizes molecules or generates free radicals that do the same.

   b. Radiation can overwhelmingly damage DNA, damage cell membranes, and cause other effects; lethal effects are primarily in the nucleus/DNA molecule (cytoplasm can withstand much higher doses of radiation than nucleus); at very high doses, lethal effects quickly occur from neurovascular damage secondary to edema.

   c. Modifiers of effects

      i. Total dose: more is worse.

      ii. Dose rate/fractionation: if spread dose over time, greater survivability.

      iii. Chemical modifiers: oxygen potentiates effects; anoxia/antioxidants are radioprotective.

      iv. Cell type: actively dividing cells more vulnerable, quiescent stem cells more resistant, and those with large volume of nucleic acids are most vulnerable. Also, those cells in mitosis are at increased vulnerability.

      v. Route of exposure: open wound, inhalation, ingestion all determine what tissues are affected, as well as the "critical organ" (the tissue or organ where radionuclide is ultimately deposited—i.e., iodine becomes concentrated in the thyroid).

       ■ In utero, radiation can cause growth retardation (esp. 3–20 weeks gestation), microcephaly, mental retardation, skeletal abnormalities, and ocular anomalies (esp. 6–11 weeks). After exposure, males initially fertile, but 35 cGy leads to 8 to 20 months of sterility; 6 Gy leads to permanent sterility. In females, do see immediate sterility, and as little as 350 cGy leads to 60% infertility.

       ■ Somatic effects include aplastic anemia, cataracts (threshold is 1.5–3 Gy for single exposure, cardiovascular, cancer.

       Leukemia (especially in children), thyroid (malignant and nonmalignant) increased rate after Nagasaki/Hiroshima. Breast cancer seen after A-bomb survivors (gamma, neutrons) and fluoroscopy patients. Bone cancer noted in radium dial painters (alpha). Lung cancer seen in uranium miners (alpha).

       Recommended dose limits: occupational = 20 mSv per year; public 1 mSv in year.

5. Acute radiation syndrome
   a. More than 0.12 Gy whole body → sperm decreases to nadir by day 45; 0.20 Gy, whole body → detectable increase in chromosomal aberrations; 0.20 to 0.50 Gy, whole body → detectable bone marrow depression with lymphocytopenia.
   b. $LD_{50/60}$ for whole-body irradiation without treatment is 3.5 to 4 Gy without treatment, increasing to 5 to 6 with supportive care (abx, transfusion) and 6 to 8 with early CSF administration.

      Worsened by coexisting trauma, nutritional deficits, infection, or chronic disease. Improved by radioprotectants (anoxia, vitamins A/E/C), partial body exposure, poorly penetrating radiation, fractionation, good medical support.
   c. Sensitivity: hematopoietic > GI > CV > CNS.
   d. Stages of acute radiation syndrome: prodrome, latent, manifest illness, recovery.
   e. Hematopoietic syndrome: dose range 1 to 6 Gy, affects dividing stem cells and progenitors for all marrow cell lines.
      i. Prodromal period: N/V, anorexia, possible diarrhea.
      ii. Latent period: asymptomatic except mild weakness for about 3 weeks.
      iii. Overt clinical period: bone marrow atrophy, hemorrhage, and infection, onset at 3 to 4 weeks. Lymphocytes show first drop in 1 to 3 days, then slowly stabilize. Neutrophils may actually increase in the first day or so, then gradually decrease to nadir within 30 to 40 days. Thrombocytes begin to decrease at 15 days, reaching minimal levels by 30 to 40 days.
   f. Gastrointestinal syndrome: dose range over 6 Gy, affects GI stem cells.
      i. Prodromal period: severe N/V, occasionally watery diarrhea and cramps, onset within hours after exposure.
      ii. Latent period: asymptomatic for 5 to 7 days.
      iii. Overt clinical period: return of severe diarrhea (progression to bloody), vomiting, fever, may develop into shock and death.
         ■ Can see malabsorption, paralytic ileus, dehydration, ARF with CV collapse, GI bleeding, anemia, and sepsis.
   g. Cardiovascular and CNS syndrome: more than 15 Gy, affects circulatory endothelium.
      i. Prodromal period: burning sensation within minutes of exposure, N/V develop within 30 minutes, with loss of balance and confusion with prostration eventually developing.
      ii. Latent period: apparent improvement for several hours.
      iii. Overt clinical period: within 5 to 6 hours, watery diarrhea, respiratory distress, and gross CNS signs.
   h. Summary of acute radiation syndrome

# Gy	Performance Loss	Injury	Survival
Hematologic Syndrome			
1	Motivational loss	Marrow	Probable
2	Fatigue, weakness	Marrow	Probable
3	Anorexia	Marrow	Likely
4	Nausea/vomiting	Severe marrow	Possible
5	Diarrhea	Severe marrow	LD_{50} w/ tx

# Gy	Performance Loss	Injury	Survival
Gastrointestinal Syndrome			
6	↑ Reaction time	Mod intestinal	Death 2–3 weeks
7	""	""	""
8	Hypotension	""	""
9	""	""	""
10	""	Severe intestinal	Death 1–2 weeks
15	Early transient incapacitation	""	""
CV/CNS			
15	""	""	Death 5–12 days
20	Loss of consciousness	Neurovascular	""
25	""	""	""
30	""	""	Death 2–5 days

    i. Managing acute radiation syndrome.
- Antiemetics: Kytril, 10 μg/kg IV, antidiarrheals, fluid replacement.
- Colloids: give through silicone central catheters.
- Blood: requires irradiation before use to prevent graft versus host reaction.
- Consider platelet transfusion if counts under 20,000/mm^3, or sooner, if bleeding and bone marrow depression progresses.
- G-CSF and Peg-G-CSF US Food and Drug Administration (FDA)-approved to prevent neutropenia. TPO mimetics and IL-11 should be considered to decrease thrombocytopenia.
- Infection control:
  Laminar flow isolation, strict-handwashing pre- and postpatient care, surgical attire for staff.
  Gut decontamination: consider neomycin or oral fluoroquinolones.
  Consider CMV prophylaxis (IV IgG, ganciclovir, acyclovir) if seronegative, and also use CMV-free blood products in those patients.
  Consider HSV prophylaxis.
  Fungal prophylaxis: fluconazole (400 mg qd, IV/PO).
  Pneumocystis carinii prophylaxis: TMP-SMX—do not begin until ANC counts are normal, given up to 6 months.
  Start empiric antibiotics with sx/sx of fever, usually weeks after exposure, and continue treatment until granulocytes > 800/mm^3.

  6. Assessing exposure and damage
ARS external irradiation
    a. Triage classification methods: prodromal effects, lymphocyte counts, physical dosimetry, biodosimetry, skin changes.
      i. Prodromal effects.

Dose (Gy)	Onset (h)	Duration (h)	Latency
0.5–2	absent to 6	<24	Absent or 3 weeks
2–3	2–6	12–24	2–3 weeks
3–5.5	1–2	24	1–2.5 weeks
>5.5	Minutes to 1	48	2–4 days

Neurologic signs indicate a nonsurvivable injury.

■ Lymphocyte assay uses cultured lymphocytes to visualize dicentrics (mutated rings) characteristic aberrant chromosomes. Sensitive to 0.1 to 0.2 Gy 1 cGy, but is not an immediate diagnostic indicator (takes about 3 days to be maximally accurate, but can interpolate—absolute lymphocyte blood cell count is a valuable indicator: small exposure: 1.5×10^9/L in 24 hours; severe exposure: 1.0×10^9/L in 24 hours, 0.5×10^9/L in 48 hours). A drop of more than 50% indicates a significant radiological injury.

■ Skin changes:

Prodromal phase: transient, atypical brief erythema, heat sensation, itching.

Acute phase: 7 to 10 days postexposure, secondary erythema and edema, blisters, moist desquamation, superficial and deep ulcers, necrosis, epilation, telangiectasias, and pigmentary changes.

Delayed phase: pigmentary changes, atrophy, subcutaneous sclerosis, keratosis, vasculitis, pain.

Gy (Local Irradiation)	Dermal Symptoms
>3	Epilation begins around day 17
~6	Erythema, minutes-weeks postexposure
>6	Edema
10–20	Blistering, 2–3 weeks postexposure
~30	Ulceration, 1–2 months postexposure
50–60	Gangrene, necrosis, deep ulceration

7. Contamination
   a. Can measure with whole-body counters, chest counters, or skin/wound monitors.
   b. Can perform swipes (skin, wound, bilateral nares) or bioassays of bile, urine, feces. Such tests can determine type of radiation. Perform early to provide baseline. Different radionuclides are excreted along different timelines through various excretion pathways—hence the need for knowing your nuclide, and repeatedly testing multiple body fluids/tissues.

8. Shielding
   a. Alpha-particles: stratum corneum of skin effectively protects but can cause intense local damage if deposited internally (inhalation, ingestion).
   b. Beta-particles: topped by aluminum foil, 30% to 55% reduction by protective clothing, high risk of skin burns.
      Neutrons: water, paraffin, oil, lithium, boron, cadmium all excellent but NOT
   c. heavy metals such as lead or bismuth
      Gamma- and x-rays: heavy metals such as lead are most protective,

    d. followed by steel, aluminum, concrete, and to a much lesser extent, earth, water.

    e. If in a building, move to the center if radiation is outside; if can move below ground, do so.

    f. As with any radiation source, the intensity falls as a function of the distance squared from the source.

9. Decontamination

    a. Treatment of life-threatening injuries always takes precedence over decontamination and dose estimation procedures; do remove person from contaminated area though if possible. In the United States, no healthcare worker has ever suffered radiation injury from emergent treatment of a contaminated patient.

    b. Decontaminate as soon as practical, but only what is necessary, and as far from contaminated area as possible.

    c. Evacuate patient to point downwind from a "clean" area. Monitor as able with meters such as "radioactivity detection, indication, and computation" (RADIAC) or multifunction survey meter.

    d. Remove and bag outer clothing and shoes (achieves 90%–90% reduction in patient contamination usually). Monitor areas again. Decontaminate skin (face and hands) with soap and water (usually produces 98% decontamination). Wash or clip hair and nails as necessary. Remonitor. Dry with absorbent material.

    e. Decontamination should come after stabilization, but precede emergency surgery, which should be followed by definitive care and treatment of radiation injuries.

10. Management

    a. Attend to life-threatening conditions first. Remember only contaminated patients are "active," not patients who are merely irradiated.

    b. Obtain history, and contact a health physicist if possible. Notify state radiation authorities. Cover entrance/floor to treatment area, remove unnecessary equipment.

    c. Mark off areas, use control points. Control air ventilation. Cover items in room.

    d. Wear surgical attire with double gloves and waterproof gowns. Procure dosimeters and check radiation background.

    e. Triage medically, then by radiation activity.

    f. In initial survey, can perform rapid assessment of contamination.

    g. Perform bilateral nasal sweeps, CBC with diff, absolute lymphocyte count.

    h. Remove patient's clothing, and wash patient with detergent (soap, betadine, phisoderm, hydrogen peroxide all useful; Dakin's solution: 0.25% sodium hypochlorite useful as may chelate particulate matter) and water (95% effective). Capture the water if possible.

    i. Drape out areas of contamination and irrigate, wash out, save irrigant.

    j. Endpoint for irrigation is 250 μrem.

    k. Do not eat/smoke/drink in controlled area.

    l. In washing patient, do not abrade skin; wash gently. Endpoints for decontamination are beta-radiation less than 1 mR/h (10 μSv/h) and alpha-radiation under 1000 disintegrations/minute.

    m. Respiratory contamination: can perform nasal irrigation and unilateral lung irrigation but do not encourage expectorants.

    n. Gastrointestinal contamination: may take 2 to 5 days to eliminate, consider stomach lavage, emetics, activated charcoal, and antacids. Among laxatives, osmotic agents such as magnesium citrate are especially good. Gaviscon is particularly useful for strontium. "Prussian blue" (ferric ferrocyanide) is not absorbed in the GI tract and has been recommended for cesium, thallium, and rubidium; dosage is 1 to 3 g, PO TID for up to 3 weeks.

o. Other specific agents:
   i. Blocking/diluting.
      ■ Iodides: can be 100% effective against I^{131} if given within 30 minutes. Dosage is 100 to 300 mg PO qd for 2 weeks.
      ■ Strontium: Ca gluconate/chloride.
      ■ Water: can use beer or water against tritium ingestion.
   ii. Mobilizing agents:
      ■ Propylthiouracil (PTU)/antithyroid medications for I^{131}.
      ■ Ammonium chloride with calcium gluconate for strontium.
   iii. Chelating agents:
      ■ May cause pain at injection site, bone marrow depression, nephrotoxicity.
      ■ DTPA for transuranics/rare earth metals, plutonium, americium, curium, californium, cobalt. Careful use in pregnancy, minors.
p. Topical agents for external contamination include titanium dioxide paste, methyl cellulose, soap and water. Anticoagulants, aerosol "lioxanol," tannin solution "baliz," hydrocortisone bandages, and wax with antibiotics have also been used.
q. Primary closure involving radiation combined injury must be completed within first 48 hours after irradiation. Reconstructive surgery must be postponed for 2 months until complete resolution of radiation injury.
r. Neutropenic fever therapy: survey for possible sources (pancultures).
   i. Antibiotics for ANC under $500/mm^3$: double beta-lactam abx such as a third-generation cephalosporin and piperacillin; monotherapy with imipenem or a third-generation cephalosporin; vancomycin plus a third-generation cephalosporin.
   ii. Add amphotericin for prolonged fever lasting 5 to 7 days after starting standard abx.
   iii. Continue abx as long as ANC under 1000.
s. Cytokine therapy: can stimulate white blood cell (WBC) production and increase hemopoiesis. FDA has approved Neupogen (granulocyte colony stimulating), TPO-mimetics, and Neumega (IL-11).
t. Radioprotection agents:
   i. Sulfur compounds: WR-2721, N-acetylcysteine, mercaptopropionylglycine.
   ii. Dietary compounds: vitamin E, vitamin A, selenium.
11. Psychological considerations
a. Anticipate considerable psychosomatic complaints. In Israeli experiences with SCUD missile attacks, the majority of emergency room visits were purely of psychological origin with no biological injury. From radiation incident in Goiania, Brazil: of the first 60,000 monitored, none was contaminated, but 5000 had psychosomatic symptoms of rash, vomiting, diarrhea which mimicked acute radiation sickness. In Three-Mile Island, no actual injuries were incurred but significant reports of headache, rash, anorexia, insomnia, aches/pains, and mood changes.
b. A "pseudo-lucid interval" may occur after radiological exposure; performance may initially decrease, then rebound to near-normal function for several hours or days before dropping again, possibly irreversibly.
12. Selected nuclides
a. Americium
   i. Am^{241} is a decay daughter of plutonium and emits primarily alpha-radiation, although 60 KeV gamma-emission allows it to be detected by standard radiacs. It is found in various instruments such as smoke detectors and in postdetonation fallout. It can cause heavy metal poisoning and whole-body irradiation in severe exposures. Dust is 75% absorbed, with 10% of particles retained in lungs. Although GI absorption is poor, it may be readily absorbed from skin wounds. It undergoes urinary and hepatic excretion.
   ii. Treatment: DTPA chelation within 24 to 48 hours of pulmonary exposure.

b. Cesium

 i. Ce^{137} is often found in medical radiotherapy instruments. A gamma- and beta-emitter, it is readily detected by gamma instruments. It is completely absorbed by lungs, GI tract, and from wounds. It is soluble in most forms and is metabolized as a potassium analog. Primary toxicity is whole-body radiation.

 ii. Treatment (internal contamination): Prussian blue (available overseas and in the United States in experimental protocols from Oak Ridge, TN) and ion exchange resins. If can intervene early after ingestion, attempt lavage and purgatives.

c. Cobalt

 i. Co^{60} is found in both medical radiotherapy devices and commercial food irradiators. Metal, nonsoluble in water, no reaction with air. It generates high-energy gamma-rays and 0.31 MeV beta; gamma-detectors readily detect this nuclide. Rapidly absorbed from the lung, between 25% and 90% of ingested cobalt will be absorbed by the GI tract, 5% liver, 45% homogenous distribution (dynamics of wound absorption is unknown). Primary toxicity will be from whole-body irradiation and acute radiation syndrome (external irradiation).

 ii. Treatment internal contamination: DTPA, Ca gluconate gastric lavage, purgatives. Severe cases might be treated by chelation with penicillamine.

d. Depleted uranium (DU; contains less than the 0.7% of U^{235} isotope as found in nature)

 i. DU emits limited alpha-, beta-, and some gamma-radiation. DU does not cause radiation threat and is found in armor-piercing ammunition, armor, and other military weaponry. It is detectable with an end-window G-M counter. Destroyed armored vehicle entry or contact with tank fires may result in inhaled DU; the salts are absorbed via inhalation. Fragments in flesh become encapsulated and are slowly metabolized, resulting in whole-body distribution, particularly to the bone and kidneys (however, no renal toxicity has been documented).

 ii. Sodium bicarbonate decreases nephrotoxicity of uranyl ion, and tubular diuretics may also be helpful. Extensive surgery undertaken only to remove DU (esp. sub-cm fragments) is not indicated. Labs include 24-h urine for U bioassay, serum BUN/Cr, beta-2-microglobulin, creatinine clearance, and LFTs.

e. Iodine

 i. $I^{131, 132, 134, 135}$ will be encountered after reactor accidents/destruction.
 Radioactive iodine (RAI) is a normal fission product found in reactor fuel rods. Most of the radiation is beta, with some gamma. Primary toxicity is to the thyroid. High levels of pediatric thyroid carcinoma arose after Chernobyl.

 ii. Treatment: If exposure is anticipated, daily intake of 130 mg of sodium iodide or potassium iodide will prevent uptake. Postexposure, 300 mg NaI or KI daily for 7 to 10 days will block thyroid uptake. Oral PTU 100 mg q8h for 8 days or methimazole 10 mg q8h for 2 days, then 5 mg q8h × 6 days, may also be used.

f. Phosphorus

 i. P^{32} generally comes from research laboratories and in medical facilities where it is used as a tracer. It has a strong beta-ray and can be detected with the beta-shield open on a beta-gamma detector. It is completely absorbed from all sites and is deposited in the bone marrow and other rapidly replicating cells. Local irradiation causes cell damage.

 ii. Treatment: lavage, aluminum hydroxide, and oral phosphates.

g. Plutonium

 i. $Pu^{238, 239}$ is produced by uranium in reactors. It is the primary fissionable material in nuclear weapons and is the predominant radioactive contaminant in nuclear weapon accidents. The primary radiation is from alpha-particles, thus rendering Pu not an external hazard. However, it is always contaminated with americium, which does have a fairly easily detectable gamma-ray by use of a thin-walled gamma-probe. Primary toxicity is from inhalation. Particles 5µ or smaller will remain in the lung and be metabolized based on the salt solubility. GI absorption will depend upon the chemical state of Pu; metal is not absorbed. Stool specimens become positive positive after 24 hours, urine after 2 weeks. Wound absorption is variable. May be washed from intact skin.

    ii. Treatment: nebulized or IV: 1 g CaDTPA within 24 hours of exposure, then day 2 and day 3, then 3 times a week, then 1 per week; followed by 1 g ZnDTPA qd, monitoring urine levels.

h. Radium

    i. Ra^{226} may be found in certain industrial and dated medical equipment. Although primary emissions are alpha particles, daughter nuclides release beta- and gamma-particles, posing a potential threat of external irradiation. Most exposure is via ingestion, with 30% being absorbed. Long-term exposure is associated with leukemia, aplastic anemia, and sarcomas.

    ii. Treatment: immediate lavage with 10% magnesium sulfate followed by saline and magnesium purgatives after ingestion. Ammonium chloride may increase fecal elimination.

i. Strontium

    i. Sr^{90} is a daughter of uranium fission. It emits beta-rays and can be an external radiation hazard (skin burn). Soluble Sr will follow calcium and is readily absorbed by both respiratory and GI routes; up to 50% will be deposited in bone.

    ii. Treatment: immediately after ingestion, oral administration of aluminum phosphate can decrease absorption by up to 85%. Administration of stable strontium can inhibit the nuclide's metabolism and increase excretion. Sodium alginate + Ca gluconate + Sr lactate. Large doses of calcium and acidification of the urine with ammonium chloride will likewise increase excretion.

j. Tritium

    i. H^3 is used in nuclear weapons and in many Western luminescent gun sights. It is unlikely to be a hazard except in a closed space, as tritium gas rapidly diffuses into the atmosphere. A beta-emitter, tritium is not a significant irradiation hazard. Tritiated water will be fully absorbed and equilibrates with body water. It is excreted in urine and can be detected within 1 hour of significant exposure. No adverse health effects have been reported from a single exposure.

    ii. Treatment: the biological half-life is 10 to 12 days. Maximally increasing oral fluids will reduce this by half.

k. Uranium

    i. U$^{238, 235, 234}$ is found, in order of increasing radioactivity, in DU, natural uranium, fuel rods, and weapons-grade material. Uranium and its daughters emit alpha-, beta-, and gamma-radiation, but DU and natural radiation are not serious irradiation threats. Chemical nephrotoxicity over 0.6 to 3 µg/g kidney. However, spent fuel rods and weapons-grade (enriched) uranium can emit significant (lethal) levels of gamma-radiation if in large enough quantities. Inhaled uranium compounds may be metabolized and excreted in the urine. Urinary levels of 100 µg% following acute exposure can cause renal failure. Absorption will be determined by the chemical state of the U. Soluble salts are readily absorbed; the metal is not.

    ii. Treatment: sodium bicarbonate makes the uranyl ion less nephrotoxic. Tubular diuretics may be beneficial. Evaluation should include urinalysis, 24-hour urine for U bioassay, serum BUN/Cr, beta-2-microglobulin, creatinine clearance, and LFTs.

13. Emergency contacts, 24 hours/d
  a. US Department of Energy—Oak Ridge REAC/TS (423) 481-1000 beeper 241
  b. US Armed Forces Radiobiology Research Institute
    DTRA-AFRRI MRAT (301) 295-0316 or 1-800-SKY-PAGE pin 8010-338

Further Reading

Armed Forces Radiobiology Research Institute 2013. *Medical Management of Radiological Casualties Handbook.* 4th ed. Bethesda, MD: AFRRI; 2013. Available at: https://www.usuhs.edu/sites/default/files/media/afrri/pdf/4edmmrchandbook.pdf.

Chambers JA, Long JN. Radiation injury and the hand surgeon. *J Hand Surg Am.* 2008;33:601–611.

Chambers JA, Purdue GF. Radiation injury and the surgeon. *J Am Coll Surg.* 2007;204(1):128–139.

Conklin JJ, Walker RI. *Military Radiobiology.* London: Academic Press; 1987.

US Army Medical Research Institute of Chemical Defense. *Medical Management of Chemical Casualties Handbook.* 5th ed. Aberdeen Proving Ground, MD: USAMRICD; 2014. Available at: https://www.cs.amedd.army.mil/Portlet.aspx?ID=a0968070-71b0-46c0-a139-9362d1b13265.

US Army Medical Research Institute of Infectious Diseases. *Medical Management of Biological Casualties Handbook.* 7th ed. Fort Detrick, Frederick, MD: USAMRIID; 2011. Available at: https://www.usamriid.army.mil/education/bluebookpdf/USAMRIID%20BlueBook%207th%20Edition%20-%20Sep%202011.pdf.

US Department of Health & Human Services. Radiation Emergency Medical Management Website. Available at: https://www.remm.nlm.gov/.

CHAPTER 15

Medical Response to Disasters

Susan Miller Briggs ■ Dennis T. Cherian ■ Alfonso C. Rosales

The demands of international disaster relief have changed over the past decade in the spectrum of threats, the field of operations, and scope of medical care. International disasters include large-scale disasters from natural events, such as earthquakes and tsunamis, and human-generated humanitarian crises, both intentional (war and terrorism) and unintentional. Today's international disasters from natural events are even more devastating because of factors such as explosive population growth, poverty, and increasing economic and social disparities. Armed conflicts increasingly involve civilians, especially vulnerable populations such as children and the elderly.[1-4]

Many of today's complex international disasters occur in "austere" environments. An austere environment is a setting where access, transport, resources or other aspects of the physical, social, economic or political environments impose constraints on the adequacy of care for the population in need. All of these factors greatly increase the challenges of international disaster relief. Civilian and military medical teams are increasingly being mobilized to respond to international disasters, which are increasing both in frequency and complexity[1,3-6] (Fig. 15.1).

Disaster medical care is not the same as conventional medical care. Disaster medical care requires a fundamental change ("crisis management care") in the care of disaster victims to achieve the objective of providing the "greatest good for the greatest number of victims." This is in contrast to the objective of conventional medical care, which is the "greatest good for the individual patient." It is important to apply the principles of crisis management care to all phases of disaster management (preparedness, mitigation, response, and recovery). Demand for resources always exceeds the supply of resources in a mass casualty incident (MCI).[1,2,5-7]

Epidemiology of Disasters

Natural disasters may be classified as sudden-impact (acute) disasters or chronic-onset (slow) disasters. Sudden-impact natural disasters generally cause significant mortality and morbidity immediately as a direct result of the primary event (e.g., traumatic injuries, crush injuries,

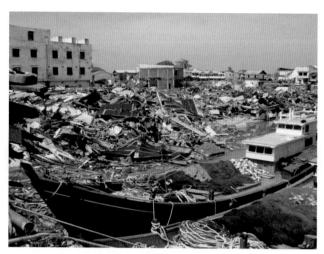

Fig. 15.1 Banda Aceh tsunami.

drowning). Chronic-onset disasters cause mortality and morbidity through prolonged secondary effects (e.g., infectious disease outbreaks, dehydration, and malnutrition). Earthquakes, tsunamis, landslides, and wildfires are examples of sudden-impact disasters. Chronic-onset disasters include famines, droughts, hurricanes, and typhoons.[1,4]

Man-made disasters may be unintentional or intentional and range from technological disasters to MCIs involving weapons of mass destruction (radioactive, biological and chemical agents).[1,5] Disasters involving weapons of mass destruction (WMD), whether accidental or man-made, are a significant challenge for medical providers for several reasons:

- WMD have the potential to produce casualties in numbers large enough to overwhelm healthcare systems.
- WMD may produce large numbers of "expectant" victims. This denotes a category of disaster victims not expected to survive because of severity of injuries or underlying diseases and/ or limited resources. This term was first used in conjunction with chemical warfare.
- WMD may produce a "contaminated" environment. Medical providers must be able to perform triage, initial stabilization, and possible definitive surgical care outside traditional healthcare facilities.
- WMD produce significant numbers of "psychogenic" casualties, greatly complicating rescue and triage efforts. Terrorists do not have to kill people to achieve their goals.

Creating a climate of fear and panic to overwhelm the medical infrastructure achieves their goals. During the sarin attack in Tokyo (1995), 5000 casualties were referred to local hospitals. Fewer than 1000 individuals were suffering from the effects of the gas. The remainder of the individuals were experiencing psychological symptoms.

PRINCIPLE 1

Medical providers cannot use traditional command structures when participating in disaster response. The Incident Command System (ICS) or Incident Management System is a modular/adaptable system for all incidents and facilities and is the accepted standard for all disaster response. Functional requirements, not titles, determine the ICS hierarchy. The organizational structure of the ICS is built around five major management activities (Incident Command, Operations, Planning, Logistics, and Finance/Administration) (Fig. 15.2). Operations directs all disaster medical personnel. The Incident Commander in international disasters may be an

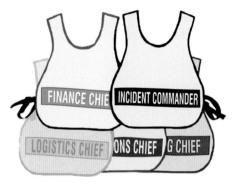

Fig. 15.2   Incident Command System organizational structure.

international organization such as the United Nations (UN) or the World Health Organization (WHO), a government military or civilian organization of the affected country, or a responding organization from outside the country.[1,5]

The structure of the ICS is the same regardless of the nature of the disaster. The difference is in the particular expertise of key personnel. Medical providers, often used to working independently, must adhere to the structure of an ICS to integrate successfully into the disaster response team and avoid many negative consequences including:

- Death of medical personnel because of lack of safety and training
- Lack of adequate medical supplies to provide care
- Staff working beyond their training.

PRINCIPLE 2

Disaster response includes basic medical and public health concerns that are the same in all disasters regardless of the etiology of the disaster (Boxes 15.1 and 15.2). A single emergency operations plan for many different situations is more effective than multiple separate disaster plans ("All Hazards Approach"), and most nations now adhere to this concept.[1,3,5] The difference in disasters is the degree of disruption of the medical and public health infrastructures and the amount of outside assistance (regional, national, or international) that is needed to meet the needs of disaster victims. Rapid assessment by experienced personnel will determine which assets are needed in the acute phase of the disaster to augment local capacity. The complexity of today's international humanitarian crises has increased the need for multidisciplinary medical and public health specialty teams as critical assets in international disaster relief. Flexibility and mobility are key assets required of all international disaster management teams, regardless of expertise.

PRINCIPLE 3

Effective "surge capacity" is not based on well-intentioned and readily available volunteers. Disaster medical responders must understand the basic principles of disaster response (ICS, disaster triage,

---

BOX 15.1 ■ Medical Concerns

- Search and rescue
- Triage
- Definitive care
- Evacuation

BOX 15.2 ■ Public Health Concerns

- Water
- Food
- Shelter
- Sanitation
- Security/safety
- Transportation
- Communication
- Endemic/epidemic diseases

---

gross decontamination) to be effective members of the disaster team. Medical providers must be willing to care for the nondisaster-related injuries/medical conditions always seen in disaster response, in addition to disaster-related injuries/diseases. Predisaster training is an essential part of disaster preparedness.

Medical Response to Disasters

Disaster medical response includes four components: (1) search and rescue; (2) triage and initial stabilization; (3) definitive medical care; and (4) evacuation. International disaster teams are designed and trained to provide specific "functional" areas of disaster care. Clinical competencies, not titles, determine the role of disaster medical responders in international disaster relief.[1-3,5]

Search and Rescue

The local population near any disaster site is the immediate search and rescue asset, but the technical equipment and expertise to facilitate extrication of victims trapped in the rubble is usually lacking. Many countries have developed specialized search and rescue teams, and acute care medical providers are part of these teams. Search and rescue teams are involved both in the rescue (extrication) and initial stabilization of victims, including field amputations and fasciotomies as necessary.[1,3,5] Search and rescue teams are generally composed of specialists in the following areas:

- Acute care specialties (surgery, emergency medicine, anesthesia)
- Technical search
- Hazardous materials
- Communications and logistics
- Trained canines and their handlers.

Disaster Triage

Triage is the process of prioritizing casualties according to the level of care they require. It is the most important, and psychologically most difficult, mission of disaster medical response, both in the prehospital and hospital phases of the disaster. Disaster triage requires a fundamental change in the approach to the medical care of victims.[1,3,5,6] The objective of conventional civilian triage is to do the greatest good for the individual patient. Severity of injury/disease is the major determinant for medical care. The objective of disaster triage is to do the greatest good for the greatest number of patients. The determinants of triage in disasters are, however, based on three parameters:

- Severity of injury
- Likelihood of survival
- Available resources (logistics, personnel, evacuation assets).

The major objective and challenge of triage is to rapidly identify the small minority of critically injured patients who require urgent life-saving interventions, including operative interventions, from the larger majority of noncritical casualties that characterize most disasters. In a mass casualty event, the critical patients with the greatest chance of survival with the least expenditure of time and resources are prioritized to be treated first.

Triage is a dynamic decision-making process of matching victims needs with available resources. Many MCIs will have multiple different levels of triage as patients move from the disaster scene to definitive medical care. Disaster medical triage may be conducted at three different levels depending on the level of casualties (injuries) to capabilities (resources).[1,4,5]

FIELD TRIAGE

Field triage, often the initial triage system used at the disaster scene in MCIs, is the rapid categorization of victims potentially needing immediate medical care where they are lying or at triage sites. Victims are designated as "acute" or "nonacute". Simplified color coding may be used. Once the victims are transported to casualty collection centers (fixed or mobile medical facilities), medical triage according to severity of injury/disease may be performed.

MEDICAL TRIAGE

Medical triage is the rapid categorization of victims, at a casualty collection site or fixed or mobile medical facilities, by the most experienced medical personnel available to identify the level of medical care needed based on severity of injury. Triage personnel must have knowledge of the medical consequences of various injuries (e.g., burn, blast, or crush injuries or exposure to chemical, biological, or radioactive agents). Color coding may be used (Fig. 15.3).

EVACUATION TRIAGE

Evacuation triage assigns priorities to disaster victims for transfer to definitive care facilities. Burns, blast and crush injuries, and pediatric trauma are among key priorities for early transfer because of the complexity of injuries and frequent need for multidisciplinary surgical teams.[8,9]

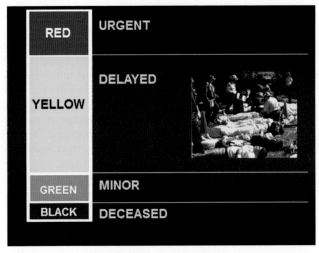

Fig. 15.3 Medical triage categories.

Definitive Care

Definitive medical care refers to care that will improve, rather than simply stabilize, a casualty's condition. Both small- and large-scale disasters may require the mobilization of disaster medical teams to participate in the field medical response or supplement capacities at facilities in the disaster region (fixed or mobile facilities). Alternatively, the evacuation of disaster victims to regional medical facilities outside the disaster regions may be required to provide definitive medical care and "surge" medical capacity may be needed.[1,5,6]

The care that medical responders deliver in disasters is significantly more austere than the care medical providers deliver on a day-to-day basis. In disasters, it is usually possible only to deliver "minimally acceptable care" in the initial phases of the disaster because of the large number of casualties, in contrast to the "maximally acceptable care" that is delivered in nondisaster situations. Difficult, and often emotional, decisions must be made as to the extent of medical care that can be delivered to patients with neglected injuries/diseases during the disaster medical response.[1,5,6,10]

Damage control surgery is frequently employed in disaster settings and is an important component of "crisis management care." In many disasters, local medical facilities are destroyed, transportation to outside medical facilities may not be feasible, or the environment may be contaminated. Damage control surgery limits surgical interventions to control of hemorrhage and contamination (Fig. 15.4). This provides the opportunity to stabilize victims of the disaster. Definitive repair of injuries can be performed at a later date. Damage control surgery was initially developed for abdominal trauma with uncontrolled hemorrhage, but has expanded to most other surgical specialties, such as orthopedic and vascular surgery.

Disaster management teams are designed and trained to provide specific "functional" capabilities such as critical care, pediatrics, obstetrics, and acute and trauma surgery, especially when the casualty load is unknown. Deployable, rapid-assembly medical facilities with the capacity for initial stabilization, operative interventions, and critical care are frequently used by both civilian and military medical teams and significantly increase the flexibility of disaster response. In recent disasters such as the Indonesian tsunami and the Haiti earthquake, hospital ships have proven valuable definitive care assets.[6–9]

International Disasters: The Players

The activation of international disaster response teams can occur in a number of ways. Generally, the affected country requests assistance via the government officials of foreign countries or organizations already in the country. For example, US aid is requested through the US embassy located in the country affected by the disaster. Other organizations such as the UN, the North Atlantic Treaty Organization (NATO), and the European Union also may forward requests for assistance to their member countries. Generally, major participants in international medical disaster relief are part of the UN organization, international organizations, governmental organizations, and nonprofit organizations.

Nonprofit organizations, especially those already working in the affected country, have an important role in both disaster preparedness and response. The response of World Vision, a worldwide nonprofit organization, to the Zika and Ebola humanitarian crises illustrates the critical role nonprofit organizations can play in both the "acute" phase of the disaster and the prevention of further mortality and morbidity. The mission and ability of nongovernmental organizations (NGOs) to engage communities, reach the unreached, and deliver solutions that are culturally acceptable are key, but also require NGOs to adapt approaches and learnings normally applied in a stable development context to a fragile context such as disaster relief. The community is paramount for effective implementation and scale up. This is where NGOs who have community relationships, understanding, and trust can best contribute to the universal effort to meet global health goals.[12]

THE ZIKA VIRUS EPIDEMIC

In May 2015, the first cases of Zika virus (ZIKV) infection were confirmed in Brazil.[13] In less than 9 months, more than 1.3 million people were infected, and the virus had spread through 41 countries and territories throughout Latin America and the Caribbean, heralding an epidemic that was anticipated to last for at least another 3 years; now an endemic disease.[14] As evidence mounted to establish a causal link between ZIKV and microcephaly, and other serious neurologic anomalies such as Guillain-Barré syndrome, the WHO declared the Zika epidemic a public health emergency of international concern in February of 2016.[15]

Although national ministries of health in affected countries led the overall response to the outbreak, the active participation of civil society has traditionally been considered important. World Vision, a civil society organization, integrated its community-based platforms into emergency national responses.

With presence in around 100 countries, World Vision is a Christian humanitarian organization dedicated to working with children, families, and their communities worldwide to reach their full potential by tackling the causes of poverty and injustice. World Vision's commitment to improving child well-being remains the same in regular work and crisis response: ensure that mothers and children are well nourished, are protected from infection and diseases, and have access to essential health services. World Vision's humanitarian health and nutrition response is based on the Sphere Minimum Standards for Health and aligns with its internal Health and Nutrition in Emergency Framework, its Do/Assure/Don't Do Framework, and the Guide to Maternal, Newborn, and Child Health and Nutrition in Emergencies. World Vision's response is complementary to and coordinated with governments' and partner agencies' efforts.

World Vision believes that it is important to focus on maternal and child health care during sudden-onset large-scale emergencies, because 60% of maternal mortality, and 45% of newborn and 53% of under-five deaths occur in humanitarian settings and crisis situations, with women and children up to 14 times more likely than men to die in disasters (source: *Renewed Global Strategy for Women Child and Adolescent Health*, 2016). World Vision does so by strengthening

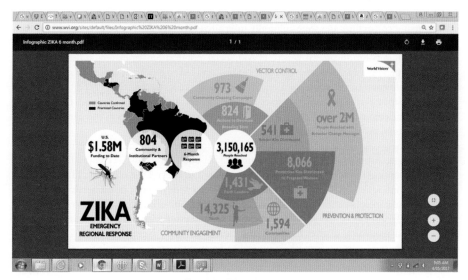

Fig. 15.4 Zika statistics.

health systems mainly at the community level, the provision of nutrition assistance, community engagement and health promotion, and the prevention of diseases with outbreak potential.

During the ZIKV outbreak, World Vision's focus was on protecting pregnant women and children in the five countries with the highest prevalence of transmission of the virus: Brazil, Colombia, El Salvador, Guatemala, and Honduras, contributing to disease surveillance in each of these countries. World Vision worked with local health authorities and other agencies to set up diagnostic facilities to ensure women and children infected with the virus could be referred to appropriate healthcare services. Mosquito nets were distributed to help prevent infection, and World Vision worked with communities to remove contaminated water and mosquito breeding grounds. Public health information was provided to communities, including basic information about the virus so that people were educated about its symptoms and how it is spread. Additionally, with financial support from Pan American Health Organization (PAHO/WHO), World Vision conducted a Knowledge, Attitudes, and Practices study in the five prioritized countries and in the Dominican Republic. The information, collected and analysed by World Vision staff, informed national communication risk programs in each of these countries and the international community via peer-reviewed journals, international conferences, and webinars.

By embedding its response in community-focused programming and utilizing established communication platforms through local and faith leaders, World Vision was able to reach over 3 million people. World Vision continues to work with these communities through ongoing programming in the region and continues to support public health efforts in relation to containing ZIKF (Fig. 15.4).

THE EBOLA VIRUS EPIDEMIC

It is widely acknowledged that the initial response to the Ebola crisis failed because of the state of healthcare systems in West Africa, which are often described as fragile and dysfunctional. A post-Ebola study commissioned by World Vision in Sierra Leone indicates that the interventions targeting the complex nature of the Ebola outbreak had varying successes. Isolation of Ebola patients and safe burials were critical in controlling the spread of the disease.[16] However, top-down approaches, particularly quarantine and body collection, were initially ineffective. Designed and implemented without buy-in and input from community leaders, they failed to address key infrastructure constraints and were culturally insensitive. This resulted in general distrust among community members, and, ultimately, underutilization of these interventions.[17] However, with the help of community healthcare workers (CHWs), social mobilization campaigns at the community level brought about awareness, changed perceptions, and led to buy-in, which then increased the use and effectiveness of these interventions. This not only points to the critical need to strengthen existing healthcare systems and integrate cultural beliefs and practices into all facets of the response, but demonstrates that community-based approaches to prevention and care can reduce Ebola transmission.[18]

NGOs that secured the trust of communities emerged as critical players in terms of changing knowledge, attitudes, and behaviors around Ebola and, ultimately, in community members accepting/adopting the lifesaving interventions required to control the outbreak. Having gained access to communities, NGOs were positioned to deliver a wide range of health services, including identifying new infections in Ebola-affected communities, providing clinical care to the critically ill in Ebola Treatment Units (ETUs), advocating for and employing survivors to assist with the response, and reopening district hospitals and health centers.[19] Nevertheless, community fears and misconceptions surrounding Ebola proved to be an even greater obstacle in controlling the outbreak. Studies show that fears and misperceptions among communities related to lack of trust in the Ebola response system may have delayed care-seeking during the country's Ebola outbreak. Consequently, it has been proven that using cultural insiders and leaders to address people's misperceptions and demonstrate accountability to the public can also enhance trust and encourage health system use.[20] Moreover, studies also demonstrate that much of the decline in the epidemic curve was driven by interventions that targeted critical behavior change within local communities rather than by international efforts that came after the epidemic had turned.[21] In circumstances like this, World Vision's experience also shows that changing peoples' behavior is never easy because it is intertwined with a complex set of social and cultural norms, and structural and faith influences.

The World Vision post-Ebola study also indicated that an integrated, multisectoral, multi-dimensional approach better responded to the needs and expectations of the community. These approaches included trainings on infection prevention and control, safe and dignified burials, household visits, hygiene and safety kit provision, religious and traditional leader engagement, food and farming assistance, small loans and grants to business traders, and close involvement of various community groups. The study demonstrates that community engagement and holistic interventions are some of many promising approaches central to greater acceptance. This approach builds community capacity, strengthens social cohesion, addresses issues of equity, and rebuilds peoples' belief and trust in their own health systems, which is fundamental to stronger demand for and utilization of healthcare services. A review of district level Ebola virus disease (EVD) records indicated that not a single Ebola-related fatality was documented among the 59,000 sponsored children or family members supported by World Vision during the outbreak, largely attributed to the comprehensive solutions provided, faith and culturally sensitive programming, and trusted relationships developed by World Vision staff in communities through long-term presence.

Summary

The goal of disaster medical response is to reduce the critical mortality associated with a disaster. Critical mortality rate is defined as the percentage of critically injured survivors who subsequently die. Numerous factors influence the critical mortality rate, including[1,2,5,10]:

- Effective use of the ICS among all organizations providing disaster relief
- Triage accuracy, particularly the incidence of over-triage of victims
- Rapid movement of disaster victims to definitive care
- Coordination of regional, national, and international disaster preparedness and response, both medical and public health, among all organizations responding to disasters.

A consistent approach to international disasters, based on an understanding of their common features and the response expertise they require, is becoming the accepted practice throughout the world. This strategy, called the MCI response, has the primary objective of reducing the mortality and morbidity associated with the disaster. All medical providers need to incorporate the key principles of the MCI response in disaster preparedness and response.

References

1. Briggs SM. *Advanced Disaster Medical Response Manual for Providers*. 2nd ed. Woodbury, CT: Cine-Med Publishing, Inc.; 2014.
2. Born CT, Cullison TR, Dean JA, et al. Partnered disaster preparedness: lessons learned from international events. *J Am Acad Orthop Surg*. 2011;19(1 suppl):S44–S48.
3. Briggs SM. Role of civilian surgical teams in response to international disasters. *ACS Bulletin*. 2010; 95:14–17.
4. Briggs SM. Natural disasters: an overview. In: Partridge RA, Proano L, Marcozzi D, Garza AG, Nemeth I, eds. *Oxford Handbook of Disaster Medicine*. US: Oxford University Press; 2012.
5. Briggs SM, Lin G, et al. Disasters. In: Meara J et al., eds. *Textbook of Global Surgery*. CRP Press, Boston, MA; 2014:443–453.
6. Lin G, Lavon H, Gelfond R, et al. Hard times call for creative solutions: medical improvisations at the Israel Defense Forces Field Hospital in Haiti. *Am J Disaster Med*. 2010;5:188–192.

7. Hasanin A, Mukhar A, Mokhtar A, Radwan A. Syrian revolution: a field hospital under attack. *Am J Disaster Med*. 2013;8:259–265.
8. Kearns R, Skarote MB, Peterson J, et al. Deployable, portable and temporary hospitals; one state's experiences through the years. *Am J Disaster Med*. 2014:195–207.
9. Sechriest 2nd VF, Wing V, Walker GJ, Aubuchon M, Lhowe DW. Healthcare delivery aboard US Navy hospital ships following earthquake disasters: implications for future disaster relief missions. *Am J of Disaster Med*. 2012;7:281–294.
10. Bartal C, Zeller L, Miskin I, et al. Crush syndrome: saving more lives in disasters, lessons learned from the early-response phase in Haiti. *Arch Intern Med*. 2011;171:694–696.
11. Latifi R, Tiley E. Telemedicine for disaster management: can it transform chaos into an organized, structure care from the distance? *Am J Dis Medicine*. 2014;9:25–37.
12. World Health Organization. *International Health Regulation (2005)*. Geneva: WHO; 2007.
13. Cardoso CW, Paploski IAD, Kikuti M, et al. Outbreak of exanthematous illness associated with Zika, Chikungunya, and Dengue viruses, Salvador, Brazil. *Emerging Infect Dis*. 2015;21:2274–2276.
14. Ferguson NM, Cucunubá ZM, Dorigatti I, et al. Countering the Zika epidemic in Latin America. *Science*. 2016;353:353–354.
15. World Health Organization. *WHO Director General Summarizes the Outcome of the Emergency Committee Regarding Clusters of Microcephaly and Guillain-Barre Syndrome* [Internet]. Geneva: WHO; [cited 2016 August 30]. Available at: http://www.who.int/mediacentre/news/statements/2016/emergency-committee-zikamicrocephaly/en/.
16. Washington ML, Meltzer ML. Effectiveness of Ebola treatment units and community care centers—Liberia, September 23–October 31, 2014. *MMWR*. 2015;64:67–69.
17. Fallah M, Dahn B, Nyenswah TG, et al. Interrupting Ebola transmission in Liberia through community-based initiatives. *Ann Intern Med*. 2016;164:367–369.
18. Pronyk P, Rogers B, Lee S, et al. The effect of community-based prevention and care on Ebola transmission in Sierra Leone. *Am J Public Health*. 2016;106:727–732.
19. Cancedda C, Davis SM, Dierberg KL. Strengthening health systems while responding to a health crisis: lessons learned by a nongovernmental organization during the Ebola virus disease epidemic in Sierra Leone. *J Infect Dis*. 2016;214(suppl 3):S153–S163.
20. Yamanis T, Nolan E, Shepler S. Fears and misperceptions of the Ebola response system during the 2014–2015 outbreak in Sierra Leone. *PLoS Negl Trop Dis*. 2016:10.
21. Kirsch TD, Moseson H, Massaquoi M, et al. Impact of interventions and the incidence of Ebola virus disease in Liberia—implications for future epidemics. *Health Policy Plan*. 2017;32(2):205–214.

CHAPTER 16

Considerations for Pandemic Preparedness and Response

Katrina Roper ■ Christian Haggenmiller

Introduction

"Although pandemics occur infrequently, planning and preparing for a pandemic is important to ensure an effective response. Planning for and responding to a pandemic is complex and pandemics can affect everyone in a community. Therefore, public health officials, health care professionals, researchers and scientists in the United States and across the world are working together to plan and prepare for possible pandemics. Many resources are available to help international, national, state and local governments, public health and health care professionals, corporations, and communities develop pandemic preparedness plans and strengthen their capabilities to respond to different pandemic scenarios"[1] (Fig. 16.1).

The Continuum of Pandemic Phases With Indicative World Health Organization Actions

PANDEMIC PLANNING AND PREPAREDNESS

Emergency preparedness and pandemic planning are continuous processes that require a commitment of resources including time, funding, and personnel, as well as political will (Fig. 16.2). This is an evolving space with increasing information to guide stakeholders to work together to plan and implement priority actions when needed.

- Every sovereign national state has the obligation to develop a strategy for a pandemic response and ensure its own emergency preparedness planning (International Health Regulations clearly describe responsibilities), which is a continuous effort. Nevertheless, epidemic and pandemic planning is a multinational and multisectoral endeavor requiring coordination among governments and international partners to address public health risks.

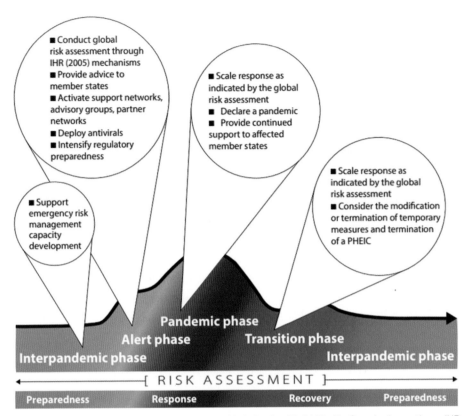

Fig. 16.1 The continuum of pandemic phases with indicative World Health Organization actions. *IHR, International Health Regulations; PHEIC, Public Health Emergency of International Concern.*

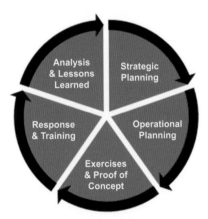

Fig. 16.2 Pandemic preparedness planning cycle. Adapted from ECDC/WHO EMRO, Guide to revision of national pandemic influenza preparedness plans.

- A pandemic transcends common public health boundaries and affects all sectors. Societies and economies are impacted in multiple ways, which can increase poverty and instability. The *Sendai Framework for Disaster Risk Reduction*[2] may be used to (1) understand disaster risk, (2) strengthen crisis management, (3) guide risk-reduction investment, and (4) enhance preparedness; it includes biological hazards such as epidemics and pandemics to help reduce mortality, increase early warning, and promote the safety of health facilities and hospitals.[3]
- Epidemic risk indicators need to include refugees and migrants living in overcrowded camps, especially in or near areas with emerging epidemics. For example, recent migrations from East Africa to Yemen were associated with a cholera outbreak facilitated by several risk factors.[4]
- Epidemic planning must be grounded on evidence-based outbreak response, lessons learned, and preparedness exercises.
- As the World Health Organization (WHO) emphasizes: "No single agency or organization can prepare for a pandemic on its own. Inadequate or uncoordinated preparedness of interdependent public and private organizations will reduce the ability of the health sector to respond during a pandemic. A concerted and collaborative effort is required by government ministries, businesses and civil society to sustain essential infrastructure and mitigate impacts of pandemic influenza on health, the economy and the functioning of society."[5]
- Pandemic preparedness plans at national or international level address five key interconnected areas: (1) strategic planning, which requires political commitment to implement into action, (2) subnational planning to create actionable plans and a defined, established network, (3) testing those plans through exercises and proofs of concept, (4) implementing the knowledge in training and emergency response, and (5) continuously analyzing and evaluating processes to feed best practices and learn.[6]

Further information:

WHO. A strategic framework for emergency preparedness. Available at: https://www.who.int/ihr/publications/9789241511827/en/.

PREPARATION OF THE RESPONDERS—INDIVIDUALS AND TEAMS

Responders to a pandemic or other humanitarian event frequently come together as rapidly formed multidisciplinary teams from different countries and cultures. Working effectively as a team can be challenging in a familiar environment with usual partners, let alone after arrival in a new environment with rapid introductions to new colleagues. As humanitarian responses frequently involve large numbers of national and international actors, coordination and collaboration can be challenging. Failures to work effectively together with a united vision and agreed path can lead to duplication of efforts or gaps in coverage.[1] However, if different organizations align too closely to improve coordination, there is the risk of losing options and innovation. Finding a balance to improve effectiveness and efficiency while retaining the ability to debate and explore avenues of response can be challenging. In the deployed situation, although external assistance may be required and requested, it is also important to remember that every person sent to a situation needs logistical support. Hence, coordinating inbound personnel is required not just to ensure the right skills are being imported, but also to adequately support additional staff without stressing an already fragile situation.

Individual and team effectiveness are optimized by:

- Being prepared and field-ready by attending appropriate deployment training and managing expectations for accommodation and support.
- Seeking terms of reference ahead of deployment to ensure a good match with your skill set.
- Upon arrival, checking in with the team and identifying partners with whom you will be working (and learning their roles). Identifying and addressing overlaps and gaps.
- Being adaptable because of the dynamic nature of the environment. Focusing on the outcomes and considering alternative methods to achieve them.

Responders often deploy individually through mechanisms such as the Global Outbreak Alert and Response Network (GOARN) or other country-registered rosters, such as UK-MED. However, in addition to rosters to fill individual billets, mechanisms exist to deploy preformed teamed. Emergency medical teams (EMTs) are an important part of the global health workforce, with a historical focus on trauma and surgery. More recently, EMTs have evolved to provide support in outbreak response. EMTs provide time-limited surge clinical capacity for affected populations. The WHO has developed a global verification system for EMTs to ensure that deployed teams meet the minimum required standards to provide quality of care that is appropriate for the context. This enables a country, when affected by a disaster or other emergency, to call on teams that have been classified at a predefined capability level.

Deployers must seek to integrate local staff—nurses, doctors, medical students, other healthcare workers—into the response team. This creates opportunities to increase local capability and capacity, a critical legacy after the event has ended. This also helps countries more effectively lead future disaster responses, even if they request external assistance.

The *Sphere Handbook* (2018)[7] guidelines provide a holistic approach to reducing public health risks, prevent disease transmission, and control disease outbreaks. Implementing hygiene standards and ensuring access to safe water help prevent outbreaks in communities. Adherence to those standards resulted in very few cholera cases in the crowded internally displaced person camps despite nearby outbreaks in Haiti (2011) and South Sudan (2014).[8]

GOARN has created "Go.Data"[9] to assist outbreak investigations; it facilitates field data collection during public health emergencies and has been successfully used in several African nations. This tool supports national public health surveillance systems which may be disrupted in crises (Fig. 16.3). Go.Data collects digital data, facilitates contact follow-up, helps visualize chains of transmission including secure data exchange, and analyzes and communicates in real-time to enable better decision-making for emergency public health and outbreak responders.

The *Health Cluster Handbook*, currently under revision, provides several planning considerations and assessments, which include other tools such as the WHO's Early Warning, Alert, and Response System (EWARS) and initial assessment reports from different organizations.[10]

Further information:

Active Learning Network for Accountability and Performance (ALNAP), a global network of nongovernmental organizations (NGOs), United Nations (UN) agencies, members of the Red Cross/Crescent Movement, donors, academics, networks, and consultants, hosts a library of evaluations of humanitarian action, making available knowledge and evidence from previous responses to assist future responses and responders. See: https://www.alnap.org/about

OpenWHO is the WHO's interactive, web-based knowledge transfer platform and provides online courses on response to health emergencies. OpenWHO also serves as a forum for the sharing of public health expertise and discussion on key issues. See: https://openwho.org

RedR Australia is an international humanitarian response agency that provides training for potential field workers. RedR Australia also manages a roster of deployable technical specialists. See: https://www.redr.org.au/training-courses/our-courses/

GOARN is a WHO network of over 250 technical institutions and networks globally that respond to acute public health events with the deployment of staff and resources to affected countries. GOARN is coordinated by an operational support team based at the WHO headquarters in Geneva and is governed by a steering committee. See: https://extranet.who.int/goarn/

UK-MED is a UK-based registered charity that trains experienced doctors, nurses, paramedics, midwives, and other health professionals to respond to disasters around the world and to work with local emergency medical teams with a view to building their resilience to future threats. See: https://www.uk-med.org

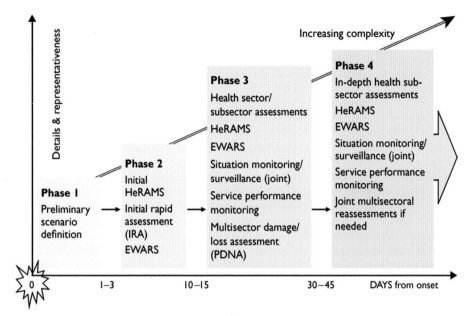

Fig. 16.3 Phases of data collection, analysis, and planning following a major, sudden-onset crisis. *EWARS, Early Warning, Alert, and Response System; HeRAMS, Health Resource Availability Mapping System; PDNA, Post-disaster needs Assessment.*

SCOPE OUT THE HEALTH SYSTEM CAPACITY AND LOCATION

Humanitarian disasters often affect already-stressed health systems with capacity gaps and endemic health challenges. However, underresourced institutions and facilities can become invaluable pillars in an outbreak response when provided support. Deployed infection prevention and control (IPC) teams should work with host institutions to help appropriate IPC. Host staff should be provided supplementary skill training if needed to ensure they are prepared to safely work in the environment. For example, during the 2014 to 2015 Ebola outbreak in West Africa, healthcare workers were provided with targeted relevant training in IPC to protect their health and ability to care for others.

An example of epidemic mapping during a complex emergency is Haiti in 2010. The nation's largest cell phone provider was able to anonymously track the movements of several million of mobile phones to inform their customers if they entered a cholera-contaminated area and simultaneously provide them advice on how to protect themselves.[11] The methodology behind this "Flowminder" can be used to slow spread during the opening phases of an epidemic when the outbreak is potentially limited to a small area.[12] Mapping and tracking health facility staffing, bed numbers, available services, and medical supply chain help determine capacity during a disaster response.

Further information:

Health Cluster Guide: https://www.who.int/hac/network/global_health_cluster

STRENGTHENING LABORATORY SUPPORT

Public health laboratories and pathology services are critical. Without the ability to provide laboratory testing of clinical samples, illnesses may be misdiagnosed and diseases newly circulating in a community may be missed. Under the 2005 International Health Regulations, member states are required to strengthen their ability to detect, assess, respond to, and report public health events. Detection of public health events requires credible and accessible laboratory services capable of providing reliable results in a timely manner.

However, in many low- and middle-income countries, laboratories remain underresourced. Many laboratories lack the capacity to do the necessary testing for endemic infectious diseases, let alone novel or rapidly expanding ones.

If one does not already exist, creation of a quality management system that complies with the requirements of the international quality standard (ISO 15189) represents a meaningful form of support. The WHO provides a range of tools developed in collaboration with the US Centers for Disease Control and Prevention (CDC) and the Clinical and Laboratory Standards Institute (CLSI) to support laboratories, suitable for low-, middle-, and upper-income countries, and includes an assessment tool, a quality manual handbook and template, and a laboratory quality implementation tool. This last tool is a website that provides a stepwise plan for laboratories to implement a quality management system in compliance with ISO 15189. These resources are free and available, some in multiple languages, at: https://www.who.int/ihr/capacity-strengthening/laboratory-improvement/en/.

Improving laboratory capacity during a public health event often involves supporting and expanding the capacities of existing laboratories, reinforcing sample transport systems for testing in reference laboratories, and potentially establishing mobile laboratories provided by international partners.

During crises, countries need to increase diagnostic testing capacity to evaluate probable cases but should also, when possible, include sentinel surveillance for asymptomatic cases. For many low- and middle-income countries, this requires assistance from major clinical diagnostic companies to produce reagents and testing kits at a large scale. Supply chains need to be agreed upon, funded, and operational. When public health events occur simultaneously in multiple countries, supply chains are at higher risk of disruption. Stakeholders should work during noncritical periods to build sustainable testing programs that are less vulnerable during stress.

Rapid point-of-care tests can be very useful, especially for countries with limited formal lab capacity. However, sensitivity and specificity parameters need to be well understood and appropriate to provide meaningful information.

For more information from WHO on diagnostic test selection:
    https://www.who.int/bulletin/volumes/95/9/16-187468/en/
For more information on laboratory quality management, regulation, biosafety, policy, and strategy: https://www.who.int/in-vitro-diagnostic/en/
For an overview of requirements for establishing good quality public health laboratory services, consider reading:
    Establishment of Public Health Laboratories in South East Asia, available at: https://apps.who.int/iris/handle/10665/274288
    Laboratory Professionals in Africa: The Backbone of Quality Diagnostics, available at: http://documents.worldbank.org/curated/en/419941468010480283/Laboratory-professionals-in-Africa-the-backbone-of-quality-diagnostics
For information on rapid malaria diagnostic tests, refer to:
    https://www.who.int/malaria/areas/diagnosis/rapid-diagnostic-tests/about-rdt/en/

CRISIS COMMUNICATION AND SOCIAL MOBILIZATION

"The right message at the right time from the right person can save lives." Barbara Reynolds, CDC Senior Crisis and Risk Communication Advisor.

The six key principles for effective crisis communication to build trust, rapport, and cooperation with the public (Crisis and Emergency Risk Communication [CERC], CDC) are:

1. Be first: communicating information quickly is crucial to engage members of the public with you as the source of information.

2. Be right: ensure credibility by delivering accurate information, including expressing what is not known and how these knowledge gaps are being addressed.
3. Be credible: always seek to be honest and truthful. Use recognized, respected people and provide clear messaging.
4. Express empathy: acknowledge the challenges that members of the public are facing.
5. Promote action: engage the community in meaningful actions. Utilize social mobilization to promote their sense of control over their situation.
6. Show respect: being respectful builds promotes cooperation with the public.

A related and equally important element of outbreak response is social mobilization. Social mobilization is the process of bringing together societal influences to raise awareness of a healthcare issue. Social mobilization becomes particularly important during outbreak response and can be a powerful tool to create necessary changes in societal behaviors. Good social mobilization empowers communities and their social networks to address and adjust behaviors and to be proactively involved in the outbreak response. Good social messaging can be used to instill in the community feelings of trust and respect for healthcare workers and to generate support for the response.

Some elements to consider when planning social mobilization activities include:

- Engage with religious leaders and build space for respectful dialogue around cultural beliefs. Find ways to incorporate scientifically valid messaging while respecting the importance of cultural beliefs and practices.
- Work with community elders to establish engagement with communities.
- Consider the education sector in particular schools. Children absorb information and take it home to their families.
- Use social media such as Instagram and Twitter, in addition to television and radio, to provide health messages in line with national public health recommendations. This can reach many more members of the community than might otherwise be reached using only official websites and traditional media.

The CERC (CDC) program provides trainings, tools, and resources to help health communicators, emergency responders, and leaders of organizations communicate effectively during emergencies. Available at: https://emergency.cdc.gov/cerc/index.asp

Additional resources:

CDC's *CERC Manual:* https://emergency.cdc.gov/cerc/manual/

WHO Guideline for Emergency Risk Communication: https://www.who.int/risk-communication/guidance/download/en/

Risk Communication and Community Engagement (RCCE): https://reliefweb.int/report/world/risk-communication-and-community-engagement-rcce-action-plan-guidance-covid-19

PREDEPLOYMENT CONSIDERATIONS: SUGGESTED PACKING ITEMS

Deploying as part of a rapid response team often entails many unknowns. Situation reports may not provide useful information for packing. Reaching out to those already in the country can help gauge what resources will be available and what might need to be brought.

Although one should be as prepared as possible, packing lightly facilitates agility, especially if it is carried on, versus checked luggage, which is vulnerable to delay or becoming lost.

If you can bring supplies for colleagues, endeavor to do so—this can mean at minimum a morale boost, and may also have significant operational impact. Also consider bringing useful supplies for the local population. Seek advice from colleagues in the country before doing this and be mindful of what you bring in—local staff should know best what to recommend and how to distribute the items without creating unintended issues.

The following items may be useful you in a deployed setting:

- 10 m of rope with a pegs/clothes pins (useful as washing line or for securing items)
- Headphones
- Small external speaker
- Silk or cotton liner in the event that you are unexpectedly billeted in a location where bed linen is not provided
- Head lamp with new batteries
- Door stop (for extra security or in the event that there is no working lock on your door)
- First aid kit with thermometer (with new batteries) and clear safety glasses
- 1 L (32 oz) clear water bottle and water purification tablets and/or small water filter—this can reduce plastic waste as well as consumption of community safe drinking water, which may be in limited supply for the local population.
- Appropriate power adapter
- Duct tape (good for making repairs to damaged luggage or tarpaulins)
- Buff headband or similar—can be a neck warmer, eye shield for sleeping, or backup mask for decreasing respiratory transmission of pathogens
- Reading device or books. Taking books means that you can share with others or opt to leave them behind to form a small library.
- Watch—a "smart" watch can provide a lot of information but will require charging and may be expensive if damaged or lost. Alternatively, a simple splashproof analog watch with date and time (e.g., a Swatch) will be robust enough for most situations and will not require reliable power.

PARTNERING WITH THE LOCAL WORKFORCE

There are several reasons to seek to employ the local workforce to advance pandemic goals. First, visiting emergency personnel create additional logistical demands. Second, local personnel best understand their culture and history and typically are able to gain trust more quickly with patients. Third, local citizens will have to manage the situation long after the visiting team has departed. Contact tracing is especially well-suited for this aim. It is resource-intensive, but during disruptive events like pandemics, there will likely be a ready supply of trainable individuals who are highly motivated to effect change.

Additional Thoughts

- Prioritize real estate for quarantine, especially for isolation patients in camp settings
- Define your plan for expansion in advance and walk through the implications
- Prioritize case definition and criteria, as well as testing protocols
- Maintain good version control of data and latest guidance/tools for data collection
- Begin intersectoral discussions early on, as soon as you realize a situation is heading toward a possible epidemic
- Standardize contact tracing protocols
- Decide early on who has what authority, especially for managing quarantine versus isolation issues
  - Understand operational needs of community—what needs to go on, and how can this be accommodated.
- Clear communication—work closely with public affairs and media
- Low threshold for protective measures
- Maintain communication with frontline medical leaders
- Lead with confidence, balance, compassion, and equanimity

- Build relationships ahead of time
- Medical personnel lead by example
- Clear communication with outside populations regarding expectations for movement into and out of your area
  - When facing crises such as pandemics, many people—including leaders—move through the five stages of grief. Logic and data alone are not always adequate to persuade, but must still always be involved in communication.

Additional Reading

Saavedra L, Knox-Clarke P. Working together in the field for effective humanitarian response. ALNAP Working Paper. London: ALNAP/ODI [Online]; 2015. Available at: https://www.alnap.org/system/files/content/resource/files/main/alnap-30-am-paper-working-together.pdf.

References

1. https://www.cdc.gov/flu/pandemic-resources/planning-preparedness/index.html.
2. https://www.undrr.org/.
3. https://www.who.int/bulletin/volumes/93/6/15-157362/en/.
4. Mystery of Yemen cholera epidemic solved. Available at: https://www.sciencedaily.com/releases/2019/01/190102140745.htm.
5. World Health Organization. Pandemic influenza risk management WHO—A WHO guide to inform & harmonize national & international pandemic preparedness and response; 2017. Available at: https://www.who.int/influenza/preparedness/pandemic/influenza_risk_management/en/.
6. https://www.ecdc.europa.eu/sites/portal/files/documents/Guide-to-pandemic-preparedness-revised.pdf.
7. https://handbook.spherestandards.org.
8. Own assessment from the IDP camp in Port au Prince, Haiti and Tomping/Juba and Bentiu in South Sudan, C Haggenmiller.
9. https://www.who.int/godata.
10. Health Cluster Guide. Available at: https://www.who.int/hac/network/global_health_cluster/chapter3.pdf.
11. The Haiti Case Study, Harvard Medical School and NATO's Joint Analysis and Lessons Learned Centre, June 2012. http://www.jallc.nato.int/products/docs/haiti_case_study.pdf.
12. Haiti Cholera Outbreak 2010. https://web.flowminder.org/case-studies/haiti-cholera-outbreak-2010.

CHAPTER 17

Strengthening and Supporting Health Systems

Margaret Ellis Bourdeaux ■ Christian Haggenmiller

Value and Challenges of Health Systems Strengthening

VALUE

There is strong global consensus on the need to strengthen health systems. "Weak health systems" are often cited as core drivers of high mortality and morbidity from disasters, poor health outcomes of a population, and the spread of outbreaks and epidemics. Health sectors in crisis-affected states are often overwhelmed with external actors with jostling agendas during acute and immediate postcrisis periods. It is imperative to prioritize during this time the effectiveness and integrity of the state's health system, both during and after the crisis.

Health development specialists concerned with addressing specific diseases or health conditions should also have a keen interest in health system integrity and functioning; the success of disease-specific interventions depends largely on the health system's capacity to implement them. For example, conflict- and crisis-affected states with weak institutions struggled in recent years to make progress in health-related Millennium Development Goals such as lowering infant and maternal mortality, and reducing the prevalence of human immunodeficiency virus/acquired immunodeficiency syndrome, tuberculosis, and malaria. In contrast, stable countries with effective health systems made relatively rapid progress.[1] Current struggles to end the Ebola outbreaks in the Democratic Republic of Congo, where trust in the health system is low after years of neglect of the health needs of the population, continued armed conflict, and political turmoil, illustrate this problematic dynamic. Initiatives to improve health security will hinge on the effectiveness of health systems.[2]

CHALLENGES

Despite its acknowledged importance, there are still significant variations in definitions, implementation frameworks, and accepted evidence for health systems strengthening (HSS).[3] Many health systems lack the capacity to measure or understand their own weaknesses and constraints, which limits policy-makers' ability to identify and address the most critical needs.[4]

A History of Health Systems Strengthening

The definition, conceptualization, boundaries, and responsibilities of health systems have featured in global health debates for more than four decades. The nature and focus of these descriptions often served the interests of those proposing them, reflecting biases in economics, political models, and other domains.[5]

Modern concepts in HSS have been strongly influenced by the Alma-Ata Declaration of 1978, which declared health as a human right and proposed that states and global health authorities focus on primary care as the foundation of health systems. The Declaration adjured governments to address "essential health care based on practical, scientifically sound, and socially acceptable methods and technology made universally accessible to individuals and families."[6] It avoided specifying which health services met these criteria, but aimed to shift the focus of health systems away from specialist-driven boutique and hospital-based care for those who could afford it to community-based health services.[7]

Critics of Alma-Ata felt its goals were too idealistic and vague. The year following Alma-Ata, the Rockefeller Foundation convened a follow-up summit in Belagio, Italy, to identify what core services health systems needed to provide. Termed "Selected Primary Care," the summit specified four health services that should be universally available—growth monitoring, oral rehydration, breastfeeding, and immunization,[8] but did not address which authorities would be responsible for implementation.

Thus, although Alma-Ata addressed the philosophical reasons states should be responsible for health systems, and the breadth of coverage and community focus, it did not specify health services for prioritized delivery or how it should be funded. Similarly, although Selected Primary Care identified a narrow set of universal programs to provide the maximum community value, it did not describe how and where these services would be provided, or by who.

Later models addressed the functional components of health systems. Frenk and Murray (2000) proposed that health systems are composed of four functions: financing, provision of health services, generation of nonfinancial resources (workforce, knowledge, infrastructure), and stewardship. They also specified three goals of health systems: improved population health; responsiveness of the health system to the expectations of the population; and financial fairness, including risk from medical bankruptcy. Mills and Ranson (2001) elaborated on these components, identifying relationships among stakeholders as important factors for success.

In 2008, Roberts et al. ("Getting Health Reform Right") attempted to create a predictive, operational model of health systems to guide policy makers in health system reform (Fig. 17.1). The World Bank adopted this model as the "Flagship Framework," conceiving health systems as a control panel with five control knobs—financing, payment, organization, regulation, and persuasion—that can be adjusted to achieve desired outcomes. For example, policymakers might consider changing the 'finance' control knob from a general tax to social insurance scheme to meet certain

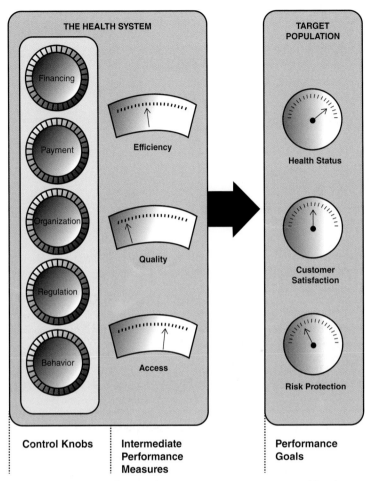

Fig. 17.1 Control Knobs Framework. From Getting health reform right: a guide to improving performance and equity by Marc J. Roberts, William Hsaio, Peter Berman and Michael R. Reich. Oxford University Press, Oxford, New York, 2004. No. of pages: 332. ISBN 0-19-516232-3.

goals. The model predicts the effect setting changes would have on health outcomes, including patient satisfaction and risk protection. This model provided two notable benefits. First, it moved beyond a descriptive framework to a mechanism for tailored action. Second, it offered researchers a better conceptual platform to analyze performance differences among health systems.

About the same time as Roberts' publication, the World Health Organization (WHO), concerned about the widening gap between the growing number of effective medical interventions and the low capacity of health systems to deliver them, proposed the "building block" model of health systems. This framework describes health systems as comprised of six "building blocks" or inputs: service delivery; health workforce; information; medical products, vaccines, and technologies; finance; and leadership, governance, and stewardship. The goal was to help researchers and policymakers more effectively categorize health system problems and discussions. The WHO model also sought consensus on four core outcomes or goals of health systems: improved

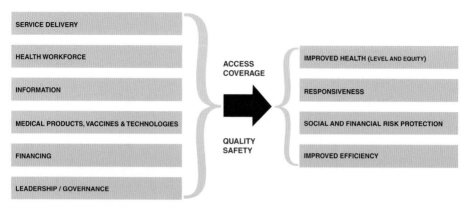

Fig. 17.2 The WHO Health System Framework. From World Health Organization, 2007. Everybody's Business: Strengthening Health Systems to Improve Health Systems WHO's framework for action.

population health; responsiveness (later often termed "customer satisfaction"); social and financial risk protection; and improved efficiency. Later models recategorized "improved efficiency" as an intermediate process goal rather than an end unto itself. Despite a high degree of consensus on these goals, the WHO's building block model (Fig. 17.2) has been criticized for its apparent inability to explain why various health systems produce different results. Some have suggested this is because although "building block" implies discrete, well-defined entities, the dynamic relationship between them is less easily understood.

Current Concepts in Health Systems Strengthening

Below are three current definitions of HSS by well-respected organizations that work in this field. For this chapter, we will focus on the WHO as it has the broadest influence.

USAID HEALTH SYSTEMS STRENGTHENING DEFINITION

The United States Agency for International Development (USAID) defines a health system as consisting of all people, institutions, resources, and activities whose primary purpose is to promote, restore, and maintain health. Strengthening a health system means initiating activities in the six internationally accepted core HSS functions—human resources for health; health finance; health governance; health information; medical products, vaccines, and technologies; and service delivery. A well-performing health system is one that achieves sustained health outcomes through continuous improvement of these six interrelated HSS functions.[9]

UNICEF HEALTH SYSTEMS STRENGTHENING DEFINITION

"UNICEF [United Nations Children's Fund] defines HSS as actions that establish sustained improvements in the provision, utilization, quality and efficiency of services delivered through the health system, and encourage the adoption of healthy behaviors and practices. These actions may also influence the health system context, including key performance drivers such as policies that impact on health in all sectors, governance, financing, management, capacity for implementation, social norms and country participation in initiatives designed to maintain national and global health security. They also implicitly improve health security by strengthening the system's resilience and its preparedness to respond efficiently and effectively in the context of emergencies."[10]

WORLD HEALTH ORGANIZATION HEALTH SYSTEMS STRENGTHENING DEFINITION

- Health systems strengthening:
  i. the process of identifying and implementing the changes in policy and practice in a country's health system, so that the country can respond better to its health and health system challenges;
  ii. any array of initiatives and strategies that improves one or more of the functions of the health system and that leads to better health through improvements in access, coverage, quality, or efficiency.
- Health system:
  i. all the activities whose primary purpose is to promote, restore, and/or maintain health;
  ii. the people, institutions, and resources, arranged together in accordance with established policies, to improve the health of the population they serve, while responding to people's legitimate expectations and protecting them against the cost of ill-health through a variety of activities whose primary intent is to improve health.[11]

As mentioned earlier in this chapter, the WHO uses a framework that identifies six building blocks/essential functions that form the foundation of a health system (which requires a functioning governing system) (Table 17.1).

TABLE 17.1 ■ **Health System Building Blocks**

Six Building Blocks	Key Components
Leadership and governance (stewardship)	• Legal framework for national multisectoral emergency management • Legal framework for health-sector emergency management • National multisectoral institutional framework for multisectoral emergency management • Institutional framework for health-sector emergency management • Health-sector emergency-management program components
Health workforce (resources)	• Human resources for health-sector emergency management
Medical products, vaccines and technology	• Medical supplies and equipment for emergency-response operations • Medical equipment and supplies for prehospital and hospital (including temporary health facilities) activities and other public health interventions
Heath information (data and data systems)	• Information-management systems for risk-reduction and emergency-preparedness programs • Information-management systems for emergency response and recovery • Risk communication
Health financing	• National and subnational strategies for financing health-sector emergency management
Service delivery	• Response capacity and capability • Emergency medical services (EMS) system and mass-casualty management • Management of hospitals in mass-casualty incidents • Continuity of essential health programs and services • Logistics and operational support functions in emergencies

Modified from World Health Organization. *Everybody's Business: Strengthening Health Systems to Improve Health Outcomes—WHO's Framework for Action*. Geneva: WHO; 2007. Available at: https://www.who.int/healthsystems/strategy/everybodys_business.pdf.

By strengthening these building blocks, the overall goal is improved health because of better access, coverage, quality, and safety. Responsiveness to changing health requirements, social and financial risk protection, and improved efficiency are additional outcomes.

WORLD HEALTH ORGANIZATION SYSTEMS THINKING

After implementing the six building blocks as a framework, many critics suggested that this framework neglected the important role of communities, essential to delivering health care where the official system stops. Therefore, the WHO initiated an additional approach to strengthening health systems by applying "system thinking."[12] This 10-step approach facilitated seeing and understanding the health system as a whole instead of one building block alone and encouraged potential synergies among different interventions.

The aim of systems thinking is to reveal the underlying characteristics and relationships of interconnected systems and fields as diverse as engineering, economics, and ecology combined with nonlinear, unpredictable, and resistant developments sometimes worsening a problem.

Within misunderstood systems, interventions—even the very simplest—often fail to achieve their goals because of the often unpredictable behavior of the system around them. As any health intervention has a direct or indirect effect on other health programs belonging to the functional areas of the building blocks, those ripple effects need to be recognized as soon as possible, to identify potential consequences—which may be symbiotic at best, competing and negative at worst (Fig. 17.3).

HEALTH SYSTEM RESILIENCE

This is defined as "the capacity of health actors, institutions, and populations to prepare for and effectively respond to crises; maintain core functions when a crisis hits; and, informed by lessons

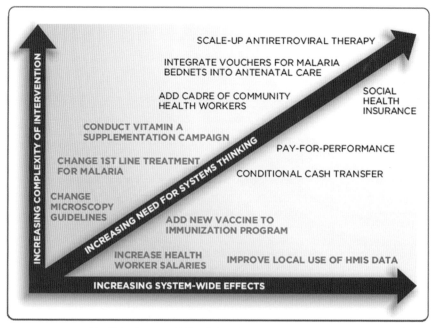

Fig. 17.3 Systems thinking for health systems strengthening.

learnt during the crisis, reorganize if conditions require it." However, additional themes are identi-fied that require further defining of the concept to simultaneously achieve sustainable transfor-mations in public health practice and health service delivery, and improve their preparedness for emergencies.[13]

HEALTH SYSTEMS STRENGTHENING IN THE CONTEXT OF FRAGILITY

The importance of understanding the strength and vulnerabilities of a health system seems to differ significantly in the context of fragility and conflict. In complex humanitarian emergencies, a key focus is needed on threats to the interface between public health provision and community processes that see community, civil society, private sector actors, and the state as key agents within a complex system adjusting to the prevailing drivers of fragility.[14]

HEALTH SYSTEMS STRENGTHENING AND DISASTER MANAGEMENT

Disaster management is being globally encouraged to improve disaster preparedness, along with growing international commitment to strengthening health systems. The WHO has pub-lished a new health emergency and disaster risk management (EDRM) framework.[15] In addi-tion to the previously describe six building blocks, this framework adds three components: Risk Communication; Community Capacities for Health EDRM; and Monitoring and Evaluation.

This framework complements the range of public health threats, including new emerging dis-eases, accidental release or deliberate use of biological, chemical, or radionuclear agents, natural disasters, human-made disasters, complex emergencies, conflicts, and other events with a poten-tially catastrophic impact on human health.

TOOLKIT

The WHO Toolkit is based on the experience and lessons of two decades of disasters, to help guidance HSS and improve disaster management capacity.[16]

Supporting Versus Strengthening Health Systems

DIFFERENCE BETWEEN A HEALTH SYSTEM AND THE HEALTH SECTOR

A health sector is the sum total of all efforts to improve the health of individuals regardless of how those efforts are or are not organized. A health system implies a centralized, deliberately governed effort to organize the health sector. Although many rightfully condemn attacks on very visible ele-ments of the health sector (i.e., clinics), more enduring but sometimes less obvious are elements of the system such as degradation of governance (leadership and decision-making capacity of trusted leadership) and its core instruments such as finance, information support, regulatory authority, policy generation, etc. Notably, some organizations consider supporting health system leadership as a political act that can worsen and fuel conflict, especially in the setting of high levels of corrup-tion. Regardless, the default position should typically be to support a nation's Ministry of Health unless there are exceptionally clear and compelling reasons for not doing so.

One may also consider the following three areas as separate but related levers for health system support—stewardship, health governance apparatus, and health delivery platform:

1. Stewardship

   Possibly the most contentious and frequently disrupted element of health systems in con-flict-affected states. Although various definitions of stewardship exist, virtually all agree on mandate, legitimacy, and authority to undertake key governing tasks with transparency and accountability. These tasks include setting priorities, deciding on strategies, regulation, and coordination.

The mandate—who gets the authority to make health system decisions—may be contested in states with political turmoil. In postconflict environments where leadership is cycling rapidly, health systems struggle to regain functionality. Priorities change and conflicting strategies emerge to address core problems regarding how, for example, service providers will be paid or services will be delivered in insecure areas. Relationships with nonhealth actors, particularly donors, are often based on personal trust in contexts where institutions are weak.

There may be pressure to choose leadership based on ethnic group affiliation rather than qualification or experience with governance. Health ministries may be a relatively "convenient" place to fill formal or informal quota agreements compared with more powerful offices. Such appointees may require extra support if they lack experience and/or support of the ruling ethnic group.

Legitimacy may be deliberately or inadvertently challenged by accusations of corruption (i.e., graft, cronyism) or perceived inability to benefit the populace.

Authority may be assumed by outside powers that have the resources to manage it. Additionally, the legal foundation of the system can be overturned by unplanned transfer of power.

A hallmark of health systems in crisis is the shearing of the relationship between stewards and the health governance apparatus, where stewards no longer effectively control policy-making or implementation, financing and disbursement, or the ability to assess performance and negotiate with actors in the system or who impact it.

2. Health governance apparatus

The health governance platform refers to the tools stewards use to raise and disburse financing; regulate processes; prioritize and organize needs; assess performance and manage relationships with nonhealth sectors.

Crises commonly impact health systems in the following ways.

a. Raising and disbursing financing
   i. Taken out of state's hands
   ii. Principal agent problem: different agendas and priorities; international donors may decide, or to cut leadership out entirely.
   iii. Shift to security
   iv. Delayed support
   v. Transaction costs

b. Interruptions of regulatory authority
   i. Erosion of trust
   ii. Cannot pay vendors
   iii. Lost oversight capability
   iv. Actively weaponized

c. Policy-making: prioritization and organization
   i. Peace dividend versus need-based care
   ii. Strong preferences on the part of international community (contracting vs. national health system). These may clash with public expectations.
   iii. Burdens of care may shift dramatically.

d. Assessing performance and managing relationships with outside actors
   i. Creates massive power differentials
   ii. "Capture" by outside interests can be a major goal of unscrupulous actors (counterfeit drugs and tenders).
   iii. Internally, the government may wish to focus exclusively on staying in power.

3. Health delivery platform

The health delivery platform is comprised of those health system elements that touch patients: the infrastructure, supply chains, medical services technologies, and health workers who deliver care. Health delivery platform elements are often the most visible in the news—clinics bombed, health workers targeted, and supply chains disrupted.

THEORETICAL FRAMEWORK

"Supporting the health system can include any activity that improves services. Support activities improve outcomes primarily by increasing inputs. By contrast, strengthening the health system is accomplished by more comprehensive changes to policies and regulations, organizational structures and relationships across the health system building blocks. Strengthening activities motivate changes in behavior and/or allow a more effective use of resources to improve (multiple) health services. Hence, health system strengthening is about making the system function better permanently, not just filling gaps or supporting the system to produce better short-term outcomes. A wide spectrum of health system strengthening interpretations exists"[17] (Box 17.1).

HSS interventions might create financial disincentives to ongoing support programs as they might compete with the same available but limited funds.[18]

True HSS interventions should have system-level effects as opposed to impacts restricted to the organizational level. Criteria[19] for HSS intervention that should be considered include:

1. Scope
2. Scale (beyond one level of the system)
3. Sustainability,
4. Effects (equity, financial risk protection, responsiveness).

SUPPORTING RATHER THAN STRESSING HEALTH SYSTEMS DURING CRISIS RESPONSE AND RECOVERY

Health system support for fragile and crisis-affected states is typically undertaken through one of the following means: as part of state-building missions to establish governing institutions in the wake of falling regimes; as part of stability missions to reduce the risk of recidivism into violence; or as "health diplomacy" to either buttress legitimacy and authority of a threatened government or that of a foreign power intervening in a state.

Despite all good intentions, before pursuing health system support during crises and recovery, the long-term rationale and ethical issues should be identified. The United Nations (UN) and several other organizations categorize crises by phases: the crisis proper, early recovery, recovery, and reconstruction. Health system interventions for the initial, early crisis period should be limited to short-term services and projects to minimize loss of life and limb. Early recovery and recovery are appropriate times to help health systems resume functioning. Recovery and reconstruction

---

BOX 17.1 ■ Criteria to Distinguish Between Health System Strengthening and Support Interventions

1. Do the interventions address policy and organizational constraints or strengthen relationships between the six World Health Organization building blocks of a health system?
2. Will the interventions produce permanent systemic impact beyond the term of the project?
3. Are the interventions tailored to country-specific constraints and opportunities, with clearly defined roles for country institutions?

Modified from Chee G, Pielemeier N, Lion, A, Connor C, "Why differentiating between health system support and health system strengthening is needed," *Int J Health Plann Manage*, 2013 Jan;28(1):85–94.

endeavors should be addressing larger capital projects and longer-term programs that help the system "build back better."

Some health system leaders in crisis-affected states have offered critiques on the previously discussed. For example, exclusive focus on short-term projects during an acute crisis deals the health system a triple blow: first, states may be pressured to shunt resources away from basic services such as health care into security; second, external actors' exclusive focus on short-term "life and limb" services often create parallel care delivery systems—money and other resources flow around the state health system, not through it to bolster its capabilities at a time where these capabilities need to be shored up; third, parallel and short-term support may draw resources out of the health system at the time of its greatest need. For example, health workers may be hired away from their primary areas of responsibility and health data may be diverted to external actors. In sum, the health system emerges from the crisis weaker and more poorly resourced.

After the crisis, development donors often delay investing in state systems out of uncertainties related to the immediate postcrisis environments. Even when willing, donors face obstacles to marshaling and disbursing resources when health system infrastructure components (staff, information systems, financial and regulatory mechanisms) have been eroded. Thus health systems may enter the reconstruction phase adrift. Clinics and facilities may be rebuilt, but without adequate experienced personnel to staff, lead, or finance them. These compounding effects create what some have termed "the Crisis Carousel." This is especially important following certain crises, such as civil war, after which deaths are often higher than during the conflict itself.[20]

Instead, critics argue, actors should focus on preserving and even expanding investments in health systems during and after crises, counter to agendas that selectively permit *dis*-integration of systems with the intent to reconstruct after the crisis. Additionally, some argue against any health system support during a crisis because of undesirable political effects.

Those sympathetic to this view assert HSS as fundamentally political, as institutions and systems are the products of negotiations among groups in society regarding how they will address collective needs, prioritize concerns, and raise and distribute resources. In conflict-affected states, these negotiations have become dysfunctional to the point of at least one party using coercive violence. Typically, the same conflicts at work in the political arena adversely impact health systems, making it challenging to achieve long-term health system benefits until the fundamental political and security needs have been stabilized and resolved. Additionally, donated funds earmarked for the health sector are often revectored or simply stolen in periods of civil disturbance.

A PROPOSED MERGER HEALTH SYSTEM MODEL FOR CRISIS-AFFECTED STATES

According to Frenk and Murray (2000), the stewards/leaders serve as the component of the health system that operates other elements—financing, regulation, organization and prioritization, performance assessment, and management of relationships in nonhealth sectors. Together, they represent the health governance apparatus of a health system (Fig. 17.4).

In contrast, four of the six WHO building blocks—information, service delivery, medical technologies, and health workforce—are not high order elements of the Flagship framework model. Rather, they are considered part of regulation and organization of the sector.* These four elements are those that actually interact with, or touch, patients. Patients receive health services from health

---

*In later works by these authors, information is unpacked to mean three different things: health information systems for governance (tracking health insurance enrollees, say, or utilization of health center services, and healthcare provider payrolls); personal health information tracking (patient records); and health data for assessing the effectiveness of the health system (health of the population, degree of risk protection) to be a cross-cutting health system element.

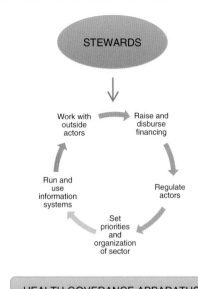

Fig. 17.4 Health governance apparatus of a health system, according to Frenk and Murray.

workers, consume medicines, and provide the health system's information. These elements that touch patients are the health delivery platform of a health system.

The implicit claim made in the Flagship framework is that the health governance apparatus—financing, organization, regulation, and generation—produce another set of health system elements of service delivery, health workforces, informational systems, and medical products and technologies. Fig. 17.5 depicts a novel health system model that merges the WHO building blocks and the Flagship framework. The outcomes of a health system consistent with both models include financial risk protection, customer satisfaction, and improved health status of the population.

This combined model suggests a reason to reflect upon the relationships among health system elements including the primacy of stewardship, the need for governance, and the distinction between inputs necessary for governance and those required for care delivery. One could thus define effective health systems as the sum of a state's governed efforts to promote the health of a specific population in a way that satisfies their demands, improves their health status, and protects them from medical bankruptcy.

A Streamlined Framework for Understanding Health Systems in Conflict-Afflicted States

The above synthesis of the Flagship Framework and WHO building blocks may be streamlined into a more streamlined novel framework.

This framework divides health systems into three components: **leaders and health policy makers; the governance apparatus;** and **the health delivery platform.** These components are hierarchical in that the former components determine and derive the later ones. In a functioning health system, leaders and policy makers utilize the governance apparatus to make and implement policies, that in turn creates and sustains the health delivery platform that delivers health services to the population. The performance goals in this framework are the same as in the WHO building

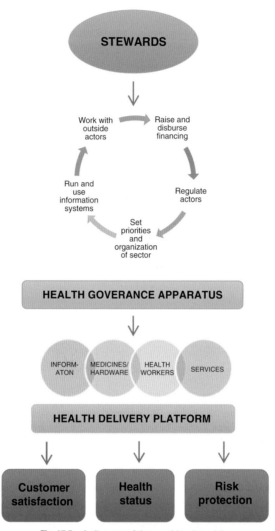

Fig. 17.5   A diagram of the combined models.

block model, but with two additional ones: health system resiliency and global health threat mitigation. In deteriorating health systems, the framework proposes, the relationships among these three components start to fray, degrading health system performance. Thus, a focus of health system strengthening efforts in conflict-affected state contexts is to shore up the relationships among these components in addition to supporting each component individually.

Leaders and Health Policy Makers: The process of conferring authority and legitimacy to lead state institutions in conflict affected states is one of the most fraught issues in state building and state stabilization missions. Leadership may be contested, rapidly changing, or aligned with violent or corrupt political factions. While some in the global health community conceive of health aid as a non-political enterprise and point to historically poor governance in conflict-afflicted states, health system strengthening needs to be undertaken and led by the public sector for it to be sustainable. Lack of capable, legitimate leadership by the state will inevitably lead to the poor health system performance.

The goal of strengthening the health system leadership component is to have a capable, well-resourced, and well-regulated leadership team that can make, implement, and refine health system policy decisions as well as liaise with leaders outside the health system and manage relationships with stakeholders. This does not imply that poor leadership should be enabled or supported, but rather clear guideposts and benchmarks should inform how health system leadership is performing and what is required to support its success, sustainability, and resilience.

Governance (Control Panel): The goal of health system governance is to provide health system leadership adequate control over policy formulation and implementation to optimally shape conditions for their population. Leaders of conflict-affected health systems often find themselves significantly dependent on international donors, diminishing their true control over priority setting, policy making, and implementation. International donors may have divergent priorities and resist giving unrestricted funds to health system leadership without being able to see the relevant "whole picture." While donors will likely always set parameters by which their grantees are measured, in a functional conflict-affected states health systems governance structure, leadership would have access to the 'control panel' described in the Flagship Framework model. Specifically, they would be able to responsibly:

- Decide how finances will be raised to fund the sector (financing)
- Decide how providers, clinics and hospitals will be paid (payment)
- Make decisions about where health services will be offered and who will provide them (organization)
- Have the legislative tools and capacities to regulate the health system (regulation)
- Have the resources and capacities to influence the health behaviors of the population and bolster health systems credibility via public health communication campaigns, transparency about health spending, hiring, strategies and standards (persuasion)

Traditionally, funding has been supported largely by international donors, especially in the immediate post-conflict period. However, options to finance the health system directly through the country's budget directly should not be overlooked. Additionally, threats to health systems financing streams can and should be anticipated and addressed. (see Overseas Development Institute, 2015).[21]

Health Delivery Platform: Health delivery platforms are the elements of a health system that involve patients directly— hospitals, clinics, and doctors' offices, pharmacies, and patient charts. These elements are defined, organized, created and sustained by health system policies.

The two core goals of strengthening health delivery platforms are (a.) linking them to health system governance and policy making processes and (b.) ensuring staff, patients, facilities, and therapeutics are protected during an acute crisis. A frequent well-intended mistake made by aid agencies and groups is to "build a clinic" or "run a training program" that has no medium- or longer-term sustainability or staffing plan and is not an integrated component of the health system. This strategy creates vulnerability by delaying the state's ability to "get back on its own two feet," and often diverts important funding from the state health system, rendering it less resilient. The staffing, funding, and regulating of health projects must align with system-wide health policy.

Outcomes and Performance Goals: As in stable states, the performance goals of a health system in a conflict-affected state should aspire to improve the health of the country's residents, satisfy the expectations of the population, and protect individuals from being driven into poverty by medical expenses. However, given the poorer health of the population, their typical erosion of trust in the public sector, and their precarious financial situation, health systems in a conflict-affected context have to perform at a higher level if these goals are to be achieved.

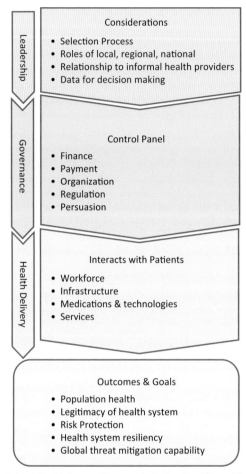

Fig. 17.6 A Health System Framework for Conflict-Affected States.

This suggests an additional set of outcomes that monitor the threats to the operations and resiliency of the health system. One example would be documenting the exodus of health workers who leave the system to work for private health facilities or calculating if health aid is 'on budget' as useful indicators to reflect the sustainability and resiliency of the health system.

Recent epidemics and the COVID-19 pandemic demonstrate how the global population as a whole is affected by every state's ability to detect and mitigate epidemics.[22,23] Measures of degrees of preparedness to keep health threats from spreading beyond a states' borders is a critical performance goal for protecting global health security. Initiatives like the Global Health Security Agenda employ a metrics-driven approach to assessment and can be incorporated into HSS frameworks (Fig. 17.6).

Conclusion

1. Currently, there is no commonly agreed definition or model framework for HSS. However, the WHO's core function of a health system is the foundation for many adaptions and interpretations.

2. Effective HSS should aim to improve preparedness for disaster and health emergency response and recovery (resilience).
3. Every intervention in a health system, either vertical or horizontal, influences the overall local and national health system. One should attempt to evaluate how the interventions are affecting the desired end state and having other, possibly unintended, consequences.
4. Outside agencies (nongovernmental organizations, international governmental organizations, governments, academia, etc.) have different strengths to offer nations seeking to strenghen health systems. Research and multilogue can help determine which potential support pieces—training, crisis surge logistics and security, surge staffing, research, host fora for conferences, compliance verification (Busan agreement, etc.), discouraging talent poaching, discouraging corruption, and so on—are most appropriate. First do no harm.
5. Respectful, transparent engagement is needed to build the trust necessary for sustained, effective results.
6. Health systems provide critical risk-mitigation to populations at risk. Their failures are impactful not just locally, but potentially globally, as recent epidemics and the COVID-19 pandemic illustrate.

Suggested Reading

Pavignani E, Colombo S. Analyzing Disrupted Health Sectors—A Modular Manual. World Health Organization; 2009. Available at: https://www.who.int/hac/techguidance/tools/disrupted_sectors/en/.

Cueto M. The origins of primary health care and selective primary health care. *Am J Public Health*. 2004;94: 1864–1874.

Harvard Global Health Institute. *Global Monitoring of Disease Outbreak Preparedness: Preventing the next Pandemic, a Shared Framework*. Harvard University; 2018.

Health Emergency and Disaster Risk Management Framework. Available at: https://www.who.int/hac/techguidance/preparedness/health-emergency-and-disaster-risk-management-framework-eng.pdf.

Marc Roberts, William Hsiao, Peter Berman, and Michael Reich; Getting Health Reform Right: A Guide to Improving Performance and Equity. Oxford University Press, Oxford; 2003.

Merson M, Black RE, Milles AJ. *Global Health Diseases, Programs, Systems, and Policies*. 3rd ed. Jones and Bartlett Publishers; 2011.

Mills A, Ranson K. The design of health systems. In: Merson, M; Black, R; MILLS, A, (eds.) International Public Health. Aspen Publishers, Gaithersburg; 2001. https://researchonline.lshtm.ac.uk/id/eprint/17796.

Organization for Economic Co-Operation and Development. 2011. *4th High Level Forum on Aid Effectiveness, Busan Partnership for Effective Development Cooperation*. 2011. Available at: https://www.oecd.org/development/effectiveness/busanpartnership.htm#:~:text=The%20Busan%20Partnership%20agreement%20sets,have%20expressed%20their%20support%20for.

Public Health Engineering in Precarious Situations. Available at: https://medicalguidelines.msf.org/viewport/MG/en/guidelines-16681097.html.

Toolkit for Assessing Health-System Capacity for Crisis Management. Available at: http://www.euro.who.int/__data/assets/pdf_file/0008/157886/e96187.pdf.

World Health Organization. *Neglected Health Systems Research: Health Policy and Systems Research in Conflict-Affected Fragile States*. WHO; 2008 Available at: http://digicollection.org/hss/documents/s15873e/s15873e.pdf.

World Health Organization. *WHO Called to Return to the Declaration of Alma-Ata*. WHO. Available at: http://www.who.int/social_determinants/tools/multimedia/alma_ata/en/. Accessed February 18, 2019.

United States Institute of Peace. *Special Report 301: Health in Postconflict and Fragile States*. 2012. Available at: https://www.usip.org/sites/default/files/SR_301.pdf.

United States Institute of Peace. *United States Army Peacekeeping and Stability Operations Institute: Guiding Principles for Stabilization and Reconstruction*. 2009. Available at: https://www.usip.org/publications/2009/11/guiding-principles-stabilization-and-reconstruction.

References

1. *Security: The Missing Bottom of the Millennium Development Goals.*
2. Harvard Global Health Institute. *Global Monitoring of Disease Outbreak Preparedness: Preventing the Next Pandemic, a Shared Framework.*
3. Witter S, Palmer N, Balabanova D, et al. Health system strengthening—reflections on its meaning, assessment, and our state of knowledge. *Int J Health Plan Mgmt.* 2019;84:e1980–e1989.
4. Systems Thinking for Health Systems Strengthening. Available at: https://www.who.int/alliance-hpsr/resources/9789241563895/en/.
5. Hsiao. What Is a Health System.
6. World Health Organization. WHO Called to Return to the Declaration of Alma-Ata.
7. Merson MH, Black RE, Milles AJ. *Global Health Diseases, Programs, Systems, and Policies.*
8. Cueto. The Origins of Primary Health Care and Selective Primary Health Care.
9. https://www.usaid.gov/sites/default/files/documents/1864/HSS-Vision.pdf.
10. https://www.unicef.org/media/60326/file.
11. https://www.who.int/healthsystems/hss_glossary/en/index5.html.
12. Systems Thinking for Health Systems Strengthening. Available at: https://www.who.int/alliance-hpsr/resources/9789241563895/en/.
13. Nuzzo J, et al. What makes health systems resilient against infectious disease outbreaks and natural hazards? Results from a scoping review.
14. Ager, et al. Health systems research in fragile settings. Bull World Health Organ.
15. *Health Emergency and Disaster Risk Management Framework.* WHO; 2019. Available at: https://reliefweb.int/report/world/health-emergency-and-disaster-risk-management-framework.
16. Toolkit for assessing health-system capacity for crisis management. Available at: https://www.euro.who.int/__data/assets/pdf_file/0008/157886/e96187.pdf.
17. Kohler, et al. Health system support and health system strengthening: two key facilitators to the implementation of ambulatory tuberculosis treatment in Uzbekistan. *Health Econ Rev.* 2016;6:28.
18. Derderian K, Philips M. Health in the service of state-building in fragile and conflict affected contexts: an additional challenge in the medical-humanitarian environment. *Conf Health.* 2015;9:13.
19. Health system strengthening—reflections on its meaning, assessment, and our state of knowledge. Available at: https://onlinelibrary.wiley.com/doi/epdf/10.1002/hpm.2882.
20. Ghoborah HA, Huth P, Russett B, "The post-war public health effects of civil conflict," *Soc Sci Med.* 2004 Aug;59(4):869–84.
21. https://www.odi.org/publications/10208-using-country-systems-fragile-states.
22. https://www.ncbi.nlm.nih.gov/pmc/articles/PMC3375795/.
23. Nuzzo J, et al. What makes health systems resilient against infectious disease outbreaks and natural hazards? Results from a scoping review.

INDEX

Page numbers followed by "*f*" indicate figures, "*t*" indicate tables, and "*b*" indicate boxes